Cumulative Trauma Disorders

Cumulative Trauma Disorders

Arminius Cassvan, M.D.
Professor of Clinical Physical Medicine and Rehabilitation, State University of
New York at Stony Brook School of Medicine Health Sciences Center; Chief of
Electrodiagnostic and Rehabilitation Medicine Center, Franklin Hospital Medical
Center, Valley Stream

Lyn Denise Weiss, M.D.
Associate Professor of Physical Medicine and Rehabilitation, State University of
New York at Stony Brook School of Medicine Health Sciences Center; Chairman of
Physical Medicine and Rehabilitation, Director of Medical Education, and Director
of Electrodiagnostic Services, Nassau County Medical Center, East Meadow

Jay Mitchell Weiss, M.D.
Assistant Professor of Physical Medicine and Rehabilitation, State University of
New York at Stony Brook School of Medicine Health Sciences Center; Medical
Director of Long Island Physical Medicine and Rehabilitation, Levittown and
Jericho; Attending Physician, Department of Physical Medicine and Rehabilitation,
Nassau County Medical Center, East Meadow

Jack L. Rook, M.D.
Medical Director, Cheyenne Mountain Rehabilitation/Cheyenne Mountain
Therapies, Colorado Springs, Colorado

Steven U. Mullens, J.D.
Attorney-at-law, Colorado Springs, Colorado

With illustrations by Omer Fast

Butterworth–Heinemann
Boston   Oxford   Johannesburg   Melbourne   New Delhi   Singapore

Butterworth–Heinemann supports the efforts of American Forests and the Global ReLeaf program in its campaign for the betterment of trees, forests, and our environment.

Library of Congress Cataloging-in-Publication Data
Cumulative trauma disorders / senior author, Arminius Cassvan ... [et al.].
    p.   cm.
  Includes bibliographical references and index.
  ISBN 0-7506-9570-6 (alk. paper)
  1. Overuse injuries. I. Cassvan, Arminius.
  [DNLM: 1. Cumulative Trauma Disorders. WE 175 C9709 1997]
RD97.6.C84 1997
617.1--dc21
DNLM/DLC
for Library of Congress   97-2667
                                      CIP

British Library Cataloguing-in-Publication Data
A catalogue record for this book is available from the British Library.

The publisher offers special discounts on bulk orders of this book.
For information, please contact:
Manager of Special Sales
Butterworth–Heinemann
313 Washington Street
Newton, MA 02158-1626
Tel: 617-928-2500
Fax: 617-928-2620

For information on all Butterworth–Heinemann publications available, contact our World Wide Web home page at: http://www.bh.com

10 9 8 7 6 5 4 3 2 1

Printed in the United States of America

To our children, with our love and gratitude, for helping us keep our perspective on what is truly important

Jeff
Audrey
Ari
Helene
Stefan
Richard
Alaina
Jordan
Jed
Scott

To our spouses, Carol, Jay, Lyn, Marlene, and Joan, for their support, humor, and encouragement

Contents

Preface

The publication of this book fills a vacuum: Cumulative trauma disorders (CTDs) have been recognized for many years, but until now, there has been no comprehensive text encompassing all their aspects. Bits and pieces may be found in different articles and a few thin and strictly specialized books. The complete picture of CTD and its related issues has been understandably difficult to grasp because each source presents only a portion, resembling the different descriptions of the same elephant given by blind men. CTDs are made up of a variety of more or less well-defined morbid entities. It is indeed unique to unite a variety of conditions under the banner of voluntary motions of the repetitive/cumulative/overuse type. This unusual situation requires a special approach to the etiology, epidemiology, pathophysiology, clinical picture, and management.

In this book most questions relating to CTDs are addressed and, it is hoped, answered. The first chapter provides an overview of general concerns, serving as the jumping-off point for the rest of the text. The historical review (Chapter 2) provides a time-based perspective. The third chapter, on neuroanatomy, acquaints the reader with the ascending pain pathways and the descending pain modulatory system, which the reader must know to understand the pain mechanism in CTD. Chapter 4 offers a pathophysiologic model for the various symptoms seen in the most intractable cases. Of particular interest is the hypothesized spreading of the activity in the dorsal horn to the ventral horn of the spinal cord with the corresponding activation of alpha motor neurons and the resulting spasm in muscles innervated by the respective spinal segment. Following the strong anatomic basis provided in Chapters 3 and 4, Chapter 5 covers the specifics of treatment with symptom management measures and includes detailed pharmaceutical descriptions of the most recommended drugs. Physical therapy modalities, psychotherapy, and behavioral/cognitive therapies are also emphasized, along with trigger point injections.

Chapter 6 provides the book's first detailed discussion of occupational hazards, particularly those to industrial workers. Beyond the physical aspect, the effects of CTDs are examined from social, legal, psychological, and economic viewpoints, recognizing the tremendous and varied impact these disorders have on our society. Ergonomics receive considerable and well-deserved attention in this chapter, as do the numerous upper-limb conditions frequently associated with CTDs.

Chapter 7 discusses entrapment neuropathies from an electrophysiologic perspective. The information provided is of interest to medical practitioners and electromyographers because of the meticulous care taken to explain each phenomenon in this area and the association of different nerve entrapments with CTDs.

Chapter 8 treats the subject of lower-extremity CTDs resulting from repetitive overloading during athletic activities. This chapter presents a more recent understanding of the condition, which has been historically confined by definition to upper limbs. As a general rule, weight-bearing plays a major role in sports and relies mostly on the antigravity effort of the lower-extremity muscles. Back injuries are the prime result of athletic activities, but this chapter thoroughly describes a host of sports-related injuries.

CTDs affecting musicians and dancers are discussed in Chapter 9. The muscle groups affected either by playing method or arm position with string instruments are clearly delineated. The chapter expands to include players of wind instruments, who require, perhaps more than other musicians, appropriate training because playing these instruments is an extremely strenuous respiratory activity. Due to the high demand placed on concert musicians, it is understandable that they seem to be affected by CTD symptomatology more than other professional groups. This also applies to dancers, especially professional dancers, in whom the physical demands of the activity are frequently conducive to injury. This chapter carefully analyzes all the elements to be taken into consideration when discussing CTDs in musicians and dancers.

The epidemic character of the industrial low-back pain syndromes renders Chapter 10, dedicated to these conditions, particularly useful when considering the associated high medical costs. The explosive increase in the occurrence of the industrial low-back pain syndromes prompts the author to speculate on the reason for its sudden rise in frequency. Studies dealing with this problem are pertinently analyzed. Prevalence of back pain, evaluation of back injuries, preventive measures, radiographic studies, ergonomics, and back-strengthening programs are covered. This chapter underscores the importance of psychosocial as well as medical considerations in the treatment of most nonspecific low-back pain injuries.

The reflex sympathetic dystrophy syndrome (RSDS) represents the worst possible scenario in CTD. This severe and frequently irreversible condition is thoroughly presented in Chapter 11: Terminology, epidemiology, clinical course, constellation of signs and symptoms, diagnostic procedures including thermography, detailed pathophysiology, and treatment related to RSDS are analyzed. This chapter presents a wealth of information in a systematic manner, enriched by comprehensive tables.

Chapter 12 is dedicated to the use of opioid analgesics, which is much less controversial than it used to be. Unfortunately, pain management remains a poorly addressed topic in most medical schools, and guidance in this area is desperately needed. This chapter includes a thorough review of the related literature, explains how opioids relieve pain as well as the concept of stimulation-produced analgesia, describes the opiate receptors and the endogenous opiates, reviews the descending pain modulating network, and delineates the indications for opioid maintenance analgesic therapy.

Chapter 13 is devoted to the intrathecal opioid pump implantation and Chapter 14 to spinal cord stimulation (SCS). Improvements in the technique and instrumentation of intrathecal opioid pump implantation have been conducive to more comfortable equipment and better outcome data, gaining wider acceptance for the procedure. The pathophysiology of SCS, patient selection criteria, technique, need for trial stimulation, permanent implantation phase, postimplantation care, goals of treatment, and complications are all discussed thoroughly.

Chapter 15 considers the important legal implications of CTDs, and is written by a lawyer experienced in this matter.

Clearly, this comprehensive text offers encyclopedic information on all aspects of CTDs, making it useful as a book to be read from beginning to end or as a reference work to be consulted from time to time in one's daily practice.

Arminius Cassvan, M.D.

Acknowledgments

We thank Karen Oberheim, Medical Editor at Butterworth–Heinemann; Sheila Slezak, secretary at Nassau County Medical Center; and Jenn Nagaj, Production Editor at Silverchair Science + Communications for their assistance in the preparation of this manuscript.

Cumulative Trauma Disorders

Chapter 1

General Considerations Regarding Cumulative Trauma Disorders

Arminius Cassvan

Terminology

Repetitive strain injuries or cumulative trauma disorders have been described as "a group of disorders that most commonly develop in workers using excessive and repetitious motions of the neck and upper extremity" [1]. In addition to workers in business and industry, these disorders may affect performing artists, athletes, and people engaged in recreational activities.

Repetitive strain injury (RSI), *cumulative trauma disorders* (CTDs), and *overuse syndrome* (OS) are three terms applied to the same group of morbid entities. These entities reflect the features of the described maladies and refer to the causative factors rather than to the specific pathologic processes affecting organs. The term *overuse syndrome* offers perhaps the best *functional* description of the effect of cumulative trauma or repetitive strain, but this term does not define the type of activity (repetitive or cumulative) that produces such an effect.

Some believe that pain syndromes in the group of morbid entities defined by the foregoing terms manifest in specific areas such as the neck and upper extremities, but in this book we also include the trunk and lower limbs. Musculoskeletal and neuropathic disorders must be carefully differentiated from "rheumatologic diseases, psychologic disorders, acute joint or tendon inflammation from other causes and single event traumatic sprains and strains" [1]. The defining characteristic of an RSI, CTD, or OS is excessive and mainly repetitious motion. Hence, no trauma caused by a single event, local inflammatory processes, or systemic diseases can be classified as any of these entities.

In view of this requirement, *repetitive strain injury*, probably the most commonly used term, appears to be adequate for defining this group of disorders. However, the word *cumulative* reflects another necessary dimension—namely that, in addition to being repetitive, the noxious agent (in this case, motion), also is accumulating, gradually increasing by successive additions [2]. The term *cumulative trauma disorders*, therefore, offers the most accurate definition.

In 1994, a new term for the same entity—*repetitive motion disorders*—was introduced [3]. This term, however, does not take into account the cumulative nature of many of these disorders. The authors of the report in which this term was coined describe the disorders as an "overuse of the joints or soft tissues of the upper extremity" [3].

Incidence

Many specific conditions may be attributed to CTDs, including cervical syndrome, tension neck syndrome, thoracic outlet syndrome, frozen shoulder syndrome, epicondylitis, carpal tunnel syndrome, and ulnar nerve entrapment. Other authors might include other entities or eliminate some of those cited here. CTDs, therefore, can comprise a large collection of pathologic conditions. Specific entities will be described in this book in terms of their relationship to different occupations or activities prone to incite CTDs.

In an article published in 1992, it was estimated that CTDs account for more than 50% of all occupational illnesses in the United States [4]. This high percentage has resulted in a loss of productivity, increased costs as a result of high medical expenses and disability payments for injured workers, and personal consequences for the employee, who suffers pain and functional impairment that sometimes necessitate a change of occupation.

A 1993 U.S. Department of Labor, Bureau of Labor Statistics report [5] revealed that in 1991 workers experienced approximately 6.3 million job-related injuries at a rate of 8.4 per 100 full-time workers. This represents a significant increase over the 1985–1986 rate of 7.9 injuries per 100 full-time workers. The factors influencing the number of reported injuries in any given year include "changes in working conditions, work practices, the number of hours worked and worker experience and training" [5]. It should be pointed out that the report refers to musculoskeletal disorders in general. Occupational CTDs, a subset of CTDs, is the major cause of disability in persons of working age (18–64 years). Louis [6] estimated that the number of annual visits made to physicians in the United States for musculoskeletal injuries and conditions is more than 12 million, with a cost in excess of $65 billion in 1984 alone. One-third of all the reported disorders were a result of upper-limb conditions.

In 1992, Schwartz [7] showed that CTDs increased fivefold since 1979 and now account for up to 47% of all workplace injuries. Schwartz found the most common diagnosed manifestations to be nerve entrapments, tendinitis, and "other soft tissue injuries." Occupational as well as nonoccupational factors contribute to the etiology of these CTDs.

Statistics show a different trend in Canada where, in 1991, there were 520,547 work-related injuries, representing a decrease of 12% as compared to 1990 [8]. The decrease was attributed mainly to a deterioration in labor-market conditions. A separate category, strains and sprains, accounted for 44% of the total number of injuries.

In Australia, a significant increase in the incidence of CTDs has been described as an epidemic for Telecom, a government organization employing 90,000 workers [9]. No fewer than 343 cases of CTDs were recorded for 1,000 keyboard telecommunication workers from 1981 to 1985. Other employees, such as clerical workers, telegraphists, and process workers also were affected. Sixteen percent of the affected employees had symptoms for more than 26 weeks, at a cost of more than $15 million.

Evaluation of the magnitude of the effect of CTDs must take into account the physical *and* psychological injuries to the patients and their families. In addition to the obvious cost of medical treatment of musculoskeletal injuries, there are hidden costs such as the loss of productivity, absenteeism, and poor performance.

Pathogenesis

Isernhagen [10] advanced our understanding of cumulative trauma by noting that, rather than affecting one joint or muscle, cumulative trauma affects several parts of the body at the same time. This explains, at least in part, the importance of a prevention program for CTDs.

In 1993, Armstrong et al. [11] presented the pathogenesis of work-related musculoskeletal disorders in the form of a conceptual model. Only a few goals were intended or attained: to demonstrate the relationship between common exposure factors and various responses, to design laboratory and field studies, and to evaluate and conceive jobs in which work-related musculoskeletal disorders are prevented. The model "contains sets of cascading exposure, dose, capacity and response variables, such that response at one level can act as dose at the next" [11]. The dynamics of the conceived model allow response to one or more doses to diminish or increase the capacity to respond to successive doses. The model is intended as a framework for studying the development of work-related muscle, tendon, and nerve diseases.

Australian researchers have shown a consistent interest in the pathogenesis of the refractory cervicobrachial syndrome. A recent article also rekindles the interest in the pathogenesis of this disorder [12]. Chapter 2 traces different hypotheses posited to explain this condition.

Causes

Among the causes of occupationally related CTDs are forceful exertions, repetitive prolonged activities, awkward postures, localized contact stresses, vibration, and cold temperatures [3]. As explained by Keyserling et al. [13], the risk of developing a CTD is directly proportional to the amount of force exerted for a certain task. Factors include pinch grips, heavy or poorly maintained tools (e.g., dull knives or scissors), and a low coefficient of friction between the hand and the respective tool handle. Wearing gloves is an impediment because it reduces tactile feedback, thereby increasing the effort the worker must make.

Silverstein et al. [14] studied 652 workers engaged in 39 jobs within seven different industrial sites. The prevalence of carpal tunnel syndrome was only 0.6% for workers in low-force, low-repetition tasks and 5.6% in employees in high-force, high-repetition tasks. The workers in the latter category were 15 times more likely to suffer than the ones in the former group. Because repetition appears to be a more important factor than force in the development of a CTD, it is conceivable that the awkward hand posture (which was not considered in Silverstein's study [14]) is a necessary ingredient for the high-force, high-repetition group and compounds the problem [3]. Armstrong et al. [15] described "tendinitis of hand and wrist," a less well-defined condition. In their study, the odds ratio for the high-force, high-repetition tasks was 29.4 greater than for the low-force, low-repetition group.

Awkward postures that result in excessive shoulder elevation, elbow motion, deviated wrist positions, and pinch grips may lead to the development of occupational CTDs involving the shoulder, elbow, wrist, and hand. Such awkward postures may affect the musculoskeletal structures, the peripheral nerves, or both [16,17].

Localized stress, or the physical contact between the worker's body and an object or tool, also plays a role in the genesis of occupational CTDs. Usually, hard or sharp tools pressing against a body part are implicated. A worker may use his or her hand as a mallet while positioning or fitting a part. Tools that press in the palm of the hand may injure the median nerve, thus producing carpal tunnel syndrome [18].

The role of vibration in the production of occupational CTDs is significant [14,16,19,20]. Grasping power tools, holding the controls of a powered machine, or using percussive tools such as hammers and chisels generates prolonged vibration exposure [15,21]. Such use of tools also results in the use of excessive force to master the vibrating tool, thus increasing the tendency to develop CTDs. Silverstein et al. [14] noted that vibration exposure was recognized in six of the 11 jobs in which a worker was suspected of having carpal tunnel syndrome. A common feature of all these jobs was high force and high repetition. Unfortunately, it was not possible to isolate the vibration factor. Nonetheless, we do know that force, repetition, and vibration can all be implicated in the genesis of carpal tunnel syndrome.

Cold temperatures are considered another risk factor for CTDs [15,21,22]. Pneumatic tools and their cold exhaust may adversely affect dexterity of the fingers and tactile sensitivity. Muscle strains and sprains may be brought about by a frigid environment that reduces the worker's ability to perform proficiently. More force is needed to achieve tasks in a cold environment than in a warm one. Armstrong et al. [15] demonstrated that normal subjects exert pressures of up to 4 pounds per square inch (psi) when using a hammer and pressing on its handle. When the hand is anesthetized, the amount of pressure needed is as high as 16 psi. Gloves can be used to protect the fingers and hands from cold temperatures, but these too have the undesirable effect of increasing the force required to perform a task because of the reduced tactile feedback.

Further study is needed to isolate the effect of each risk factor so that the etiology of CTDs can be better understood.

Manifestations

Kroemer [23] has developed a table of entities considered to be manifestations of CTDs (Table 1-1). A logical sequence for the list of 15 conditions was not established. Kroemer [23] cites activities such as soldering, buffing, grinding, polishing, and sanding as factors that contribute to the development of CTDs and to the rare pronator (teres) syndrome. In addition to these activities, sawing, cutting, butchering, using pliers, turning controls, inserting screws in holes, forceful hand wringing, and operating a punch press may produce tenosynovitis/tendovaginitis, disorders that affect tendons "that are inside tendon sheaths" and characterized by swelling of the respective sheath [23].

Thoracic outlet syndrome, a condition that is difficult to diagnosis neurogenically, is frequently men-

Table 1-1. Common Repetitive Strain Injuries to Nerves, Tendons and Tendon Sheaths, Muscles, or Blood Vessels

Disorder (type)	Description	Typical Activities
Carpal tunnel syndrome (writer's cramp, neuritis, median neuritis) (N)	The result of compression of the median nerve in the carpal tunnel of the wrist. This tunnel is an opening under the carpal ligament on the palmar side of the carpal bones. Through this tunnel pass the median nerve, the finger flexor tendons, and blood vessels. Swelling of the tendon sheaths reduces the size of the opening of the tunnel and pinches the median nerve and, possibly, blood vessels. The tunnel opening is also reduced if the wrist is flexed or extended or pivoted ulnarly or radially.	Buffing, grinding, polishing, sanding, assembly work, typing, keying, cashiering, playing musical instruments, performing surgery, packing, housekeeping, cooking, butchering, hand washing, scrubbing, hammering.
Cubital tunnel syndrome (N)	Compression of the ulnar nerve below the notch of the elbow. Tingling, numbness, or pain radiating into the ring or little fingers.	Resting forearm near elbow on a hard surface or sharp edge; also when reaching over an obstruction.
de Quervain's disease (T)	A special case of tenosynovitis that occurs in the abductor and extensor tendons of the thumb, where they share a common sheath. This condition often results from combined forceful gripping and hand twisting, as in wringing clothes.	Buffing, grinding, polishing, sanding, pushing, pressing, sawing, cutting, performing surgery, butchering, using pliers, turning controls such as on a motorcycle, inserting screws in holes, forceful hand wringing.
Epicondylitis (tennis elbow) (T)	Irritation of the tendons attaching to the epicondyle (the lateral protrusion at the distal end of the humerus bone). This condition is often the result of impacting or jerky throwing motions, repeated supination and pronation of the forearm, and forceful wrist extension movements. It is well known among tennis players, pitchers, bowlers, and people who hammer. A similar irritation of the tendon attachments on the inside of the elbow is called *medial epicondylitis* ("golfer's elbow").	Turning screws, assembling small parts, hammering, meat cutting, playing musical instruments, playing tennis, pitching, bowling.
Ganglion (T)	A tendon-sheath swelling filled with synovial fluid or a cystic tumor at the tendon sheath or a joint membrane. The affected area swells up and creates a bump under the skin, often on the dorsal or radial side of the wrist. (Because in the past this bump occasionally was smashed by striking with a Bible or heavy book, it was also called a *Bible bump*.)	Buffing, grinding, polishing, sanding, pushing, pressing, sawing, cutting, playing musical instruments, playing tennis, pitching, bowling.
Neck tension syndrome (M)	An irritation of the levator scapulae and trapezius group of muscles of the neck, commonly occurring after repeated or sustained overhead work.	Conveyor-belt assembly, typing, keying, assembling small parts, packing, load carrying in hand or on shoulder.
Pronator (teres) syndrome (N)	Result of compression of the median nerve in the distal third of the forearm, often where it passes through the two heads of the pronator teres muscle in the forearm. This condition is common with strenuous flexion of the elbow and wrist.	Soldering, buffing, grinding, polishing, sanding.

Shoulder tendinitis (rotator cuff syndrome or tendinitis, supraspinous tendinitis, subacromial bursitis, subdeltoid bursitis, partial tear of the rotator cuff) (T)	Shoulder disorder at the rotator cuff. The cuff consists of four tendons that fuse over the shoulder joint, where they pronate and supinate the arm and help to abduct it. The rotator cuff tendons must pass through a small bony passage between the humerus and the acromion, with a bursa as cushion.	Soldering, buffing, grinding, polishing, sanding.
Tendinitis (tendinitis) (T)	Inflammation of a tendon, often associated with repeated tension, motion, bending, being in contact with a hard surface, or vibration. The tendon becomes thickened, bumpy, and irregular on its surface. Tendon fibers may be frayed or torn apart. In tendons without sheaths, such as within the elbow and shoulder, the injured area may calcify.	Punch-press operations, assembly work, wiring, packaging, core making, using pliers.
Tendonitis (tendinitis) (T)	An inflammation of a tendon. Often associated with repeated tension, motion, bending, being in contact with a hard surface, or vibration. The tendon becomes thickened, bumpy, and irregular on its surface. Tendon fibers may be frayed or torn apart. In tendons without sheaths, such as within the elbow and shoulder, the injured area may calcify.	Punch-press operations, assembly work, wiring, packaging, core making, use of pliers.
Tenosynovitis (tendovaginitis) (T)	Disorder of tendons inside synovial sheaths. The sheath swells, impeding movement of the tendon within the sheath and causing pain. The tendon surfaces can become irritated, rough, and bumpy. If the inflamed sheath presses progressively onto the tendon, the condition is called *stenosing tenosynovitis*. de Quervain's disease is a special case occurring in the thumb; the trigger-finger condition occurs in flexors of the fingers.	Buffing, grinding, polishing, sanding, punch-press operation, sawing, cutting, performing surgery, butchering, using pliers, turning controls such as on a motorcycle, inserting screws in holes, forceful hand wringing.
Thoracic outlet syndrome (neurovascular compression syndrome, cervicobrachial disorder, brachial plexus neuritis, costoclavicular syndrome, hyperabduction syndrome) (V, N)	Disorder resulting from compression of nerves and blood vessels between the clavicle and first and second ribs at the brachial plexus. If this neurovascular bundle is compressed by the pectoralis minor muscle, blood flow to and from the arm is reduced. This ischemic condition makes the arm numb and limits muscular activities.	Buffing, grinding, polishing, sanding, overhead assembly, overhead welding, overhead painting, overhead auto repair, typing, keying, cashiering, wiring, playing musical instruments, performing surgery, truck driving, stacking, material handling, postal letter carrying, carrying heavy loads with arms extended.
Trigger finger or thumb (T)	Special case of tenosynovitis in which the tendon becomes nearly locked, so that its forced movement is not smooth but is in a snapping, jerking manner. This is a special case of stenosing tenosynovitis crepitans, a condition usually found with digit flexors at the A1 ligament.	Operating a finger trigger, using hand tools with sharp edges that press into the tissue or whose handles are too far apart for the user's hand, so that the end segments of the user's fingers are flexed while the middle segments are straight.

Table 1-1. *Continued*

Disorder (type)	Description	Typical Activities
Ulnar nerve entrapment (Guyon's tunnel syndrome) (N)	Results from entrapment of the ulnar nerve as it passes through Guyon's tunnel in the wrist. It can occur from prolonged flexion and extension of the wrist and repeated pressure on the hypothenar eminence of the palm.	Playing musical instruments, carpentering, bricklaying, using pliers, soldering, hammering.
White finger ("dead finger," Raynaud's syndrome, vibration syndrome) (V)	Stems from insufficient blood supply, bringing about noticeable blanching (finger turns cold and numb and tingles); sensation and control of finger movement may be lost. The condition is due to closure of the digit's arteries caused by vasospasms triggered by vibrations. A common cause is continued forceful gripping of vibrating tools, particularly in a cold environment.	Chainsawing, jackhammering, using a vibrating tool, sanding, paint scraping, using a tool that is too small for the hand, often in a cold environment.
Ulnar artery aneurysm	Weakening of the wall of the ulnar artery as it passes through Guyon's tunnel in the wrist; often from pounding or pushing with heel of the hand. The resulting "bubble" presses on the ulnar nerve in Guyon's tunnel.	Assembly work.

N = nerve disorder; T = tendon disorder; M = muscle disorder; V = vessel disorder.
Source: Reprinted with permission from KHE Kroemer. Avoiding cumulative trauma disorders in shops and offices. Am Ind Hyg Assoc J 1992;53:599.

tioned in relation to CTDs. Any activity that requires one to maintain the arms above the head may lead to thoracic outlet syndrome. String instrument players, overhead painters, and postal and auto repair workers are among those who might be affected.

Kroemer [23] also lists trigger finger or thumb (defined as a special case of tenosynovitis in which the tendon becomes nearly locked), distal ulnar nerve entrapment, white finger (Raynaud's syndrome), and ulnar artery aneurysm as possible manifestations of CTDs. Kroemer's classification emphasizes the fact that CTDs comprise heterogeneous conditions (see Table 1-1).

A manifestation of cumulative trauma in physical fitness and sporting activities is so-called overtraining. Like other forms of cumulative trauma, overtraining increases the demands on the musculoskeletal system and results in clinical, functional, and biomechanical adaptations that are potentially detrimental to sport performances [24]. Overtraining injuries may be overt, preventing the patient from engaging in any sport activities for some time, or subclinical, being detected rarely. As a rule, however, overtraining injuries decrease performance. A thorough evaluation of an athlete before performance should be conducted. Subtle signs of maladaptation in terms of strength and flexibility may reflect undertraining or overtraining and increased chance of injury. The best antidote for overtraining-related adaptations is an effective sport-specific conditioning program, aimed at giving the athlete a "strong musculoskeletal base on which to build athletic skills" [24]. In addition, a maintenance conditioning program of long duration may be important for maintaining fitness throughout the entire athletic season.

Symptoms

The initial symptoms of CTDs might be tenderness, pain, swelling, weakness, sensation loss or disturbance, and temperature change [6,20]. Although symptoms generally have a gradual onset, occasionally a patient may become aware of them suddenly. This usually portends a subclinical, gradual development of symptoms that do not present until the involved tissue becomes overloaded.

Muscle damage by exercise is far from rare [25]. Overuse at the muscular level and subsequent struc-

tural damage of the contractile elements is manifested clinically by delayed-onset muscular soreness (DOMS). From a pathologic viewpoint, an initial insult is followed by an inflammatory response, which in turn is followed by regeneration. The details of the process are not yet understood fully. Although it is assumed calcium plays a major role in the development of DOMS, the inflammatory changes in humans do not correlate with biopsy data, so DOMS remains unexplained.

It is known that one session of eccentric exercises has a prolonged protective effect against damage provoked by a second session of exercises [25]. It was demonstrated experimentally that this adaptive phenomenon may be explained in part by an increase in connective tissue. Gender differences also influence exercise-induced plasma creatine kinase. Here, sex hormone–dependent differences in sarcolemmal permeability account for variability in the plasma creatine kinase activity, considered to be a marker for the extent of muscle damage. However, the plasma creatine kinase level does not necessarily reflect the amount of structural damage [25].

Management

Prevention of CTDs through safer work environments, early diagnosis, and appropriate therapy are advocated as the best ways to decrease the number of CTDs in the workplace. Management of CTDs emphasizes prevention as the cornerstone of successful intervention. Rest and rehabilitation are paramount in effective treatment [26].

Peate [27], in a review of workplace injuries or illnesses caused by mechanical stress, strain, sprain, vibration, or irritation, reported that conservative treatment of CTDs consists of ice or heat packs, protective devices such as splints, nonsteroidal anti-inflammatory drugs, and progressive strengthening exercises. Ergonomics and specific work practices are considered useful tools in managing musculoskeletal conditions. Specific work practices call for attention to and revision of workplace conditions, psychosocial factors, and special worker training in the use of active modalities such as exercise and a progressive increase in activities of daily living. These methods are preferred over the more passive measures such as bedrest and traction.

Of 176 musicians referred to the author for overuse injury syndromes, 41 had not been prescribed rest, refused to rest, or quit rest treatment early. Of 45 of the referred patients prescribed a modified rest management program, 87% were cured of symptoms [26]. Ninety of the patients were prescribed "radical rest treatment" [26], for whom the success rate also was 87%. The relative amount of rest must be individualized.

Ergonomic interventions are emphasized in an overview published in 1992 [19]. Occupational risk factors were identified as forceful exertion, repetitiveness, vibration, cold, and "extreme postures." The author stressed the need to evaluate the efficacy of ergonomic interventions using the same methods used to identify problems initially.

The clinical presentations of injuries incurred in physical fitness and sporting activities must be understood so that the exact point at which training becomes overtraining can be recognized, a prospective determination that is very difficult. An effort to define the anatomic parameters and amount of exercise responsible for overtraining will be a task of the future, as will be devising physical fitness examinations and training programs to allow maximal performance with minimal overtraining risk. Adaptations occur in muscles, tendons, and bones as a reaction to high training loads, with detrimental effect on performance and increased risk of injury. Because the exact optimal exercise dose remains unknown, careful evaluation of these adaptations, of noninjured areas, and of rehabilitated areas is necessary.

Meeusen and Borms [28] looked at gymnastic injuries and the relationship of such injuries to overtraining. For gymnasts, as for many other athletes, the ankle is statistically the most injured body part. Upper-limb and back injuries are also common in these athletes. In gymnastics, the upper limbs characteristically are used as weight-bearing extremities, and the high-impact loads are distributed through the elbow and wrist. Activities specific to gymnasts, such as vaulting and hyperextension, may be conducive to back injuries as a result of single or repeated episodes of microtrauma. Early detection of injury plays an important role in the management of these conditions, especially in the elbow, wrist, and back. It is critical to allow the injured gymnast enough time for complete rehabilitation [28] before he or she

returns to full-time practice. There seems to be a correlation between the rate of maturation and predisposition to injury; an individual is at especially high risk for injury during intense training following periods of rapid growth.

References

1. Guidotti TL. Occupational repetitive strain injury [review]. Am Fam Physician 1992;45:585.
2. Webster's Dictionary: The New Lexicon. New York: Modern Publishing, 1987.
3. Williams R, Westmorland M. Occupational cumulative trauma disorders of the upper extremity [see comments]. Am J Occup Ther 1994;48:411.
4. Rempel DM, Harrison RJ, Barnhart S. Work-related cumulative trauma disorders of the upper extremity. JAMA 1992;267:838.
5. Bureau of Labor Statistics. Occupational Injuries and Illnesses in the United States by Industry. Washington, DC: US Department of Labor, Bureau of Labor Statistics, 1991.
6. Louis D. Cumulative trauma disorders. J Hand Surg [Am] 1987;12:823.
7. Schwartz RG. Cumulative trauma disorders [review]. Orthopedics 1992;15:1051.
8. Statistics Canada, Labour Division. Work Injuries 1989–91. Ottawa, Ontario: Statistics Canada, Labour Division, 1992.
9. Hocking B. Epidemiological aspects of "repetition strain injury" in Telecom, Australia. Med J Aust 1987;147:218.
10. Isernhagen SJ. Principles and prevention for cumulative trauma. Occup Med 1992;7:147.
11. Armstrong TJ, Buckle P, Fine LJ, et al. A conceptual model for work-related neck and upper limb musculoskeletal disorders. Scand J Work Environ Health 1994;19:73.
12. Cohen ML, Arroyo JF, Champion GD, et al. In search of the pathogenesis of refractory cervicobrachial pain syndrome. A deconstruction of the RSI phenomenon [review]. Med J Aust 1992;158:432.
13. Keyserling WM, Armstrong TJ, Punnett L. Ergonomic job analysis. A structured approach for identifying risk factors associated with overexertion injuries and disorders. Appl Occup Environ Hyg 1991;6:353.
14. Silverstein B, Fine IJ, Armstrong TJ. Occupational factors and carpal tunnel syndrome. Am J Ind Med 1987;11:343.
15. Armstrong TJ, Fine LJ, Goldstein SA, et al. Ergonomic considerations in hand and wrist tendinitis. J Hand Surg [Am] 1992;12:830.
16. Armstrong TJ. Ergonomics and cumulative trauma disorders. Hand Clin 1986;3:533.
17. Johnson SI. Ergonomic tool design. Hand Clin 1993;9:299.

18. Szabo RM, Gleberman RH. The pathophysiology of nerve entrapment syndromes. J Hand Surg [Am] 1987;12:880.

19. Frederick IJ. Cumulative trauma disorders: an overview. AAOHN J 1992;40(3):13.

20. Chatterjee DS. Repetitive strain injury: a recent review. Occup Med 1987;37:100.

21. Falkenburg SA, Schultz DJ. Ergonomics for the upper extremity. Hand Clin 1993;9:263.

22. Sheifer RE, Kok R, Lewis MI, et al. Finger skin temperature and manual dexterity: some intergroup differences. Appl Ergon 1984;15:135.

23. Kroemer KHE. Avoiding cumulative trauma disorders in shops and offices. Am Ind Hyg Assoc J 1992;53:593.

24. Kebler WB, Chandler TJ, Stracener ES. Musculoskeletal adaptations and injuries due to overtraining. Exerc Sport Sci Rev 1992;20:99.

25. Kuipers H. Exercise-induced muscle damage. Int J Sports Med 1994;15:132.

26. Fry HJ. The treatment of overuse injury syndrome. Md Med J 1993;42:277.

27. Peate WF. Occupational musculoskeletal disorders [review]. Prim Care 1994;21:313.

28. Meeusen R, Borms J. Gymnastic injuries [review]. Sports Med 1992;13:337.

Chapter 2
Historical Review of Cumulative Trauma Disorders

Arminius Cassvan

Organic Versus Functional Theories of Cumulative Trauma Disorder Pathogenesis

Although cumulative trauma disorders (CTDs) emerged as a by-product of modern technology, it is not a new phenomenon. In the seventeenth century, Ramazzini [1] first recognized work as a cause of musculoskeletal disorders due to "violent motions of the body." Severe and persistent arm pain associated with other sensory symptoms were described in scriveners, men whose occupation demanded incessant writing. Their affliction was referred to as *scrivener's palsy*, a condition at times so severe that the affected patients had to give up their profession. The condition was described in 1864 and 1867 by Solly, Senior Surgeon at St. Thomas's Hospital in London [2,3]. The sensations were described as burning or aching pain in the arm and numbness and pins and needles in the fingers. The arm felt fatigued and cold. Only one of Solly's patients [3] complained early in the course of the disease of cramp in the entire hand after too much writing. The cramp later was replaced by severe pain of the hand and arm and tingling in the fingers. Pain and fatigue required this patient to stop writing altogether. Solly [3] hypothesized that injury, through excessive work, to a center located either in the spinal cord or the cerebellum was creating the symptoms.

A few years later, another London physician, Reynolds [4], considered the condition synonymous with writer's cramp, as the diagnosis of this latter morbid entity was based solely on the presence of involuntary spasmodic symptoms (cramp). Reynolds recognized that abnormal sensations in the affected area, such as numbness, cold, heaviness, and pain, occurred in only a few of the patients suffering from writer's cramp. A pathologically related disease was described also in artists, musicians, seamstresses, smiths, and milkmaids.

New York clinician Austin Flint [5] ascribed much less importance to this so-called writer's cramp, describing it as a "local spasmodic affection" not deserving of taxonomic efforts.

George Vivian Poore [6–10] invested a great amount of time and effort in attempting to understand this and related disorders. In an initial article [6], he described the management of only one patient suffering from the spasmodic form of the cramp. The condition at first was considered a "curious sample of a most rare and difficult disorder." From 1872 to 1875, Poore [7] collected 42 cases demonstrating a common feature, the patient's loss of the ability to write. In more than one-third of patients, this was believed to be due to the fatigue of a few muscles overused in the process of incessant writing. However, this phenomenon involving agonist and, at times, antagonist groups of muscles occurred relatively infrequently. In fact, the majority of patients studied suffered from a condition called *sine materia*, in which there was no evidence of either cramp or paralysis but instead a kind of idiopathic "impotence." Of special interest was the case of a renowned pianist who developed this type of neuralgic pain when playing her instrument.

Poore [8] next published a study of 75 cases in 1878. Different manifestations of the same condition were noted and classified into six categories: paralytic, spasmodic, degenerative, neuritic or neuralgic, "true" writer's cramp, and an anomalous group including entities such as locomotor ataxia. The paralytic group, which included patients with paralysis of muscles secondary to definite peripheral nerve lesions, appeared to be one of the most objective. The second group included a case of focal dystonia after excessively long hours of incessant writing. A case of hemiplegia, possibly hemiparesis, is also included in the second group. Tremors of the upper extremities made writing impossible for the patients classified in the third group, and this symptom heralded the initial stage of severe degenerative central nervous system (CNS) disease.

Patients in the fourth and fifth groups resembled the ones described by Solly [2,3]. Symptoms in these patients included neuralgic or fatigue pain related to any activity of the affected upper limb, inability to find a comfortable position for the same during sleep, and numbness and cramping of the affected hand. On physical examination, tenderness on radial nerve palpation was often found. Objectively, faradism disclosed an exaggerated irritability of the radial nerve and of the muscles supplied by it. There were manifestations of muscle weakness as well, such as difficulty with forearm supination and flexion of the respective thumb. Pain and dysesthesia on the dorsum of the hand were also noted.

The number of cases presented by Poore [9] increased to 117 by 1887. Excluded from these were cases bearing little similarity to writer's cramp, such as the cases classified in the paralytic and degenerative categories [10]. Loss of writing ability was again the common denominator. In this series of cases, tenderness was noted mainly along the median rather than radial nerve. The faradic irritability was depressed rather than increased for a number of muscles. The change in irritability was attributed to muscle fatigue, whereas nerve tenderness was attributed to overuse. Contrary to Solly, Poore believed that these patients were the victims of a peripheral neuromuscular disorder rather than of a more central neurologic disease.

In 1887, Poore [10] reported on 21 piano players who experienced inability to perform due to pain. The most constant finding among these musicians was nerve trunk tenderness. Even slight stretching of the tender nerves frequently was very painful. In this article, Poore [10] described specific stretching tests for each major nerve of the forearm (median, ulnar, and radial).

Poore received support for his views on the pathogenesis of CTDs from the American clinician Beard [11] who, in 1874, studied 125 patients with writer's cramp and related conditions and concluded that the pain originated from local involvement of upper-limb nerves and muscles.

More than 100 years later, an electrophysiologic approach to the spasmodic form of writer's cramp was initiated by Nakashima et al. [12]. The authors studied the H reflex in the flexor carpi radialis muscle and found a disturbance of reciprocal inhibition in the forearm flexor muscles, with cocontraction of agonist and antagonist muscles during the voluntary act of writing. There was, in addition, an overflow of contraction to remote muscles. It is interesting to note that the same findings were described in the dystonic upper limb of patients with symptomatic hemidystonia, a condition secondary to structural brain lesions, as well as in certain patients with hemiparesis resulting from cerebrovascular accidents. The conclusion was that, in all these cases, a basal ganglia dysfunction could be identified. Such a disease affected the descending control of those spinal interneurons that mediate the group I presynaptic inhibition of afferent terminals in the spinal cord.

The impact made by Poore and Beard in understanding a peripheral etiology for these conditions was reversed by a number of articles published in the sixth and seventh decades of the nineteenth century, in which the spasmodic, paralytic, and neuralgic syndromes described by Poore were considered clinical symptoms of an underlying dysfunction within the CNS [4,13]. A prominent English physician, Gowers [14,15], was aware of Poore's research and, following the German trend, addressed all these upper-limb disorders as "occupation neuroses" (from the German *Beschaftigung Neurosen*). By definition, the term *neurosis* was considered by German students such as Cassirer [16] to mean "devoid of any underlying lesion of the nervous system." In his intentional use of the term, Gowers related the occupation neuroses to a "nervous" temperament and considered this an important predisposing factor. He divided the occupation neuroses into motor (spasmodic) and sensory (neuralgic) varieties and postulated that dysfunction of a central cortical center was responsible for affected repetitive or cumulative activity. Gowers recognized, however, the added contribution of any local upper-limb disease or injury.

In an attempt to unify his views and the previous contributions by Poore and Beard, Gowers [15] acknowledged the possibility of secondary pathologic changes in sensory nerves and attributed these changes to pain of CNS origin. He considered reflex pain mechanisms responsible for secondary changes in the irritability and nutrition of the muscles of the affected limb. Gowers considered that any predisposing factor for cramp was able to lower the tone of the nervous system. His favorite example was anxiety, a symptom found in many of his patients as a result of family or professional troubles. The same factors were noted by Reynolds [4], who did not consider them nearly as important as did Gowers.

The most powerful supporter of the CNS theory in explaining occupation neuroses was the German neurologist Oppenheim [13]. According to him, "continued emotion" was the causative factor. Writer's cramp, he postulated, was a functional disorder, a so-called exhaustion neurosis, originating in centers in the central apparatus responsible for associative action of the muscles involved in writing. Oppenheim claimed that a neuropathic predisposition was present in most of his patients. Related conditions found in these patients were neurasthenia, hemicrania, neuralgia, epilepsy, stuttering, tabes, and agoraphobia. Cassirer [16] concurred with Oppenheim's views. He considered most of the cases of writer's cramp to be related to neurasthenia, a fashionable condition at that time, considered to reflect a congenital or acquired neuropathic disposition.

The CNS theory for explaining occupational neuroses was attacked by Boston neurologist W.E. Paul in 1911 [17], who argued that proponents of that theory paid the most attention to a rarely encountered symptom, namely cramping. Indeed, in his extensive clinical study of 200 patients, Paul [17] found no patient with this symptom to whom he could attribute a CNS origin. The symptomatology described in his patient population included upper-limb pain in 177 patients (pain in muscles, joints, and adjacent areas), numbness in 38 patients, and weakness in 26 patients. He concluded that the entire collection of entities known as *CTDs* can be explained by local injuries to muscles or peripheral motor nerves innervating them or to tendons, fascia, or joints, caused by repetitive or cumulative impacts and tensions of short duration.

Another peripheral nervous system (PNS) theory was based on evidence of chronic myositic nodules as noted by Norstrom in 1904 [18]. These nodules were found in the posterior muscles of the neck and were deemed responsible for the headaches suffered by his patients. Later he noted the same nodules in muscles of the head, arm, and forearm in 34 of 47 patients suffering from the spasmodic form of writer's cramp. The cramp was believed to be secondary to "chronic myositis," which Norstrom treated mostly with massage. Norstrom [18] recognized that a neurotic disposition preceding or following the "cramp" could worsen the prognosis and indicated this association by using the term *reflex irritability*. Another move toward unifying the CNS and PNS etiologies was to consider the cases of cramp without myositic nodules to be of CNS origin, as the cause in these cases could be a disturbance of the centers for the coordination of motion.

As early as 1898, Monell [19,20] cited chronic fatigue as the cause of CTDs. He believed that the rapid repetitive movements required by certain occupations did not give the muscles damaged by their own metabolism the time to regenerate, especially if there were only short periods of rest. He described a progression of symptoms from acute muscle fatigue to a persistent, chronic stage at which the patients experienced pain but also "lameness," heaviness of the arm, and marked weakness. With the progression of symptoms, significant deficiency in nutrition of the tissues took place and, consequently, even more prolonged rest periods became increasingly less effective.

Additional Theories of Cumulative Trauma Disorder Pathogenesis

In the early years of the twentieth century, it became increasingly evident that CNS or PNS theories could not explain all the cases of CTDs. Paul's views [17] were addressed at the Thirty-Seventh Annual Meeting of the American Neurological Association [21] at which the noted neurologist Ramsay-Hunt mentioned the existence of 50–60 different types of occupation "neuritis." He recommended distinguishing these conditions from true cramp or spasm-type pain.

The taxonomic concern displayed by some authors regarding occupational neuritis is of interest. In a four-group classification proposed in 1912, the first group consisted of patients with direct repeated trauma to the nerves caused by the type of work, whereas the second group was composed of those exposed to such poisonous substances as lead [22]. In the third group, which bears the most similarity to CTDs, were patients in whom a nerve lesion was produced by fatigue of certain muscle groups or by entrapment neuropathies. Finally, the fourth group included alcoholic patients or those suffering from infectious conditions.

A New York clinician, Charles Dana from Cornell, contributed another article addressing the heterogeneity of the occupational neuritic conditions [23]. His 100 patients, drawn from a large variety of occupations such as writing, telegraphing, stenography, typing, musical performing, pressing, ironing, and tailoring, suffered mainly upper-limb symptomatology related to their occupations. More than half of the patients, according to the author, suffered from occupational neuralgias and neuritides. Another 23 patients experienced true occupationally induced cramps, whereas cramps were associated with brachialgia or neuritis in six patients. Dana's theory for the origin of these patients' pain had a symptomatic basis: If there was major pain in the arm, tenderness along the course of the affected nerves, tingling, numbness, and pins-and-needles sensations, the condition definitely was primarily peripheral in nature and secondarily attributable to an existing neuritis [23].

Windscheid [24], a German physician who did not believe that neurologic deficits represented a necessary ingredient in the definition of the term *neuralgia*, theorized that overstrain caused by various occupations could predispose to "neuralgia of the nerves of the cervical and brachial plexus." Other authors, too, found an anatomic basis for occupational neuroses [25]. Discrete peripheral nerve lesions of the upper limbs were described as being related to occupational factors. In his retrospective view of previously published materials, Spaans [25] asserted that many conditions termed *occupational neuroses* in the older literature were, in fact, caused by lesions of peripheral nerves.

Despite the aforementioned contributions concerned with the organic nature of writer's cramp and similar disorders, the functional view continued well into the twentieth century [26]. The nineteenth-century opinion that "nervous diseases are the consequence of the innate vulnerability of the human nervous system to the stresses and strains of civilization" continued to play an important role in the understanding of CTDs [15].

In 1879, contrary to the idea that a "vulnerable" nervous system could explain the various CTDs, Beard [11] believed that the "writer's cramp" was essentially a peripheral neuromuscular disease occurring "mostly in those who are of strong, frequently of very strong, constitution, and is quite rare in the nervous and delicate."

If occupational neuralgia and neuritis had their share of opposing views regarding their pathogenesis, the spasmodic form of writer's cramp offered the same considerable challenge. *Psychasthenia* was the term used by Janet [27], the prominent French neuropsychiatrist, to describe this rather rare condition. In his classification of psychoneuroses, which included the spasmodic form of writer's cramp, he also included phobias, compulsions, and anxiety. Definite hysteria was excluded. Very popular at the beginning of the twentieth century, psychasthenia was considered to result from a lowering of psychic energy, or nervous exhaustion.

Williams [28] attributed the lack of coordination that characterized the spasmodic form of writer's cramp to the influence of "mental processes" preceding the occupational act. He was skeptical about therapeutic measures to prevent fatigue and improve the general health of workers: He maintained that as long as those measures did not address themselves to the "ideational seeds" that must be prevented from germinating in the "minds of workers" [28], they could not succeed.

The role of a disordered CNS in producing the cramp was denied by Culpin in 1931 [29,30]. His arguments included the great variety of symptoms included in the syndrome called *cramp*, the fact that certain patients displayed the symptoms only when observed, and the occurrence of cramp among workers in jobs that did not demand excessive writing.

More recently, psychological explanations were given for the occupationally related cramp, such as conversion reaction [31] and psychosomatic disorder in obsessional and dependent patients [32]. A primary psychogenic etiology was considered in Brain's textbook [33], whereas others described the spasmodic form of writer's cramp as a form of localized dystonia [34].

Conclusion

In summary, there are three general theories regarding the etiology of CTDs: the neurogenic theory, muscle overuse, and psychogenic or psychosocial hypotheses. Arguments favoring the neurogenic hypothesis center around the fact that the clinical features of CTDs mimic those found in the neuralgic form (considered the true form) of writer's cramp [6–9]. The condition that resembles CTDs most is considered by some authors to be brachial neuritis [5,14,15]. In view of this, CTDs were labeled by a few authors as an integral part of a neurogenic pain syndrome. According to them, increased mechanosensitivity of the upper-limb peripheral neural tissues, as a consequence of their exposure to excessive forces of friction or tension generated during the performance of repetitive (and cumulative) manual work, is responsible for the pain and other sensory symptoms related to these activities. Quintner [35,36], an Australian clinician favoring the neurogenic theory, is credited with providing the basis for the present historic perspective.

Ferguson, another Australian scholar [37], supported the "muscle-overuse hypothesis," which stems from the clinical observation that "the majority of cases of repetition strain injury are not localized syndromes, but of a more diffuse disorder, apparently of muscles" [37]. The same author described in 1971 an "occupational myalgia," a synonym for the same condition, in a number of telegraphists. Many studies agreed with this hypothesis [38–42]. Similarities were noted between CTDs and primary fibromyalgia [43,44]. As mentioned earlier, Norstrom [18] diagnosed and treated chronic myositic nodules in the upper-limb muscles in a number of his patients suffering from the spasmodic form of writer's cramp.

Lucire [45] was among the supporters of the psychogenic or psychosocial hypothesis. She considered CTD to be psychogenic, with elements of both somatization and conversion [46]. Lucire argued against the muscle-overuse hypothesis primarily on the basis of her opinion that any condition affecting a group of muscles for only a particular intentional activity but not for another could not be organic. Lucire drew an analogy between CTD and the spasmodic forms of writer's or telegraphist's cramp. Not unlike Williams [28], Lucire considered the "idea" of injury as generating the neurosis, referring to an actual or potential pathologic event. Other authors shared this psychogenic hypothesis for explaining CTDs [47–51]. Together with Lucire [46], they contributed to creating a proposed model for a psychosocial dimension of the condition. To any "stressful life situation" able to generate a "conflict about working" and the "so-called everyday aches and pains (fatigue) during the performance of repetitive manual work," they added a psychosocial element such as a strong belief that "repetitive movements can injure upper limb tissues." This belief was reinforced by fellow workers and other components of a litigation- and compensation-prone society. If one adds to an easily accessible workers' compensation insurance system a valid medical diagnosis of work-related injury without well-defined physical signs, a purely psychogenic condition becomes a recognized compensable collection of morbid entities.

Despite the rich literature on the topic, the etiology of CTDs remains a medical enigma. Neurotics and organic elements compete equally in the search for the real basis for this multifaceted ailment. However, it is possible that what appears psychogenic today might be attributed to an organic origin tomorrow if the responsible lesion is recognized.

References

1. Ramazzini B. Diseases of Workers (WC Wright, trans). New York: Hafner, 1964. (Original work published in 1700 and 1713.)
2. Solly S. Scrivener's palsy, or the paralysis of writers. Lancet 1864;2:709.
3. Solly S. On scrivener's palsy. Lancet 1867;1:561.
4. Reynolds JR. Writer's Cramp. In JR Reynolds (ed), A System of Medicine, Vol 2. London: Macmillan, 1872;243.
5. Flint A. Clinical Medicine: A Systematic Treatise on the Diagnosis and Treatment of Diseases. London: Churchill Livingstone, 1879;615.
6. Poore GV. On a case of "writer's cramp," and subsequent general spasm of the right arm, treated by the joint use of the continuous galvanic current and the

rhythmical exercise of the affected muscles. Practitioner 1872;9:129.

7. Poore GV. Electricity in spasmodic affections and "writer's cramp." Lancet 1875;1:115.

8. Poore GV. An analysis of seventy-five cases of "writer's cramp" and impaired writing power. Med Chir Trans 1878;61:114.

9. Poore GV. An analysis of 93 cases of "writer's cramp" and impaired writing power, making, with 75 cases previously reported, a total of 168 cases [abstract]. Proceedings of the Royal Medical and Chirurgical Society. Lancet 1887;2:935.

10. Poore GV. Clinical lecture on certain conditions of the hand and arm which interfere with performance of professional acts, especially piano playing. BMJ 1887;1:441.

11. Beard GM. Conclusions from the study of one hundred and twenty-five cases of writer's cramp and allied affections. Med Rec 1879;15:244.

12. Nakashima K, Rothwell JC, Day BL, et al. Reciprocal inhibition between forearm muscles in patients with writer's cramp and other occupational cramps, symptomatic hemidystonia and hemiparesis due to stroke. Brain 1989;112:681.

13. Oppenheim H. Diseases of the Nervous System. London: Lippincott, 1901;807.

14. Gowers WR. Remarks on two cases of writer's cramp. Med Times Gazette 1877;2:536.

15. Gowers WR. A Manual of Diseases of the Nervous System (2nd ed). London: Churchill Livingstone, 1892;97.

16. Cassirer R. Occupation Neuroses. In A Church (ed), Diseases of the Nervous System. London: Sidney Appleton, 1908;1149.

17. Paul WE. The etiology of the occupation neuroses and neuritides. J Nerv Ment Dis 1911;38:449.

18. Norstrom G. A study of the affection "writer's cramp." N Y Med J Phila Med J 1904;79:491.

19. Monell SH. The cure of writer's cramp and telegrapher's paralysis. Med Rec 1898;54:121.

20. Monell SH. Writer's cramp: what is it and how can it be treated by the family physician? Med Rec 1908;72:101.

21. Society proceedings: Thirty-Seventh Annual Meeting of the American Neurological Association, Baltimore. J Nerv Ment Dis 1911;38:610.

22. Mirowsky M. Occupation Neuritis. In HT Patrick, P Bassoe (eds), The Practical Medicine Series, Vol 10: Nervous and Mental Diseases. Chicago: Year Book, 1912;162.

23. Dana CL. The occupational neuroses. A clinical study of one hundred cases. Med Rec 1912;81:451.

24. Windscheid F. The Prevention of Disease of the Nervous System. In HT Bulstrode (ed), The Prevention of Disease [translated from the German]. Westminster: Archibald Constable, 1902;507.

25. Spaans F. Occupational Nerve Lesions. In PJ Vinken, GW Bruyn (eds), Handbook of Clinical Neurology, Vol 7: Diseases of Nerves. Amsterdam: North-Holland, 1970;326.

26. Hunter D. The Diseases of Occupation (5th ed). London: Hodder & Stoughton,1975;839.

27. Janet P. Psychological Healing, Vol 2. New York: Macmillan, 1925;710.

28. Williams TA. Occupation neuroses: their true nature and treatment. Med Rec 1913;83:464.

29. Culpin M. Recent Advances in the Study of the Psychoneuroses. London: Churchill Livingstone, 1931;175.

30. Culpin M. Mental Abnormality: Facts and Theories. London: Hutchinson's University Library, 1948;59.

31. Cameron N. Personality Development and Psychopathology. Boston: Houghton Mifflin, 1963;317.

32. Crisp AH, Moldofsky HA. A psychosomatic study of writer's cramp. Br J Psychiatry 1965;111:841.

33. Walton JN. Brain's Diseases of the Nervous System (8th ed). Oxford: Oxford University Press, 1977;1200.

34. Lance JW. A Physiological Approach to Clinical Neurology. London: Butterworth, 1970;135.

35. Quintner J. The RSI syndrome in historical perspective. Int Disabil Studies 1991;13:99.

36. Quintner JL. The pain of RSI: the central issue. Aust Fam Physician 1989;8:1542.

37. Ferguson D. An Australian study of telegraphists' cramp. Br J Ind Med 1971;28:280.

38. Stone WE. Repetitive strain injuries. Med J Aust 1983;2:616.

39. Crockett JE. RSI, "Kangaroo paw" or what [letter]? Med J Aust 1985;142:376.

40. Fry HJH. Overuse syndrome of the upper limb in musicians. Med J Aust 1986;144:182.

41. Dennett X, Fry HJH. Overuse syndrome: a muscle biopsy study. Lancet 1988;1:905.

42. Wigley RD. Repetitive strain syndrome—fact not fiction. N Z Med J 1990;103:75.

43. Champion GD, Cornell J, Browne CD, et al. Clinical observations in patients with the syndrome "repetition strain injury." J Occup Health Safety Aust N Z 1986;2:107.

44. Miller MH, Toplis DJ. Chronic upper limb pain syndrome (repetitive strain injury) in the Australian workforce: a systematic cross-sectional study of 229 patients. J Rheumatol 1988;15:1705.

45. Lucire Y. Neurosis in the workplace. Med J Aust 1986;145:323.

46. Lucire Y. Social iatrogenesis of the Australian disease "RSI." Community Health Studies 1988;12:146.

47. Brooks PM. Regional pain syndrome—the disease of the '80s. Bull Postgrad Commun Med Univ Sydney 1986;42:55.

48. Morgan RG. RSI [letter]. Med J Aust 1986;144:56.

49. Awerbuch M. Regional pain syndrome [letter]. Med J Aust 1987;147:59.

50. Ireland DCR. Psychological and physical aspects of occupational arm pain. J Hand Surg [Br] 1988;13:5.

51. Bell DS. "Repetition strain injury": an iatrogenic epidemic of simulated injury. Med J Aust 1989;151:284.

Chapter 3

Neuroanatomy: Ascending Pain Pathways and the Descending Pain Modulatory System

Jack L. Rook

Most patients with repetitive upper-extremity injuries (cumulative trauma disorders) recover with rest, analgesics, physical therapy, and ergonomic modifications. Occasionally, a worst-case scenario develops, characterized by a progressively worsening or migrating pain syndrome that may evolve despite aggressive attempts at treatment. Early focal upper-extremity pain and paresthesias may give rise to diffuse upper-extremity and trunk myofascial discomfort, in association with headaches, depression, sleep disturbance, and other symptoms commonly seen in chronic pain syndromes.

Chapters 4, 5, 11, 12, 13, and 14 are devoted to discussion of this worst-case scenario. In this chapter, we review the neuroanatomy of the pain pathway. This background will be useful to the reader's understanding of the pathophysiologic model for cumulative trauma disorder (Chapter 4), the rationale for medication management of symptoms (Chapter 5), and the pathophysiologic abnormalities that result in the reflex sympathetic dystrophy syndrome (Chapter 11).

Ascending Pain Pathways

Pain Fibers

Painful impulses are transmitted from the periphery to the central nervous system (CNS) via nociceptive C and A delta afferent nerve fibers [1–4]. The most complete knowledge of these nociceptive fibers comes from research on cutaneous afferents, which are easily accessible in superficial sensory and mixed nerves. Less is known about pain fibers from muscle and joint structures, even though the most commonly occurring type of pain is musculoskeletal. Both joint and muscle are innervated by A delta and C primary afferents [5–7]. Musculoskeletal structures presumed to be innervated by primary nociceptors include joint capsules, ligaments, tendons, muscles, periosteum, and bone.

Activation of C and A Delta Fibers

The major class of C fiber (unmyelinated) nociceptor is the C polymodal nociceptor, so named because it responds to noxious thermal, mechanical, and chemical stimuli. A delta (thin, myelinated) nociceptors are of two types, the A delta mechanical nociceptors, which are particularly sensitive to sharp, pointed instruments, and A delta mechanothermal nociceptors, which respond to heat [8,9].

The function of a sensory receptor is to respond to a particular type of stimulus while remaining relatively insensitive to all other types. For example, C and A delta nociceptors are sensitive to intense mechanical and thermal stimuli and to irritant chemicals. Somehow, the presence of such stimuli leads to the generation of nociceptive nerve impulses. The process by which noxious stimuli depolarize the nociceptor is called *transduction*. It is not known exactly how transduction occurs [10]. Possibly, the nociceptor terminals are chemosensitive in that they are activated by pain-producing substances that accumulate near the terminals following tissue injury. At least three sources of these noxious compounds are known: (1) They may leak out from damaged cells, (2) they may be synthesized locally by enzymes—either those gleaned from substrates released by cell damage or those that enter the damaged area secondary to plasma extravasation, and (3) they may be released by activity in the nociceptor itself [10].

Damaged tissue cells will produce leakage of intracellular contents. Released chemicals that either activate or sensitize nociceptors include acetylcholine, serotonin, adenosine triphosphate, potassium, and histamine.

Transducing or sensitizing agents synthesized by enzymes in the area of tissue damage include bradykinins and metabolic products of arachidonic acid (prostaglandins and leukotrienes). Prostaglandins are formed from arachidonic acid by the action of the enzyme fatty acid cyclooxygenase. Several of the prostaglandins sensitize primary afferent nociceptors. That these metabolic intermediaries in the cyclooxygenase pathway of arachidonic acid metabolism play an important role in nociception is supported by the fact that cyclooxygenase inhibitors (aspirin and other nonsteroidal antiinflammatory drugs) have significant analgesic potency [10–21].

In addition to chemical mediators that are released from damaged cells or synthesized in the region of damage, the nociceptors themselves release a substance or substances that enhance nociception. The exact material has not yet been determined, but substance P, an 11–amino acid polypeptide, is believed to be a likely constituent. Substance P, a potent vasodilator, causes the release of histamine from mast cells and promotes the formation of edema. Histamine, which activates nociceptors, also can produce vasodilatation and edema [22–25] (Figure 3-1).

Thus, tissue damage results in transduction of nociceptive stimuli. There is subsequent *transmission* of these impulses to the CNS. Without appropriate treatment, there may be further sensitization and spread of this nociceptive process.

Peripheral Nerves

Major peripheral nerves are made up of different types of afferent and efferent nerve fibers (Figure 3-2). Afferent fibers include C and A delta nociceptors and large myelinated A alpha mechanoreceptor sensory fibers. Efferent fibers include unmyelinated sympathetic nervous system fibers and large myelinated alpha motor neurons. The majority of peripheral nerve axons are primary afferents and, of these, three-fourths are unmyelinated C fibers. Thus, C fiber afferents are the most common element in most peripheral nerves, and the overwhelming majority of C fibers are believed to be nociceptors [26,27]. Nociceptive impulses are transmitted by A delta and C fibers into the dorsal horn of the spinal cord.

Dorsal Horn

The spinal cord gray matter is organized into sheets that are elongated in the rostrocaudal axis. This laminar organization, first described by Rexed [28], now is generally accepted. Rexed divided the gray matter of the spinal cord into 10 laminae on the basis of the microscopic appearance of the neurons: their size, orientation, and density (Figure 3-3). He numbered the laminae sequentially from dorsal to ventral. Important layers with respect to ascending pain pathways include layers I, II, and V. In layer I is the nociceptor-specific pain transmission cell (NSPTC). In layer II, there are interneurons that project to other layers. In layer V is the large wide dynamic-range neuron (WDRN) (Figure 3-4). The second-order pain transmission cells (NSPTCs and WDRNs) in layers I and V project to the thalamus.

A delta and C fibers terminate in the dorsal horn. In general, A delta afferents terminate directly on second-order nociceptive projection neurons in layers I and V, whereas the C nociceptors terminate on small interneurons in layer II [29]. These interneurons make local connections to other laminae, particularly to the projection neurons in layer I.

The NSPTC in layer I responds maximally to noxious stimuli and tends to have a smaller receptive field than the WDRN. It receives input from A delta fibers directly and from C fibers indirectly via

Damaged Tissue

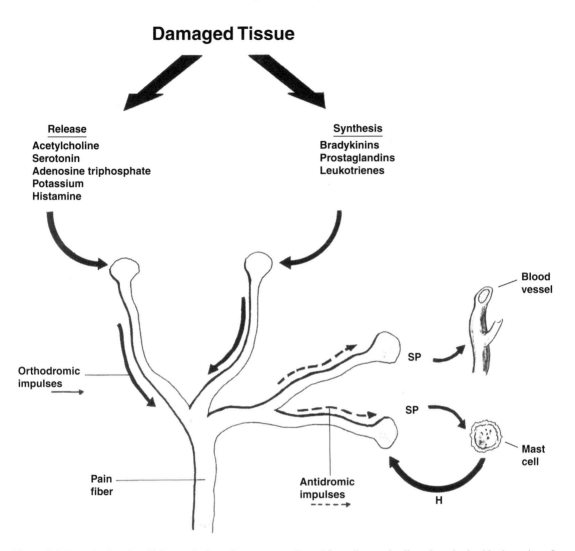

Figure 3-1. Transduction, in which transducing substances are released from disrupted cells and synthesized in the region of damage. Orthodromic impulses travel via C and A delta nociceptive fibers toward the spinal cord dorsal horn. Antidromic impulses within nociceptive nerve terminals promote release of substance P (SP), which promotes edema formation by its effects on mast cells (histamine release) and blood vessels (vasodilatation). Histamine (H) is also a transducing substance.

the interneurons from lamina II. The NSPTC projects to the thalamus.

The WDRN in layer V receives both nociceptive (A delta and C) and non-nociceptive (A alpha) afferent information. In contrast to the NSPTC, the WDRN has a wider range of functions, responding to both noxious and non-noxious stimuli. The A alpha and A delta fibers directly synapse on the WDRN, whereas the C fibers innervate this cell indirectly via interneurons from lamina II. The WDRN has a larger receptive field than does the

NSPTC. Stimulation of this cell ultimately results in poorly localized pain. The WDRN also projects to thalamic nuclei (see Figure 3-4) [30].

Spinothalamic Tract and Anterolateral Quadrant

Axons from each class of second-order projection neuron cross to the contralateral anterolateral quadrant, forming the spinothalamic tract (STT), the major pathway for ascending nociceptive transmis-

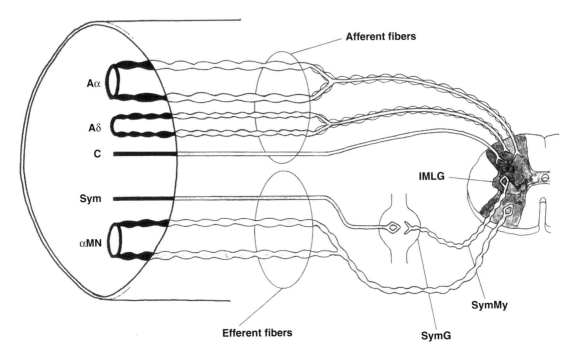

Figure 3-2. Major mixed nerve in cross-section, demonstrating both afferent (A alpha [Aα], A delta [Aδ], C) and efferent (sympathetic postganglionic [Sym] and alpha motor neuron [αMN]) fibers. The nociceptive C and sympathetic postganglionic fibers are unmyelinated. All other fibers are myelinated. (SymMy = sympathetic preganglionic myelinated fiber; SymG = sympathetic ganglion; IMLG = intermedial lateral gray.)

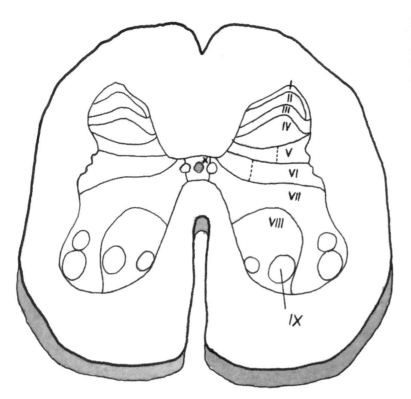

Figure 3-3. Rexed [28] divided the spinal cord gray matter into 10 laminae, on the basis of the microscopic appearance of the neurons.

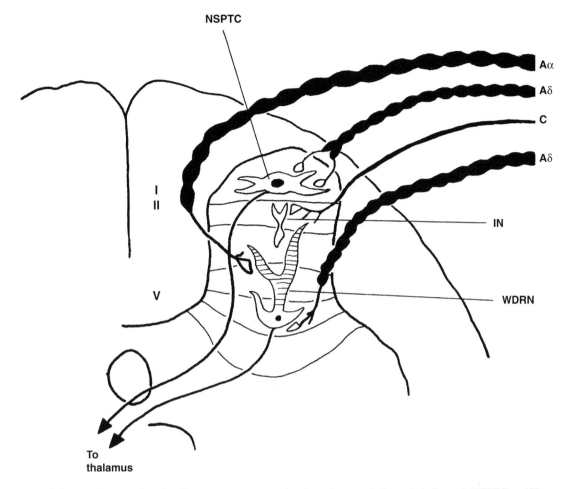

Figure 3-4. The primary nociceptive fibers synapse on second-order pain transmission cells in layers I (NSPTC) and V (WDRN) and on interneurons (INs) in layer II. The interneurons project to other layers. The second-order pain transmission cells project to the thalamus. (NSPTC = nociceptor-specific pain transmission cell; WDRN = wide dynamic-range neuron; Aα, Aδ, and C = A alpha, A delta, and C nociceptor fibers.) (Adapted from HL Fields. Pain. New York: McGraw-Hill, 1987;55.)

sion to target nuclei in the brain stem and thalamus [30–34]. The STT is somatotopically organized, with the WDRN fibers occupying a medial location and the NSPTC producing the more lateral fibers of this tract (Figure 3-5) [35].

Pain Pathways Within the Brain

This somatotopic fiber organization of the STT continues at the brain stem level, where two distinct pathways have been identified anatomically and are believed to have evolved phylogenetically. A medial, more primitive pathway, the paleospinothalamic tract, courses to medial thalamic nuclei stimulating third-order cells, which project to the frontal cortex, limbic system, and reticular formation of the brain stem. The nociceptive neurons in this portion of the thalamus have highly convergent input from large areas of skin and deep tissues and no obvious topographic arrangement [33,36,37]. Activity in this pathway leads to poorly localized pain (WDRN contribution), with emotional connotations, possibly depression, anxiety, sleep disturbances, and other features seen in the chronic pain syndrome. According to Fields, Melzack and Casey [38] "proposed that this paramedian path-

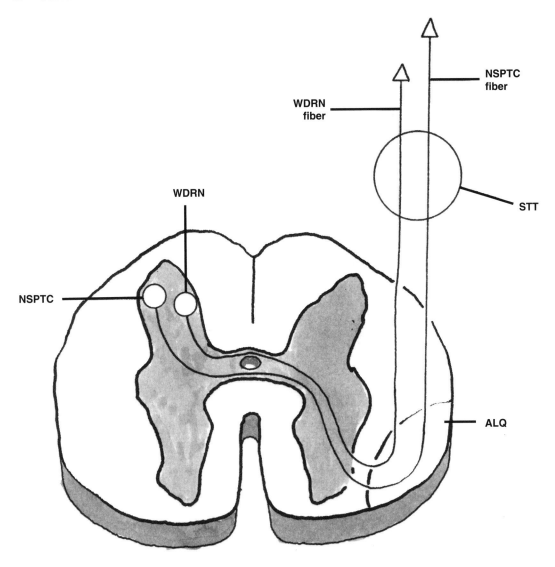

Figure 3-5. Axons from second-order pain transmission cells cross to the contralateral anterolateral quadrant (ALQ) to form the spinothalamic tract (STT). The STT is somatotopically organized, with wide dynamic-range neuron (WDRN) fibers occupying a more medial position than nocieptor-specific pain transmission cell (NSPTC) fibers.

way, with its diffuse projection to the limbic system and to the frontal lobe, subserves the affective-motivational aspects of pain" [33].

The lateral pathway, which projects to lateral thalamic nuclei, is known as the *neospinothalamic tract*. Input to lateral thalamic third-order neurons comes principally from the NSPTCs in layer I of the contralateral spinal cord. These third-order cells have smaller receptive fields and help to localize the noxious input. The lateral thalamic nuclei give rise to a dense projection restricted to the somatosensory cortex (Figure 3-6).

With the evolution of increased encephalization, the lateral thalamic projection made its appearance, reaching its greatest development in primates. Some of the STT neurons that project to the lateral thala-

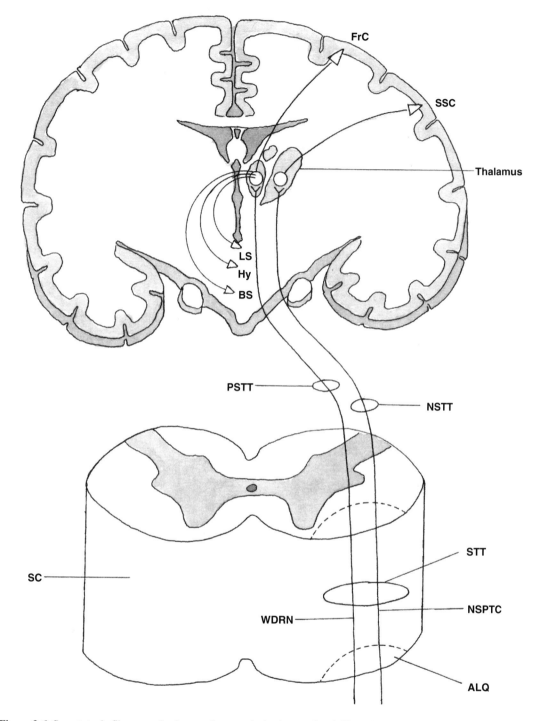

Figure 3-6. Somatotopic fiber organization continues at the brain stem level. The paleospinothalamic tract (PSTT) courses to medial thalamic nuclei, stimulating third-order cells, which project to the frontal cortex (FrC), limbic system (LS), hypothalamus (Hy), and reticular formation of the brain stem (BS). This paramedian pathway, with its diffuse projection to the limbic system and frontal lobe, subserves the affective-motivational aspects of pain. The lateral pathway, which projects to lateral thalamic nuclei, is known as the *neospinothalamic tract* (NSTT). The lateral thalamic nuclei give rise to a dense projection restricted to the somatosensory cortex (SSC). (STT = spinothalamic tract; SC = spinal cord; ALQ = anterolateral quadrant; WDRN = wide dynamic-range neuron; NSPTC = nociceptor-specific pain transmission cell.)

mus also send collateral branches to the medial thalamus, suggesting a strong functional link between the two systems. However, the striking differences in receptive field organization of the neurons in the two regions, and their distinct efferent projections, suggest that the paleospinothalamic and neospinothalamic tract pathways make functionally distinct contributions to nociception [33].

Descending Pain Modulatory Pathways

Analgesia via Midbrain Stimulation

The concept of an independent and specific CNS network that modified pain sensation was first suggested by the observation that electrical stimulation of the midbrain in rats selectively repressed responses to painful stimuli [39,40]. This phenomenon, termed *stimulation-produced analgesia*, was confirmed in humans when neurosurgeons placed electrodes in homologous midbrain sites and demonstrated that stimulation produced a striking and selective reduction of severe clinical pain [41–43]. Stimulation-produced analgesia is elicited by stimulation of the midbrain in the region of the periaqueductal gray matter (PAG), the periventral gray matter of the hypothalamus, and the rostroventral medulla (RVM) [44–47]. The RVM includes the midline serotonin-containing nucleus raphe magnus [48,49].

The analgesic effect of midbrain stimulation is due to activation of a pain-modulating circuit that projects via the medulla to the spinal cord dorsal horn. This descending pain modulatory circuit, which contains high concentrations of endogenous opioid peptides, can be activated by opiate analgesics such as morphine and by certain kinds of stress. Major sources of input to the PAG come from frontal cortical, hypothalamic, and limbic system structures, suggesting that cognitive and emotional input plays a role in pain modulation.

The RVM receives its major input from the PAG. The pain-inhibiting effect of PAG stimulation is relayed to the spinal cord through the RVM. Stimulation of the PAG has a predominantly excitatory effect on RVM cells that project to the spinal cord (Figure 3-7) [48].

Thus, the RVM gives rise to a major projection to the spinal cord via the dorsolateral funiculus

(DLF) (Figure 3-8). The terminals of DLF fibers concentrate in dorsal horn laminae I, II, and V, where there are synaptic connections with terminals of nociceptive primary afferents, opioid-secreting interneurons, and cell bodies of STT neurons (the second-order pain transmission cells). Stimulation of either the PAG or RVM inhibits nociceptive neurons in these laminae [50,51].

Another major brain stem projection to the spinal cord via the DLF arises from the dorsolateral pons (see Figure 3-8). These spinally projecting neurons are noradrenergic [52–54]. Application of norepinephrine directly to the spinal cord selectively inhibits nociceptive dorsal horn neurons [55,56].

In contrast to this noradrenergic system, the RVM contains a high percentage of spinally projecting serotoninergic neurons [49]. In fact, the RVM is the major, if not the sole, source of serotonin in the dorsal horn [57]. Serotonin inhibits dorsal horn nociceptive neurons, including STT cells [58]. Spinally projecting serotoninergic neurons from the RVM contribute to analgesia by inhibiting dorsal horn pain transmission neurons in one of three ways: (1) by direct postsynaptic inhibition; (2) by activating an inhibitory opioid-secreting interneuron that then postsynaptically inhibits the transmission cell; and (3) by presynaptic inhibition of the terminals of nociceptive primary (C and A delta) afferent fibers (Figure 3-9) [59–64].

Hence, there are two descending pain modulatory pathways, one (noradrenergic) originating from the dorsolateral pons and the other (serotoninergic) from the RVM. Both travel via the DLF to the superficial layers of the spinal cord, where there is inhibition of nociceptive transmission.

Opiate Activation of the Descending Pain Modulatory System

Opiates produce analgesia by directly affecting the CNS. The injection of small amounts of opiates directly into the brain can produce potent analgesia [65,66]. The brain stem regions that produce analgesia when electrically stimulated largely overlap those at which opiate microinjection produces analgesia. It has been possible to map the distribution of opiate receptors in the brain using radioactively labeled opiates. Dense concentrations of opiate-binding sites have been localized to the midbrain

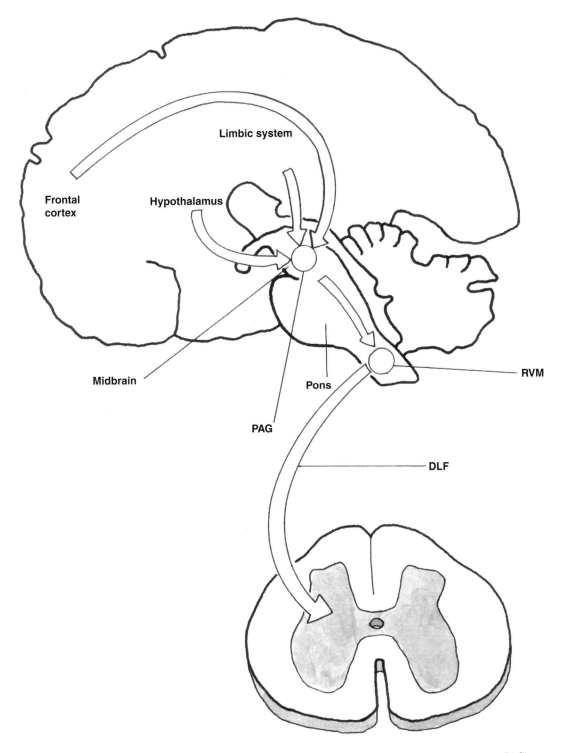

Figure 3-7. The descending pain modulatory system. Major sources of input to the periaqueductal gray matter (PAG) come from frontal cortical, hypothalamic, and limbic system structures. The rostroventral medulla (RVM) receives its major input from the PAG. Stimulation of the PAG has a predominantly excitatory effect on RVM cells that project to the spinal cord via the dorsolateral funiculus (DLF).

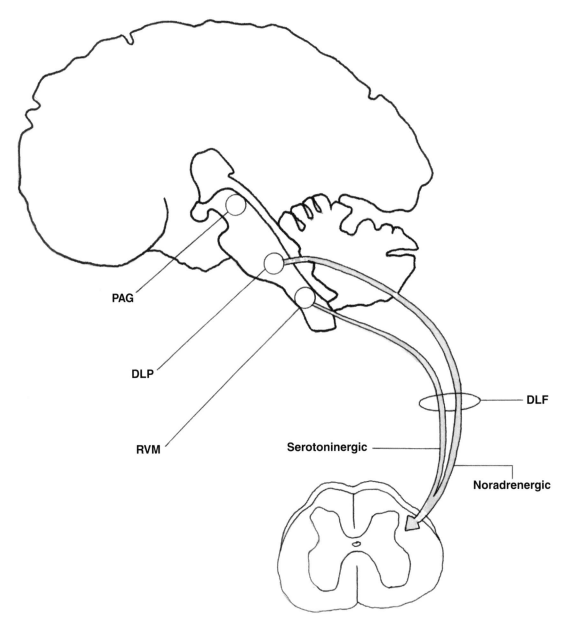

Figure 3-8. The dorsolateral funiculus (DLF). The rostroventral medulla (RVM), which gives rise to a major projection to the spinal cord via the DLF, contains a high percentage of spinally projecting serotoninergic neurons. Another major brain stem projection to the spinal cord via the DLF arises from the dorsolateral pons (DLP). These spinally projecting neurons are noradrenergic. (PAG = periaqueductal gray matter.)

PAG, the RVM, and the superficial dorsal horn of the spinal cord [59,67–69].

Once the opiate receptor had been identified, researchers began searching for endogenous opioid ligands to bind at these highly specific receptor sites.

The first major breakthrough occurred when Hughes et al. [70] reported that they had isolated two endogenous opioids from the brain, the pentapeptides leu- and met-enkephalin. Since the discovery of the enkephalins, a number of other endogenous

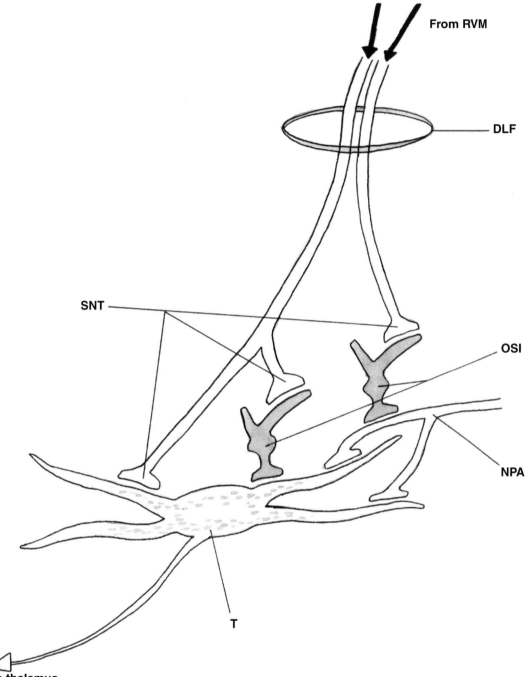

Figure 3-9. Spinally projecting serotoninergic neurons from the rostroventral medulla (RVM) contribute to analgesia by inhibiting dorsal horn pain transmission neurons in one of three ways: (1) by direct postsynaptic inhibition, (2) by activating an inhibitory opioid-secreting interneuron (OSI) that postsynaptically inhibits the transmission cell, or (3) by presynaptically inhibiting the terminal of the nociceptive primary afferent (NPA) fibers. (DLF = dorsolateral funiculus; SNT = serotoninergic nerve terminals; T = second-order pain transmission cell.)

opioid peptides have been discovered, including beta-endorphin, the most potent endogenous opioid yet discovered, and the dynorphin peptides.

The enkephalins, beta-endorphin, and the dynorphins are all present in the PAG. The enkephalins and dynorphins are also present in the RVM and in regions of the spinal dorsal horn involved in nociception. Thus, all the known opioid peptide families are present in structures identified with nociceptive modulation, and it is believed that they normally function to relieve pain [71,72]. Furthermore, systemically administered narcotic analgesics produce analgesia by mimicking the action of endogenous opioid peptides in the PAG, RVM, and spinal cord.

References

1. Bessou P, Perl ER. Response of cutaneous sensory units with unmyelinated fibers to noxious stimuli. J Neurophysiol 1969;32:1025.
2. Beitel RE, Dubner R. Response of unmyelinated (C) polymodal nociceptors to thermal stimuli applied to monkey's face. J Neurophysiol 1976;39:1160.
3. LaMotte RH, Campbell JN. Comparison of responses of warm and nociceptive C-fiber afferents in monkey with human judgements of thermal pain. J Neurophysiol 1978;41:509.
4. Campbell JN, Meyer RA. Primary Afferents and Hyperalgesia. In TL Yaksh (ed), Spinal Afferent Processing. New York: Plenum, 1986;59.
5. Freeman MAR, Wyke B. The innervation of the knee joint. An anatomical and histological study in the cat. J Anat 1967;101:505.
6. Langford LA, Schmidt RF. Afferent and efferent axons in the medial and posterior articular nerves of the cat. Anat Rec 1983;206:71.
7. Stacey JJ. Free nerve endings in skeletal muscle of the cat. J Anat 1969;105:231.
8. Adriaensen H, Gybels J, Handwerker HO, et al. Response properties of thin myelinated (A delta) fibers in human skin nerves. J Neurophysiol 1983;49:111.
9. Georgopoulos AP. Functional properties of primary afferent units probably related to pain mechanisms in primate glabrous skin. J Neurophysiol 1974;39:71.
10. Fields HL. The Peripheral Pain Sensory System. In HL Fields (ed), Pain. New York: McGraw-Hill, 1987;13.
11. Juan H, Lembeck F. Action of peptides and other algesic agents on paravascular pain receptors of the isolated perfused rabbit ear. Naunyn Schmiedebergs Arch Pharmacol 1974;283:151.
12. Perl ER. Sensitization of Nociceptors and Its Relation to Sensation. In JJ Bonica, D Albe-Fessard (eds),

Advances in Pain Research and Therapy, Vol 1. New York: Raven, 1976;17.
13. Beck PW, Handwerker HO. Bradykinin and serotonin effects on various types of cutaneous nerve fibers. Pflugers Arch 1974;347:209.
14. Bisgaard H, Kristensen JK. Leukotriene B_4 produces hyperalgesia in humans. Prostaglandins 1985;30:791.
15. Burgess PR, Perl ER. Cutaneous Mechanoreceptors and Nociceptors. In A Iggo (ed), Handbook of Sensory Physiology, Vol 2: Somatosensory System. Berlin: Springer, 1973;29.
16. Lembeck F. Sir Thoma Lewis's nocisensor system, histamine and substance-P-containing primary afferent nerves. Trends Neurosci 1983;6:106.
17. Levine JD, Lau W, Kwiat G, et al. Leukotriene B_4 produces hyperalgesia that is dependent on polymorphonuclear leukocytes. Science 1984;225:743.
18. Hagermark O, Hokfeld T, Pernow B. Flare and itch induced by substance P in human skin. J Invest Dermatol 1978;71:233.
19. Keele CA. Measurement of Responses to Chemically Induced Pain. In AVS De Reuck, J Knight (eds), Touch, Heat, and Pain. Boston: Little, Brown, 1966.
20. Moucada S, Flower RJ, Vane JR. Prostaglandins, Prostacyclin, Thromboxane A_2 and Leukotrienes. In AG Gilman, LS Goodman, A Gilman (eds), The Pharmacological Basis of Therapeutics (7th ed). New York: Macmillan, 1985.
21. Vane JR. Inhibition of prostaglandin synthesis as a mechanism of action for aspirin-like drugs. Nat New Biol 1971;231:232.
22. Chahl LA, Ladd RJ. Local edema and general excitation of cutaneous sensory receptors produced by electrical stimulation of the saphenous nerve in the rat. Pain 1976;2:25.
23. Chapman LF, Ramos AO, Goodell H, et al. Neurohumoral features of afferent fibers in man. Arch Neurol 1961;4:617.
24. Otsuka M, Konishi S, Yanagisawa M, et al. Role of substance P as a sensory transmitter in spinal cord and sympathetic ganglia. Ciba Found Symp 1982;91:13.
25. LaMotte RH, Thalhammer JG, Robinson CJ. Peripheral neural correlates of magnitude of cutaneous pain and hyperalgesia: a comparison of neural events in monkey with sensory judgments in human. J Neurophysiol 1983;50:1.
26. Ochoa J, Mair WGP. The normal sural nerve in man: I. Ultrastructure and numbers of fibers and cells. Acta Neuropathol 1969;13:197.
27. Torebjork HE. Afferent C units responding to mechanical, thermal, and chemical stimuli in human nonglabrous skin. Acta Physiol Scand 1974;92:374.
28. Rexed B. A cytoarchitectonic atlas of the spinal cord in the cat. J Comp Neurol 1952;96:415.
29. Cervero F, Iggo A. The substantia gelatinosa of the spinal cord. A critical review. Brain 1980;103:717.

30. Willis WD. The Pain System. Basel, Switzerland: Karger, 1985.
31. Willis WD, Kenshalo DR Jr, Leonard RB. The cells of origin of the primate spinothalamic tract. J Comp Neurol 1979;188:543.
32. Willis WD, Trevino DL, Coulter JD, et al. Responses of primate spinothalamic tract neurons to natural stimulation of hindlimb. J Neurophysiol 1974;37:358.
33. Fields HL. Pain Pathways in the Central Nervous System. In HL Fields (ed), Pain. New York: McGraw-Hill, 1987;41.
34. Albe-Fessard D, Berkley KJ, Kruger L, et al. Diencephalic mechanisms of pain sensation. Brain Res Rev 1985;9:217.
35. Hooshmand H. Pathophysiology of the Sympathetic System. In H Hooshmand (ed), Reflex Sympathetic Dystrophy Prevention and Management. Boca Raton, FL: CRC Press, 1993;33.
36. Jones EG, Leavitt RY. Retrograde axonal transport and the demonstration of non-specific projections to the cerebral cortex and striatum from thalamic intralaminar nuclei in the rat, cat, and monkey. J Comp Neurol 1974;154:349.
37. Kaufman EFS, Rosenquist AC. Efferent projections of the thalamic intralaminar nuclei in the cat. Brain Res 1985;335:257.
38. Melzack R, Casey KL. Sensory, Motivational, and Central Control Determinants of Pain. A New Conceptual Model. In D Kenshalo (ed), The Skin Senses. Springfield, IL: Thomas, 1968;423.
39. Fields HL, Basbaum AI. Brainstem control of spinal pain transmission neurons. Annu Rev Physiol 1978;40:217.
40. Mayer DJ, Price DD. Central nervous system mechanisms of analgesia. Pain 1976;2:379.
41. Baskin DS, Mehler WR, Hosobuchi Y, et al. Autopsy analysis of the safety, efficiency, and cartography of electrical stimulation of the central gray in humans. Brain Res 1986;371:231.
42. Hosobuchi Y, Adams JE, Linchitz R. Pain relief by electrical stimulation of the central gray matter in humans and its reversal by naloxone. Science 1977;197:183.
43. Richardson DE, Akil H. Pain reduction by electrical brain stimulation in man. J Neurophysiol 1977;47:178.
44. Abols IA, Basbaum AI. Afferent connections of the rostral medulla of the cat: a neural substrate for midbrain-medullary interactions in the modulation of pain. J Comp Neurol 1981;201:285.
45. Beitz AJ. The organization of afferent projections to the midbrain periaqueductal gray of the rat. Neuroscience 1982;7:133.
46. Mantyh PW. The ascending input to the midbrain periaqueductal gray of the primate. J Comp Neurol 1982;211:50.
47. Zorman G, Hentall ID, Adams JE, et al. Naloxone-reversible analgesia produced by microstimulation in the rat medulla. Brain Res 1981;219:137.
48. Fields HL, Heinricher MM. Anatomy and physiology of a nociceptive modulatory system. Philos Trans R Soc Lond B Biol Sci 1985;308:361.
49. Bowker R, Westlund KN, Coulter JD. Origins of serotonergic projections of the spinal cord in rat: an immunocytochemical retrograde transport study. Brain Res 1981;226:187.
50. Fields HL, Basbaum AI, Clanton CH, et al. Nucleus raphe magnus inhibition of spinal cord dorsal horn neurons. Brain Res 1977;126:441.
51. Willis WD. Control of Nociceptive Transmission in the Spinal Cord. New York: Springer, 1982.
52. Westlund KN, Bowker RM, Ziegler MG, et al. Descending noradrenergic projections and their spinal terminations. Prog Brain Res 1982;57:219.
53. Westlund KN, Bowker RM, Ziegler MG, et al. Origins and terminations of descending noradrenergic projections into the spinal cord of the monkey. Brain Res 1984;292:1.
54. Reddy SVR, Yakah TL. Spinal noradrenergic terminal system mediates antinociception. Brain Res 1980;189:391.
55. Belcher G, Ryall RW, Schaffner R. The differential effects of 5-hydroxytryptamine, noradrenaline, and raphe stimulation on nociceptive and non-nociceptive dorsal horn interneurons in the cat. Brain Res 1978;151:307.
56. Duggan AW. Pharmacology of descending control systems. Philos Trans R Soc Lond B Biol Sci 1985;308:375.
57. Dahlstrom A, Fuxe K. Evidence for the existence of monoamine neurons in the central nervous system: II. Experimental demonstration of monoamines in the cell bodies of brainstem neurons. Acta Physiol Scand Suppl 1964;232:1.
58. Jordan LM, Kenshalo DR, Martin RF, et al. Depression of primate spinothalamic tract neurons by iontophoretic application of 5-hydroxytryptamine. Pain 1978;5:135.
59. Fields HL. Central Nervous System Mechanisms for Control of Pain Transmission. In HL Fields (ed), Pain. New York: McGraw-Hill, 1987;99.
60. Glazer EJ, Basbaum AI. Axons which take up [³H]serotonin are presynaptic to enkephalin immunoreactive neurons in cat dorsal horn. Brain Res 1984;298:389.
61. Ruda MA. Opiates and pain pathways: demonstration of enkephalin synapses on dorsal horn projection neurons. Science 1982;215:1523.
62. Fields HL, Emson PC, Leigh BK, et al. Multiple opiate receptor sites on primary afferent fibers. Nature 1980;284:351.
63. Hiller JM, Simon EJ, Crain SM, et al. Opiate receptors in culture of fetal mouse dorsal root ganglia (DRG) and spinal cord: predominance in DRG neurites. Brain Res 1978;145:396.
64. Mudge AW, Leeman SE, Fischbach GD. Enkephalin inhibits release of substance P from sensory neurons in culture and decreases action potential duration. Proc Natl Acad Sci U S A 1979;76:526.

65. Leavens ME, Hill CS Jr, Cech DA, et al. Intrathecal and intraventricular morphine for pain in cancer patients: initial study. J Neurosurg 1982;56:241.

66. Nurchi G. Use of intraventricular and intrathecal morphine in intractable pain associated with cancer. Neurosurgery 1984;15:801.

67. Chang KJ. Opioid Receptors: Multiplicity and Sequelae of Ligand-Receptor Interactions. In PM Conn (ed), The Receptors, Vol 1. Orlando, FL: Academic, 1984;1.

68. Martin WR. Pharmacology of opioids. Pharmacol Rev 1984;35:283.

69. Snyder SH, Matthysse S. Opiate receptor mechanisms. Neurosci Res Prog Bull 1975;13:1.

70. Hughes J, Smith TW, Kosterlitz HW, et al. Identification of two related pentapeptides from the brain with potent opiate agonist activity. Nature 1975;258:577.

71. Khachaturian H, Lewis ME, Watson SJ. Enkephalin systems in diencephalon and brainstem of the rat. J Comp Neurol 1983;220:310.

72. Palkovits M. Distribution of neuropeptides in the central nervous system: a review of biochemical mapping studies. Prog Neurobiol 1984;23:151.

Chapter 4
Pathophysiologic Model of Cumulative Trauma Disorders

Jack L. Rook

Most patients with cumulative trauma disorders recover with rest, analgesics, physical therapy, and ergonomic modifications. However, occasionally, patients develop chronic intractable symptoms that persist despite aggressive attempts at treatment. Such symptoms may include pain (due to persistent tendinitis, nerve irritation or damage, or myofascial pain syndrome [MPS] involving arm, thoracic outlet, neck, and upper back muscles) and other problems often seen in conjunction with chronic pain (sleep disturbances and depression).

Currently, there is no fully accepted pathophysiologic model to explain the constellation of symptoms seen in these intractable cases. The following proposed model, based on current knowledge of pain pathways, has been broken down into six distinct stages, which parallel patterns of disease progression:

- Peripheral injury
- Opening of the gate
- Livingston's vicious circle (development of myofascial pain)
- Migration of the myofascial pain
- Development of headaches
- Chronic pain syndrome

Peripheral Injury

The peripheral nociceptive process may include a non-neurogenic injury (chronic strain, tendinitis, or bursitis), a peripheral nerve compression syndrome, or a combination of neurogenic and non-neurogenic pathologic processes. An acute or chronic musculoskeletal injury, with associated tissue cell damage and leakage of intracellular contents, will cause activation and sensitization of peripheral C and A delta nociceptor fibers (transduction). The C and A delta fiber information is transmitted into the dorsal horn of the spinal cord (layers I, II, and V), where there is stimulation of second-order pain transmission cells (nociceptor-specific pain transmission cells [NSPTCs] and wide dynamic-range neurons [WDRNs]). At this point, information is predominantly from the NSPTCs, whose axons travel across the spinal cord to the anterolateral quadrant, ascend toward the brain via the spinothalamic tract (STT), and terminate in the lateral thalamus. Ultimately, there are third-order projections to the somatosensory cortex, inciting localized or regional pain perception.

Activity in the dorsal horn may spread to the ventral horn via interneurons, causing activation of alpha motor neurons and reactive spasm in muscles innervated by the respective spinal segment (Figure 4-1) [1,2]. Nociceptive input for upper-extremity pathologic processes will involve one or more spinal segments from C4 through T1. Reactive spasm in C4 through T1 myotomes could involve forearm muscles, proximal arm muscles, and muscles of the thoracic outlet, neck, and upper back (Table 4-1). Increased tone in forearm, arm, and thoracic outlet muscles can result in chronic pressure on peripheral nerves and the brachial plexus,

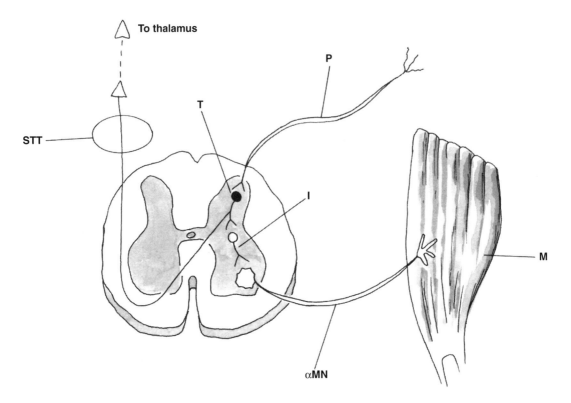

Figure 4-1. Reflex muscle spasm. Activity in the dorsal horn may spread to the ventral horn via interneurons (I), causing activation of alpha motor neurons (αMNs) and reactive spasm in muscles (M) innervated by the respective spinal segment. (P = peripheral C or A delta nociceptors; T = second-order pain transmission cell; STT = spinothalamic tract.) (Adapted from HL Fields. Pain. New York: McGraw-Hill, 1987;153.)

respectively. Such a situation can also develop with peripheral nerve entrapment syndromes (carpal tunnel syndrome, cubital tunnel syndrome, radial tunnel syndrome, superficial radial nerve entrapment) and the thoracic outlet syndrome. Large A alpha fibers are most sensitive to compression, whereas the smaller, unmyelinated C fiber nociceptors continue functioning until compression becomes much more severe. Mild to moderate compression of peripheral nerves and the brachial plexus can lead to selective compression of A alpha fibers and loss of their input at the dorsal horn level of the spinal cord [3–6]. It is the loss of A alpha input that leads to the next stage, opening of the gate.

Opening of the Gate

A revised version of the gate-control hypothesis has been described by Melzak and Wall. According to this theory, there is down-regulation of the second-order pain transmission cell by an inhibitory interneuron that is activated by large, myelinated A alpha fibers [7]. If peripheral nerve compression causes dropout of A alpha fibers, while activity in unmyelinated C nociceptors continues, there is resultant loss of activity of the inhibitory interneuron, which causes an uninhibited excitatory effect by the nociceptor on the second-order pain transmission cell (Figure 4-2). Over time, the second-order pain transmission cells are sensitized, and pain ensues from nonpainful stimuli (e.g., range of motion of the involved joint within a normal range). There may even be pain while the joint is at rest.

Impulses from second-order pain transmission cells (NSPTCs and WDRNs) travel via the STT to the brain. Increased activity in the WDRN is transmitted via the medial pathway (the paleospinothalamic tract [PSTT]). Over time, increased activity in this pathway can lead to depression, anxiety, and

Table 4-1. Muscles that Might Be Involved by Reactive Spasm in C4 Through T1 Myotomes

Region	Muscle	Nerve Root Innervation
Arm	Deltoid	C5, C6
	Biceps	C5, C6
	Brachialis	C5, C6
	Brachioradialis	C4, C5, C6
	Extensor carpi radialis longus and brevis	C4, C5, C6
	Triceps	C7, C8
	Supinator	C6, C7
	Extensor carpi ulnaris	C7, C8
	Extensor digitorum	C7, C8
	Extensor digiti minimi	C7, C8
	Abductor pollicis longus	C7, C8
	Extensor pollicis longus	C7, C8
	Extensor pollicis brevis	C7, C8
	Extensor indicis	C7, C8
	Pronator teres	C6, C7
	Flexor carpi radialis	C6, C7
	Palmaris longus	C7, C8
	Flexor digitorum sublimis	C7, C8, T1
	Flexor pollicis longus	C7, C8
	Flexor digitorum profundus	C7, C8
	Pronator quadratus	C7, C8
	Flexor carpi ulnaris	C7, C8
	Hand intrinsics	C8, T1
Neck and upper back	Cervical paraspinals	C4–T1
	Rhomboids	C4, C5
	Levator scapulae	C4, C5
	Supraspinatus	C5, C6
	Infraspinatus	C5, C6
	Teres minor	C5
	Teres major	C5, C6
Chest	Serratus anterior	C5, C6, C7
	Pectoralis major	C4–T1
	Pectoralis minor	C7–T1
	Latissimus dorsi	C7–T1

sleep disturbances. In general, this vicious cycle results in increased activity in the spinal cord dorsal horn, which brings us to the next stage, Livingston's vicious circle.

Livingston's Vicious Circle: Development of Myofascial Pain Syndrome

Thus far, we can see how peripheral nociceptive input feeds into the dorsal horn and causes sensitization of second-order pain transmission cells. Increased dorsal horn activity spreads to alpha motor neurons in the ventral horn via interneurons.

The activation of alpha motor neurons results in muscle spasm, a painful phenomenon that activates the muscle's own nociceptive C and A delta fibers, which then feed back to the spinal cord to sustain the spasm. Therefore, the original noxious stimulus sets in motion a spreading and potentially self-sustaining process first described by Livingston (Figure 4-3) [1,2]. The myofascial pain may persist even if the peripheral injury heals.

Upper-extremity structures are generally supplied by peripheral nerves emanating from the brachial plexus, which, in turn, is formed by nerve roots C4 through T1. Reactive spasm that occurs at the C4 through T1 level might involve muscles

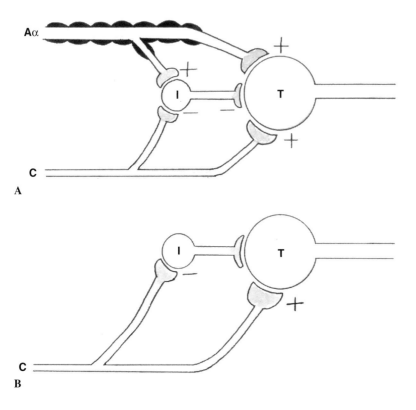

Figure 4-2. Revised gate-control hypothesis. A. There is down-regulation of the second-order pain transmission cell (T) by an inhibitory interneuron (I) that is activated by large myelinated A alpha fibers (Aα). B. If peripheral nerve compression causes dropout of A alpha fibers, continued activity in unmyelinated nociceptor C fibers (C) produces an uninhibited excitatory effect by the nociceptor on the second-order pain transmission cell. (Adapted from H Fields. Pain. New York: McGraw-Hill, 1987;139.)

of the hands, arms, neck, chest, and back (see Table 4-1). Such reflex spasm causes myofascial pain that, over time, might constitute an MPS. Clinical features of such a syndrome include (1) continuous, dull, deep aching pain; (2) pain produced by pressure on tender spots or bands (trigger points) in muscles; (3) pain relieved by inactivation of trigger points; (4) restricted range of motion in affected muscle; (5) local muscle twitch produced by trigger-point stimulation; and (6) patient startle or jump sign with trigger-point pressure [8–11].

Peripheral noxious input from any source can, by reflex action, induce muscle contraction [12]. Furthermore, muscle contraction will produce a more severe and sustained secondary pain if the contracting muscle contains a latent trigger point. Travell and Simons [11] believe that MPS occurs when latent trigger points are activated. Trigger points have particularly sensitive muscle nociceptors. The nociceptor input from trigger points feeds back to the spinal cord to cause further muscle contraction and to sustain the pain [13].

In patients with upper-extremity pain secondary to nerve injury, tendinitis, or arthritis, MPS may add to the pain's severity and to its resistance to therapy. In addition, spasm or tightness in the scalene muscles, the pectoralis minor muscle, and forearm (pronator and supinator) muscles could irritate or compress underlying nerves (brachial plexus, median, and radial nerves, respectively), further perpetuating this cycle.

Migration of Myofascial Pain

It is common knowledge that irritated trigger points refer pain to various locations. This can lead to activation of latent trigger points in other muscles, with gradual migration of the myofascial pain [9,11]. In addition, spread of impulses in the spinal cord may occur in a cephalad-caudal direction as well as segmentally. Such impulse propagation could lead to activation of alpha motor neurons at adjacent spinal segments, causing

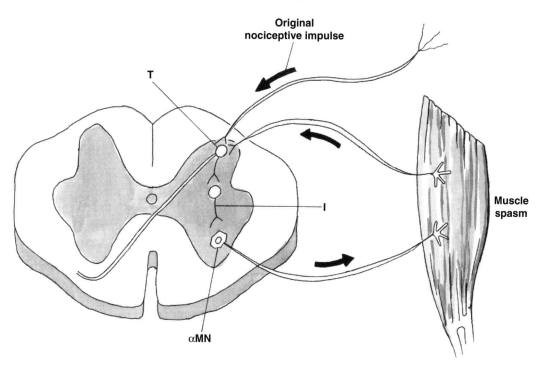

Figure 4-3. Livingston's vicious circle. Increased dorsal horn activity spreads to alpha motor neurons (αMNs) in the ventral horn via interneurons (I). The activation of alpha motor neurons results in muscle spasm. The painful muscle's own nociceptive fibers feed back to the spinal cord to sustain the spasm. (T = second-order pain transmission cell.) (Adapted from HL Fields. Pain. New York: McGraw-Hill, 1987;153.)

spread of myofascial pain due to activity within the central nervous system.

Development of Headaches

As pain spreads from the arms to the neck and upper back, patients may develop headaches. The etiology will vary from patient to patient. Three principal types may occur secondary to the spread of myofascial pain: (1) headaches secondary to temporomandibular joint (TMJ) dysfunction, (2) occipital neuralgia, and (3) vascular headaches.

Headaches Secondary to Temporomandibular Joint Dysfunction

Cervical MPS can refer pain to facial (pterygoid and masseter) muscles, thereby activating latent trigger points (Figure 4-4). Over time, MPS may develop in these muscles, and chronic muscle contraction may cause slight alteration of the TMJ. Slight malalignment of the jaw could cause chronic tension of the temporal muscle tendon, which attaches to the coronoid process of the mandible (Figure 4-5). This chronic strain could lead to muscle-contraction headaches.

Travell and Simons [14] have pointed out that pterygoid muscle trigger points may develop as satellites in response to trigger-point activity of the neck muscles. Furthermore, the masseter muscles are among the first to contract in patients who are extremely emotionally tense, intensely determined, or desperate, and they often remain contracted for abnormally long periods in patients who develop the temporomandibular pain and dysfunction syndrome [15,16]. Unfortunately, the emotional component of pain is sometimes overemphasized while the myofascial trigger-point contribution to internal derangements of the TMJ is neglected [17].

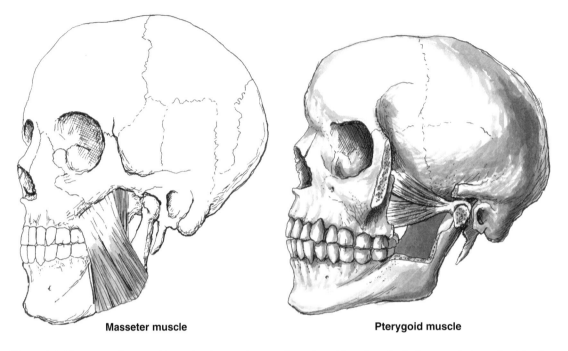

Masseter muscle   **Pterygoid muscle**

Figure 4-4. Masseter and pterygoid muscle trigger points may be activated by referred pain from cervical myofascial pain syndrome.

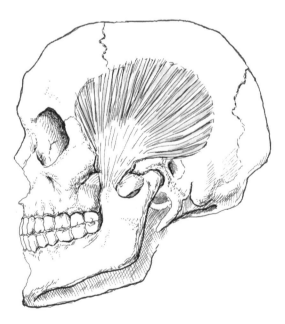

Figure 4-5. Slight malalignment of the jaw could cause chronic tension of the temporal muscle tendon, which attaches to the coronoid process of the mandible.

Occipital Neuralgia

Chronic cervical muscle contraction can result in entrapment or irritation of the occipital nerves (Figure 4-6). The C1 through C3 nerve roots coalesce to form the four occipital nerves, two greater and two lesser nerves, which supply sensation to the scalp. Entrapment of any of these nerves within tight musculature could lead to chronic tension headaches [18–22].

Vascular Headaches

Nociceptive impulses from head and neck structures are relayed to the nucleus caudalis, possibly effecting a situation that leads to the development of migraine headaches. The nucleus caudalis is analogous to the spinal cord dorsal horn. It occupies a similar location in the brain stem and actually extends caudally into the upper cervical cord. In fact, in view of its association with nociceptive transmission and its structural and functional similarities to the spinal cord dorsal horn, the nucleus caudalis has been termed the *medullary dorsal horn* (Figure 4-7) [23–26].

The exact pathophysiology of vascular headaches has never been elucidated completely. However, extensive research since 1983 seems to implicate as important factors in the pathogenesis of migraine an ascending serotoninergic neural system from midbrain raphe nuclei and the release of substance P and calcitonin gene–related polypeptide (CGRP), neuropeptides from trigeminal nerve peripheral nociceptor terminals that innervate cerebral blood vessels [27,28].

The first step in the development of vascular headaches is the convergence of nociceptive information from head and neck structures onto second-order pain transmission cells in the nucleus caudalis. In the neck, nociceptive information from cervical MPS or irritated occipital nerves (C1–C3) travels via C and A delta fibers into the upper spinal cord portion of the nucleus caudalis. Likewise, nociceptive impulses from cranial structures (masseter, pterygoid, and temporal muscles and the TMJ) are transmitted via C and A delta fibers of cranial nerve V to the brain stem nucleus caudalis.

Animal experiments have indeed demonstrated extensive convergence of neural input from neck and jaw musculature onto second-order pain transmission cells in the nucleus caudalis. Sessle et al. [23] showed that stimulation of high-threshold (nociceptive) afferents from cat jaw, tongue, and neck muscles caused excitation of WDRNs and NSPTCs in the nucleus caudalis.

In addition to this nociceptive input, neurons in the nucleus caudalis of the trigeminal nuclear complex also may integrate both excitatory and inhibitory supraspinal impulses. Supraspinal impulses generated by tension, stress, anxiety, and depression probably have an excitatory effect on the trigeminal nucleus caudalis projection neuron (Figure 4-8). Over time, the convergence of noxious and supraspinal impulses may sensitize second-order pain transmission cells [29]. Activity in these second-order cells activates the ascending pain pathway (outlined extensively in Chapter 3), which travels toward the thalamus via the STT. However, before this pathway reaches the thalamus, neural connections at midbrain raphe nuclei stimulate an ascending serotoninergic system that travels toward cerebral blood vessels, ultimately releasing serotonin at the blood vessel level. It is the release of serotonin that may underlie the vascular

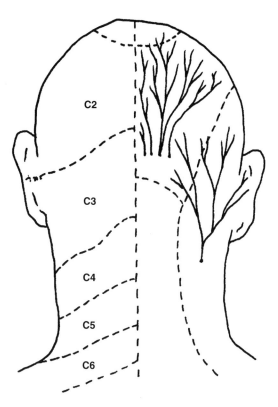

Figure 4-6. Chronic cervical muscle contraction can result in entrapment or irritation of the occipital nerves C2–C6, which may lead to chronic tension headaches.

abnormalities seen in migraine headaches (Figure 4-9). Therefore, some discussion of serotonin receptors is warranted.

There are at least four classes of serotonin (5-hydroxytryptamine, or 5-HT) receptors—5-HT_1 through 5-HT_4—and subtypes of these classes. The 5-HT_1 receptors are inhibitory, whereas the other types are excitatory. In humans, there are at least three 5-HT_1 receptor subtypes: 5-HT_{1A}, 5-HT_{1C}, and 5-HT_{1D}. The 5-HT_{1D} receptor is the most widespread serotonin receptor in the brain and functions as an autoreceptor modulating neurotransmitter release. Presynaptic 5-HT_{1D} receptor activation *inhibits* the release of 5-HT, norepinephrine, acetylcholine, CGRP, and substance P. Moreover, postsynaptic 5-HT_{1D} receptors are found on cerebral blood vessels. Agonist action of these receptors appears to produce vasoconstriction [30,31].

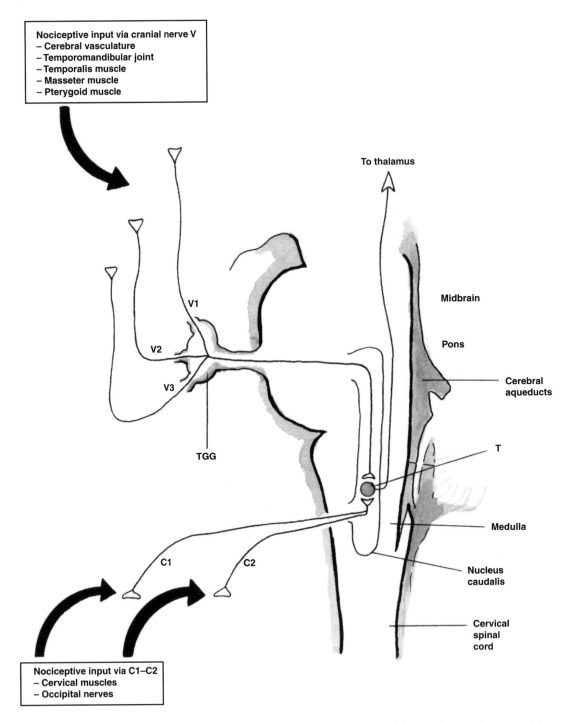

Figure 4-7. Pathophysiology of vascular headaches. Nociceptive impulses from head (via cranial nerve V) and neck (via C1–C2 nerve roots) structures are relayed to second-order pain transmission cells (T) in the nucleus caudalis (medullary dorsal horn). Transmission cells relay the information to thalamic nuclei. (V1, V2, V3 = three divisions of trigeminal nerve; TGG = trigeminal ganglion.)

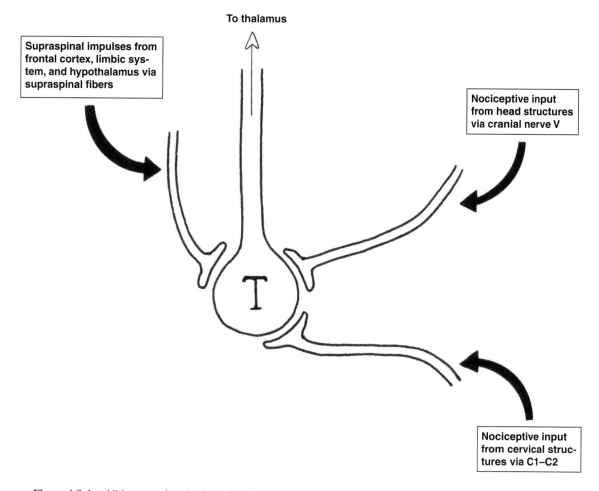

Figure 4-8. In addition to nociceptive input from head and neck structures, transmission neurons (T) in the nucleus caudalis also may integrate both excitatory and inhibitory supraspinal impulses.

The serotonin released from the ascending system binds to 5-HT receptors on nerve terminals of C and A delta fibers surrounding the cerebral blood vessels (the trigeminal vascular system). The binding of serotonin to these nociceptive nerve terminals causes release of various neurotransmitters, including substance P, CGRP, and other neuropeptides. The released neuropeptides interact with the blood vessel wall, producing dilatation, plasma extravasation, and sterile inflammation. Released substance P is postulated to increase vascular permeability and dilate cerebral blood vessels. Substance P has been shown to activate macrophages to synthesize thromboxanes, to activate lymphocytes, and, at high concentrations, to degranulate mast cells, with resultant local release of histamine. Local inflammation ensues. The presence of pain-producing substances causes orthodromic conduction of nociceptive impulses along trigeminal nerve fibers, toward the second-order pain transmission cells in the nucleus caudalis, thereby perpetuating this cycle [27,28].

Many of the drugs effective in treating migraine are believed to work in one of two ways. Some of the medications—including ergot, amitriptyline, propranolol (Inderal), dihydroergotamine (DHE), and verapamil—possess serotonin receptor–blocking properties and are useful in both the prophylaxis

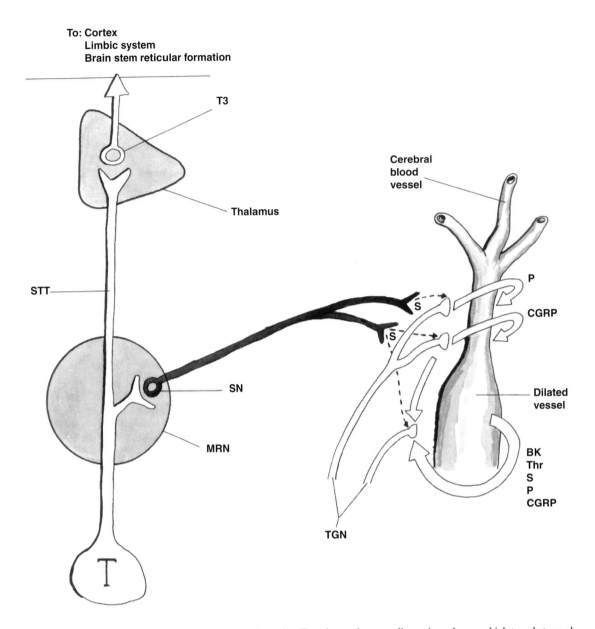

Figure 4-9. Activity in second-order pain transmission cells (T) activates the ascending pain pathway, which travels toward the thalamus via the spinothalamic tract (STT). Before this pathway reaches the thalamus, neural connections at midbrain raphe nuclei (MRN) stimulate an ascending serotoninergic system that travels toward cerebral blood vessels, ultimately releasing serotonin (S) at the blood vessel level. It is the release of serotonin that may underlie the vascular abnormalities seen in migraine headaches. Refer to the text for details. (T3 = third-order pain transmission cell; SN = serotoninergic neuron; BK = bradykinins; Thr = thromboxanes; TGN = trigeminal nerve fibers; P = substance P; CGRP = calcitonin gene–related polypeptide.)

and short-term treatment of migraine. Calcium ions are essential for neurotransmitter release, and calcium channel blockers therefore may owe some of their effectiveness to this action on perivascular sensory nerve fibers [27,32,33]. DHE 45 and sumatriptan (Imitrex) interact at 5-HT_{1A} and 5-HT_{1D} receptors, which, as mentioned previously, are inhibitory. They prevent the release of vasoactive neuropeptides from the nociceptive nerve terminals by having an inhibitory rather than a stimulatory (serotoninergic) effect on these receptors [30].

Understanding the foregoing pathophysiologic model will be helpful in formulating a plan for treatment of vascular headaches. Efforts to decrease nociceptive input to the nucleus caudalis should be made. Physical modalities and medications aimed at decreasing such noxious input from the TMJ, cervical muscles, occipital nerves, and facial structures might prove helpful. In addition, it would be beneficial to decrease supraspinal influences that may be up-regulating the nucleus caudalis projection neurons. To diminish such influences will require psychotherapeutic techniques and medications aimed at treating depression, tension, and anxiety. Finally, medications that prevent the release of serotonin at the cerebral blood vessel level (Imitrex, DHE 45, verapamil), as well as medications that block the effect of serotonin (tricyclic antidepressants, ergotamines, Inderal), also have proven efficacious in the treatment of vascular headaches.

Chronic Pain Syndrome

We are aware of many sources of chronic nociceptive input, among them musculoskeletal upper-extremity pain; irritated or damaged peripheral nerves; MPS in proximal shoulder, neck, and upper-back muscles; and headaches. Over time, there is sensitization of second-order pain transmission cells in the dorsal horn, with resultant relay of nociceptive information to third-order cells in the thalamus via the STT.

Increased activity in the PSTT (mediated principally by WDRNs) results in chronic pain syndrome symptomatology. Third-order cells in the PSTT make connections with the frontal lobes, limbic system, reticular activating system, and brain stem. Increased activity in these areas results in characteristic features of chronic pain syndrome, including anxiety, depression, diffuse or poorly localized pain (WDRNs), and sleep disturbance.

References

1. Fields HL. Painful Dysfunction of the Nervous System. In HL Fields (ed), Pain. New York: McGraw-Hill, 1987;133.
2. Livingston WK. Pain Mechanisms. New York: Macmillan, 1943.
3. Fowler TJ, Ochoa J. Unmyelinated fibres in normal and compressed peripheral nerves of the baboon: a quantitative electron microscopic study. Neuropathol Appl Neurobiol 1975;1:247.
4. Ochoa J. Pain in Local Nerve Lesions. In WJ Culp, J Ochoa (eds), Abnormal Nerves and Muscles as Impulse Generators. New York: Oxford University Press, 1982;568.
5. Ochoa J, Noordenbos W. Pathology and disordered sensation in local nerve lesions: an attempt at correlation. Adv Pain Res Ther 1979;3:67.
6. Stewart JD, Aguayo AH. Compression and Entrapment Neuropathies. In PJ Dyck, PK Thomas, EH Lambert, et al. (eds), Peripheral Neuropathy, Vol 2 (2nd ed). Philadelphia: Saunders, 1984;1435.
7. Melzack R, Wall PD. The Challenge of Pain. New York: Basic Books, 1982.
8. Gutstein M. Diagnosis and treatment of muscular rheumatism. BMJ 1938;1:302.
9. Kellgren JH. A preliminary account of referred pains arising from muscle. BMJ 1938;1:325.
10. Simons DG, Travell JG. Myofascial origins of low back pain. Postgrad Med 1983;73:66.
11. Travell JG, Simons DG. Myofascial Pain and Dysfunction: The Trigger Point Manual. Baltimore: Williams & Wilkins, 1983.
12. Lewis T, Kellgren JH. Observations relating to referred pain, visceromotor reflexes and other associated phenomena. Clin Sci (Colch) 1939;4:47.
13. Fields HL. Evaluation of Patients with Persistent Pain. In HL Fields (ed), Pain. New York: McGraw-Hill, 1987;205.
14. Travell JG, Simons DG. TMJ Dysfunction. In JG Travell, DG Simons (eds), Myofascial Pain and Dysfunction: The Trigger Point Manual. Baltimore: Williams & Wilkins, 1983;260.
15. Wolff HG. Wolff's Headache and Other Head Pain [revised by DJ Dalessio] (3rd ed). Oxford: Oxford University Press, 1972;550.
16. Yemm K. Temporomandibular dysfunction and masseter muscle response to experimental stress. Br Dent J 1969;127:508.
17. Millstein-Preutky S, Olson RE. Predictability of treatment outcome in patients with myofascial pain dysfunction (MPD) syndrome. J Dent Res 1979;58:1341.

18. Bovim G, Fredriksen TA, Stolt-Neelsen A, et al. Neurolysis of the greater occipital nerve in cervicogenic headache. Headache 1992;32:175.

19. Bogduk N. The anatomy of occipital neuralgia. Clin Exp Neurol 1981;17:167.

20. Edmeads J. Headaches and head pains associated with diseases of the cervical spine. Med Clin North Am 1978;62:533.

21. Hammond SR, Danta G. Occipital neuralgia. Clin Exp Neurol 1978;15:258.

22. Hunter CR, Mayfield FH. Role of the upper cervical roots in the production of pain in the head. Am J Surg 1949;78:743.

23. Sessle BJ, Hu JW, Amano N, et al. Convergence of cutaneous, tooth pulp, visceral, neck and muscle afferents onto nociceptive and non-nociceptive neurons in trigeminal subnucleus caudalis (medullary dorsal horn) and its implications for referred pain. Pain 1986;27:219.

24. Gobel S, Hockfield S, Ruda MA. Anatomical Similarities Between Medullary and Spinal Dorsal Horns. In Y Kawamura, R Dubner (eds), Oral-Facial Sensory and Motor Functions. Tokyo: Quintessence, 1981;211.

25. Hoffman DS, Dubner R, Hayes RL, et al. Neuronal activity in medullary dorsal horn of awake monkeys trained in a thermal discrimination task: I. Responses to innocuous and noxious thermal stimuli. J Neurophysiol 1981;46:409.

26. Hu JW, Dostrovsky JO, Sessle BJ. Functional properties of neurons in cat trigeminal subnucleus caudalis (medullary dorsal horn): I. Response to oral-facial noxious and non-noxious stimuli and projections to thalamus and subnucleus oralis. J Neurophysiol 1981;45:173.

27. Moskowitz MA. The neurobiology of vascular head pain. Ann Neurol 1984;16:157.

28. Silberstein SD. Advances in understanding the pathophysiology of headache. Neurology 1992;42(suppl 2):6.

29. Olesen J. Clinical and pathophysiological observations in migraine and tension-type headache explained by integration of vascular, supraspinal, and myofascial inputs. Pain 1991;46:125.

30. Saper JR, Silberstein S, Gordon CD, et al. Mechanisms and Theories of Head Pain. In JW Pine (ed), Handbook of Headache Management. Baltimore: Williams & Wilkins, 1993;16.

31. Raskin NH. Serotonin receptors and headache. N Engl J Med 1991;325:353.

32. Amery WK. Flunarizine, a calcium channel blocker: a new prophylactic drug in migraine. Headache 1983;23:70.

33. Diamond S, Schenbaum H. Flunarizine, a calcium channel blocker, in the prophylactic treatment of migraine. Headache 1983;23:39.

Chapter 5
Symptom Management

Jack L. Rook

Most patients who develop a cumulative trauma disorder (CTD) will recover with timely and appropriate treatment. Such treatment should include (1) early identification of the problem, followed by (2) relative rest (from the activity that has caused the problem) or absolute rest of the involved extremity or extremities, (3) anti-inflammatory analgesics, (4) physical and occupational therapy appropriate to the patient's needs, and (5) appropriate work-site modifications so that return to work after recovery does not result in recurrence of the problem.

The goal of such treatment is to eliminate as quickly as possible the peripheral nociceptive input to the dorsal horn pain transmission cells, so as to prevent the development of vicious cycles, myofascial pain, nerve irritation, and sensitization of the projection neurons. Unfortunately, a small percentage of patients develop chronic unrelenting unilateral or bilateral upper-extremity pain, and, occasionally, physicians are faced with full-blown chronic pain problems characterized by the following:

- Headaches
- Sleep disturbance
- Depression and anxiety
- Proximal myofascial pain syndrome (MPS) involving neck, upper-back, and thoracic outlet muscles
- Multiple nerve irritations or neurogenic pain

Treatment of this worst-case scenario involves symptom management, job modification, and, possibly, vocational retraining.

Headaches

As mentioned in Chapter 4, different types of headaches can develop in the face of a CTD, including tension muscle-contraction headaches, occipital neuralgia, headaches secondary to temporomandibular joint (TMJ) dysfunction, and vascular headaches. More than one type of headache can coexist, in which case treatment will be more challenging.

Tension Headaches, Occipital Neuralgia, and Headaches Secondary to Temporomandibular Joint Dysfunction

For patients who suffer from muscle-contraction headaches or occipital neuralgia, treatment modalities that promote relaxation of head and neck musculature might reduce headaches by relieving pressure on the involved occipital nerves. Modalities available include physical therapy, massage therapy, and psychotherapy (biofeedback and behavioral and cognitive therapies). Among headache sufferers are some with clear evidence of psychiatric, stress-induced, and behavioral disturbances that contribute to, or occur as a response to, the headaches or chronic pain. Biofeedback, stress management, and behavioral and cognitive therapies can constitute primary, effective intervention in many patients with headache, even those without psychological problems or evident distress. These therapies also serve as adjunctive interventions in patients who suffer frequent headaches for which medications are required. Use of these therapies, which should be administered by expert professionals well versed in headache disorders, is recommended whenever appropriate [1–4].

Patients who suffer headaches associated with TMJ dysfunction must undergo a dental evaluation. Treatment might include trigger-point injections and massage therapy for head, neck, and facial (pterygoid and masseter) musculature. Often, such treatment in combination with dental splinting is sufficient to alleviate headaches associated with TMJ dysfunction.

Vascular Headaches

As noted in Chapter 4, a vascular or migraine headache syndrome may develop as a response to the chronic nociceptive input from head and neck structures. The vascular component of the headache syndrome will vary from case to case. Some patients will suffer mild, chronic daily vascular headaches, whereas others will experience intermittent classic migraine attacks interspersed among chronic daily musculoskeletal headaches. Identification of mild, chronic daily vascular headaches is difficult; these often are not diagnosed until patients respond to symptomatic or prophylactic migraine medications.

Treatment of vascular headaches includes pharmacologic and nonpharmacologic interventions. Medications usually are described as being either symptomatic or preventive [5].

Pharmacologic Treatment

Symptomatic Therapy. The symptomatic treatment of head pain involves the use of agents that reverse, abort, or reduce pain once it has begun or is anticipated. Symptomatic treatment should be considered when attacks are infrequent (two or fewer per week). Many symptomatic headache medications are combinations of vasoconstrictive agents and muscle relaxants, aspirin, acetaminophen, narcotics, tranquilizers, or caffeine. Caffeine produces vasoconstriction, enhances analgesia, and increases gastrointestinal absorption. Whereas modest caffeine intake might have no adverse effect on headache patients and might even help

some, excessive caffeine intake can aggravate or induce headaches. High daily intake greater than 500 mg per day can produce dependency, leading to withdrawal headaches 8–16 hours after the last dose. The total daily caffeine intake of headache patients should be calculated or at least carefully estimated (Table 5-1), as caffeine overuse can be an important contributing factor in some cases [1,6,7].

Symptomatic headache treatment medications include traditional analgesics, combination analgesics, opioids, antiemetics, ergotamine derivatives, steroids, and the injectable migraine medications (Table 5-2). Opioids may be necessary for symptomatic relief of intermittent migraine headaches. Most patients respond to oral opioids of mild to moderate strength. Parenteral opioids (meperidine [Demerol], morphine, butorphanol [Stadol]) are occasionally required for severe intractable migraines in the emergency-room setting. Prochlorperazine (Compazine), promethazine (Phenergan), and metoclopramide (Reglan) may aid in the treatment of nausea and vomiting that frequently occurs with severe vascular headaches.

Ergotamine derivatives remain the drugs of first choice for moderate to severe migraine headaches. Cafergot and dihydroergotamine (DHE 45) are the most commonly used agents. Proposed mechanisms for the ergotamines include agonist action on 5-HT_{1A} and 5-HT_{1D} receptors (inhibiting release of substance P and calcitonin gene–related polypeptides from trigeminal nerve endings), agonist action at alpha-adrenergic receptors, and reuptake inhibition of norepinephrine at sympathetic nerve endings (both producing vasoconstriction of involved cerebral vessels). Recommended use of ergotamine derivatives includes moderate to severe migraine, intractable migraine, and intractable chronic daily headache. Cafergot is appropriate for initial treatment of acute attacks of migraine. DHE 45 (intravenously, intramuscularly, or subcutaneously) is appropriate for more severe attacks or for prolonged intractable attacks [1,5,8–11].

Steroids are occasionally useful adjuncts in the treatment of severe vascular headaches, helping to reduce inflammation within the involved cerebral vessels [1].

Imitrex, a selective 5-HT_1 agent, is considered useful for symptomatic treatment of acute migraine headache. This drug produces vasoconstriction and

Table 5-1. Caffeine Content of Foods, Beverages, and Drugs

	Serving Size or Dose	Caffeine (mg)
Beverages		
Coffee, drip	5 oz	110–150
Coffee, perked	5 oz	60–125
Coffee, instant	5 oz	40–105
Coffee, decaffeinated	5 oz	2–5
Tea, 5-min steep	5 oz	40–100
Tea, 3-min steep	5 oz	20–50
Tea, 1-min steep	5 oz	9–33
Hot cocoa	5 oz	2–10
Coca-Cola	12 oz	45
Canned iced tea	12 oz	22–36
7-Up/Diet 7-Up	12 oz	0
Diet Pepsi	12 oz	34
Dr. Pepper	12 oz	38
Fresca	12 oz	0
Ginger ale	12 oz	0
Mountain Dew	12 oz	52
Pepsi-Cola	12 oz	37
Tab	12 oz	44
Foods		
Milk chocolate	1 oz	1–15
Bittersweet chocolate	1 oz	5–35
Chocolate cake	1 slice	20–30
Baking chocolate	1 oz	35
Chocolate candy bar	1 oz	25
Over-the-counter drugs		
Anacin, Empirin, or Midol (analgesics)	2 tablets	64
Excedrin (analgesic)	2 tablets	130
NoDoz (stimulant)	2 tablets	200
Aqua-Ban (diuretic)	2 tablets	200
Dexatrim (weight-control aid)	1 tablet	200
Vanquish (analgesic)	1 tablet	33
Vivarin tablets (stimulant)	1 tablet	200
Prescription drugs		
Darvon (propoxyphene)	1 tablet	32.4
Esgic (butalbital, acetaminophen, caffeine)	1 tablet	40
Fioricet (butalbital, acetaminophen, caffeine)	1 tablet	40
Fiorinal (butalbital, aspirin, caffeine)	1 tablet	40
Norgesic (orphenadrine, aspirin, caffeine)	1 tablet	30
Norgesic Forte (orphenadrine, aspirin, caffeine)	1 tablet	60
Synalgos-DC (dihydrocodeine, aspirin, caffeine)	1 tablet	30

reverses neurogenic inflammation. It is available with a convenient injector system that enables patients to self-inject as needed [12]. Recently, it has also become available in tablet form (25- and 50-mg strengths).

Preventive Therapy.   For frequent attacks of migraine, a combination of preventive and symptomatic treatment is often necessary. Preventive (prophylactic) treatment is used to reduce the frequency and severity of headache events [5]. It is appropriate

Table 5-2. Symptomatic Medications in the Treatment of Migraine

Trade Name	Generic Name
Traditional analgesics	
Tylenol	Acetaminophen
Bufferin, Ecotrin, etc.	Acetylsalicylic acid
Anaprox, Naprosyn, Ibuprofen, Motrin, etc.	Nonsteroidal anti-inflammatory drugs
Combination analgesics	
Esgic	Butalbital 50 mg + acetaminophen 325 mg + caffeine 40 mg
Esgic with codeine	Butalbital 50 mg + acetaminophen 325 mg + caffeine 40 mg + codeine 30 mg
Fioricet	Butalbital 50 mg + acetaminophen 325 mg + caffeine 40 mg
Fiorinal	Butalbital 50 mg + aspirin 325 mg + caffeine 40 mg
Fiorinal with codeine #3	Butalbital 50 mg + aspirin 325 mg + caffeine 40 mg + codeine 30 mg
Midrin	Isometheptene mucate 65 mg + dichloralphenazone 100 mg + acetaminophen 325 mg
Phrenilin	Butalbital 50 mg + acetaminophen 325 mg
Phrenilin Forte	Butalbital 50 mg + acetaminophen 650 mg
Phrenilin with codeine #3	Butalbital 50 mg + acetaminophen 325 mg + codeine phosphate 30 mg
Opioids	
Bancap HC	Hydrocodone bitartrate 5 mg + acetaminophen 500 mg
Darvocet-N 100	Propoxyphene napsylate 100 mg + acetaminophen 650 mg
Darvocet-N 50	Propoxyphene napsylate 50 mg + acetaminophen 325 mg
Darvon Compound	Propoxyphene HCl 32 mg + aspirin 389 mg + caffeine 32.4 mg
Darvon Compound-65	Propoxyphene HCl 65 mg + aspirin 389 mg + caffeine 32.4 mg
Darvon with ASA	Propoxyphene HCl 65 mg + aspirin 325 mg
Darvon-N	Propoxyphene napsylate
Darvon-N with ASA	Propoxyphene napsylate 100 mg + aspirin 325 mg
Demerol (tablets or injectable)	Meperidine HCl
Dilaudid	Hydromorphone
DHC Plus	Dihydrocodeine bitartrate 16 mg + acetaminophen 350 mg + caffeine 30 mg
Dolophine HCl (tablets)	Methadone HCl
Empirin with codeine #2	Codeine 15 mg + aspirin 325 mg
Empirin with codeine #3	Codeine 30 mg + aspirin 325 mg
Empirin with codeine #4	Codeine 60 mg + aspirin 325 mg
Levo-Dromoran	Levorphanol tartrate
Lorcet	Hydrocodone bitartrate (5, 7.5, 10 mg) + acetaminophen (500 or 650 mg)
Lortab	Hydrocodone bitartrate (2.5, 5, 7.5 mg) + aspirin 500 mg
Mepergan	Meperidine HCl + promethazine HCl
MS Contin (tablets)	Morphine sulphate
MSIR (tablets or oral solution)	Morphine sulphate
Percocet	Oxycodone 5 mg + acetaminophen 325 mg
Percodan	Oxycodone HCl 4.5 mg + oxycodone terephthalate 0.38 mg + aspirin 325 mg
Stadol (injectable or nasal spray)	Butorphanol tartrate
Synalgos-DC	Dihydrocodeine bitartrate 16 mg + aspirin 356.4 mg + caffeine 30 mg
Talacen	Pentazocine HCl 25 mg + acetaminophen 650 mg
Talwin compound	Pentazocine HCl 12.5 mg + aspirin 325 mg
Talwin NX	Pentazocine HCl 50 mg + naloxone HCl 0.5 mg
Tylenol #2	Acetaminophen 300 mg + codeine 15 mg
Tylenol #3	Acetaminophen 300 mg + codeine 30 mg
Tylenol #4	Acetaminophen 300 mg + codeine 60 mg
Tylox	Oxycodone 5 mg + acetaminophen 500 mg
Vicodin	Hydrocodone bitartrate 5 mg + acetaminophen 500 mg

Steroids

Decadron (tablets and suspension)	Dexamethasone
Deltasone (tablets)	Prednisone
Medrol (tablets)	Methylprednisolone
Medrol Dosepak	Methylprednisolone
Solu-Medrol (parenteral)	Methylprednisolone

Antiemetics

Antivert	Meclizine
Compazine	Prochlorperazine
Phenergan	Promethazine HCl
Reglan	Metoclopramide HCl
Tigan	Trimethobenzamide HCl

Ergotamine derivatives

Cafergot (suppositories)	Ergotamine tartrate 2 mg + caffeine 100 mg
Cafergot (tablets)	Ergotamine tartrate 1 mg + caffeine 100 mg
Ergomar (sublingual tablets)	Ergotamine tartrate 2 mg
Ergostat (sublingual tablets)	Ergotamine tartrate 2 mg
Wigraine (suppositories)	Ergotamine tartrate 2 mg + caffeine 100 mg + tartaric acid 21.5 mg
Wigraine (tablets)	Ergotamine tartrate 1 mg + caffeine 100 mg

Injectable migraine medications

Imitrex	Sumatriptan
DHE 45	Dihydroergotamine mesylate

when attacks of acute pain occur more than two times per week, when the severity or duration of infrequent attacks justifies the use of preventive treatment, when symptomatic medications are ineffective for infrequent attacks, and to enhance the efficacy of symptomatic medications. Preventive medications include beta blockers, calcium channel blockers, antidepressants, and anticonvulsants (Table 5-3).

Beta blockers are the group of prophylactic agents most widely used for migraine and related headaches. In 60–80% of cases, they are effective in reducing the frequency of headache by at least 50%. They should be administered initially in small, divided doses, titrating upward to tolerance. Two-, three-, or four-times-daily dosing is superior to once-daily dosing. Selected major untoward reactions to beta blockers include fatigue, depression, memory disturbances, impotence, hypotension, bradycardia, weight gain, peripheral vasoconstriction, bronchospasm, and adverse influence on cholesterol and lipid metabolism. Contraindications to beta-blocker use include congestive heart failure (CHF), asthma, significant diabetes or hypoglycemia, bradycardia, hypotension, and moderate to

Table 5-3. Medications Used for Headache Prophylaxis

Drug	Recommended Dose
Tricyclic antidepressants	
Nortriptyline hydrochloride	10–125 mg/day
Amitriptyline hydrochloride	10–300 mg/day
Doxepin hydrochloride	10–50 mg/day
Antidepressants	
Fluoxetine hydrochloride	20–80 mg/day
Calcium channel blockers	
Verapamil hydrochloride	240–720 mg/day
Nifedipine	30–180 mg/day
Nimodipine	60 mg four times daily
Diltiazem hydrochloride	120–360 mg/day
Beta blockers	
Propranolol hydrochloride	40–320 mg/day
Atenolol	50–150 mg/day
Nadolol	40–240 mg/day
Timolol maleate	10–30 mg/day
Anticonvulsants	
Valproate	250–750 mg/day
Phenytoin sodium	200–400 mg/day

Table 5-4. Foods That Should Be Avoided by the Headache Patient

1. Salt on an empty stomach (e.g., snacks of potato chips, popcorn, peanuts)
2. All cheeses except American, cottage, and Velveeta
3. Real sour cream (imitation sour cream acceptable)
4. Live yogurt cultures
5. Fresh breads, raised coffee cakes, raised donuts
6. Beans of any sort—navy, lima, pinto, and so on, and pea pods
7. All nuts, including peanut butter
8. All preserved meats, including sausage, hot dogs, ham, bacon; all deli meats, including chicken and turkey
9. Oranges, orange juice, and other citrus foods, bananas, pineapple
10. Anything pickled, fermented, or marinated
11. Chocolate
12. Monosodium glutamate in any form
13. Excessive caffeine intake
14. Alcoholic beverages

severe hyperlipidemia. Beta-blocker therapy must be individualized. Underdosing is a major cause of therapeutic failure. When discontinuing beta blockers after extended usage, a gradual reduction program is necessary.

Verapamil is the calcium channel blocker most widely used for the treatment of vascular headache. It is appropriate when contraindications to beta blockers exist. As with beta blockers, a small, divided dose should be used initially and then titrated upward to tolerance. High-dose verapamil (160 mg three to four times per day) may be necessary for beneficial effects in some patients. Selected major untoward reactions to verapamil include constipation, atrioventricular block, CHF, hypotension, and reflex tachycardia. Contraindications include CHF, heart block, moderate to severe bradycardia, hypotension, sick sinus syndrome, atrial flutter or fibrillation, and severe constipation [1,10].

Tricyclic antidepressants (TCAs) are particularly valuable prophylactic agents in patients who suffer chronic daily headache or intermittent migraines, with or without depression. TCAs are sedating, and so patients with associated sleep disturbances will enjoy an added benefit of using these agents. Generally, TCAs should be administered as a single dose at bedtime. The major TCAs for headache include amitriptyline, nortriptyline, doxepin, desipramine, and protriptyline. Untoward

reactions to TCAs include weight gain, dizziness, subtle cognitive impairment, and anticholinergic symptoms (drowsiness, dry mouth, constipation, urinary retention, blurry vision, and tachycardia). Contraindications to TCA use include significant cardiac arrhythmia, glaucoma, and urinary retention [13–16].

Anticonvulsants such as phenytoin (Dilantin), carbamazepine (Tegretol), and valproate (Depakote) occasionally benefit migraine sufferers. They also might help patients who suffer chronic daily headache and occipital neuralgic syndromes. The membrane-stabilizing effects of these drugs might be useful in occipital neuralgia, a condition characterized by entrapment or irritation of the occipital nerves in tight paracervical musculature. Anticonvulsants must be administered carefully, beginning with small, divided doses.

Dilantin is administered in doses of 100–400 mg per day. Tegretol should be given in doses beginning at 100–200 mg two to three times per day, with gradual increase to tolerance or efficacy. Depakote should be started at a dose of 125–250 mg three to four times per day. Doses should be increased gradually to a maximum dose of 1–2 g per day [5,17–19]. Blood level monitoring is advisable in all patients taking anticonvulsants. Also, periodic evaluation of hematologic and liver function is recommended, per standard protocol.

Nonpharmacologic Treatment

Nonpharmacologic interventions for headache sufferers include applying ice; resting in a cool, quiet, dark environment; practicing biofeedback and relaxation techniques; discontinuing smoking; and exercising regularly. Furthermore, the patient will benefit from keeping activities the same from day to day, insofar as this is possible, and from avoiding foods (Table 5-4) and circumstances that might provoke headache [1].

Sleep Disturbance

Sleep disturbance, like headaches, is another problem commonly associated with chronic pain syndromes. It is characterized by (1) difficulty falling asleep; (2) restlessness and nocturnal myoclonus, to the extent that the patient frequently kicks the covers off the bed; (3) inability to find a comfortable position; (4) frequent awakening with discomfort; (5) inability to enter deeper stages of sleep; and (6) daytime fatigue, ranging from bothersome tiredness to overwhelming exhaustion.

Restlessness at night causes increased pain and discomfort during the day. Pain in conjunction with chronic fatigue can lead to impaired cognitive processes. Therefore, sleep disturbance in this context needs to be addressed.

Conservative treatment might include behavioral and cognitive techniques such as relaxation training or listening to relaxing cassette tapes, which should be attempted at bedtime by patients who have difficulty falling asleep. However, pharmacologic management of sleep disturbances is often necessary. Such management includes the use of TCAs, conventional hypnotics, muscle relaxants, and the drug clonazepam (Klonopin).

Important concerns when choosing sedatives and hypnotics should include effectiveness of the drug, cost, side effects (including daytime fatigue and hangover effect), and presence or absence of nocturnal myoclonus or muscle spasm. Occasionally, combinations of different classes of medications prove most helpful (e.g., a low-dose TCA with Klonopin).

Tricyclic Antidepressants

TCAs play an important role in the treatment of patients with chronic pain [13–16,20–25]. These agents offer the chronic pain patient three potentially useful effects: analgesia, sedation, and antidepressant actions. TCAs relieve pain and help promote sleep at lower dosages, at lower plasma levels, and in a shorter period of time than normally are required for treatment of depression. For example, chronic pain sufferers often benefit from low-dose amitriptyline (Elavil, 10–75 mg), in whom the drug's positive analgesic and hypnotic effects are seen within days. On the other hand, the severely depressed patient will require higher doses (100–150 mg), and several weeks usually will go by before a therapeutic effect is realized [26]. Of the TCAs (Table 5-5), amitriptyline and imipramine are the most sedating. Trazodone also is quite sedating, although structurally it is not a true TCA (Figure 5-1).

Table 5-5. Commonly Used Tricyclic Antidepressant Drugs

Drug (Trade Name)	Usual Daily Dose (mg)
Amitriptyline HCl (Elavil)	75–150
Desipramine HCl (Norpramin)	75–200
Doxepin HCl (Adapin, Sinequan)	75–150
Imipramine HCl (Tofranil)	50–200
Nortriptyline HCl (Pamelor)	75–100
Trazodone HCl (Desyrel)	150–200

Hypnotics

If TCAs are tolerated poorly or if there are contraindications to TCA use, conventional hypnotics are frequently helpful. Among these are over-the-counter medications, benzodiazepines (temazepam [Restoril], flurazepam [Dalmane], triazolam [Halcion], quazepam [Doral], Klonopin), or nonbenzodiazepine hypnotics (zolpidem tartrate [Ambien]). Klonopin (0.5–2.0 mg at bedtime) is useful in decreasing nighttime restlessness (nocturnal myoclonus); patients tend to feel more rested during the day if this phenomenon is lessened. Cyclobenzaprine HCl (Flexeril), which is structurally similar to the TCAs, may be helpful in promoting sleep in patients whose muscle spasms contribute to their chronic pain syndrome. The administration of hypnotic medications must be individualized.

Depression

Depression in the CTD patient may occur secondary to functional losses, the chronic unrelenting pain, inability to engage in vocational or avocational pursuits, financial worries, and family stressors.

When depression is mild, psychological counseling, perhaps in conjunction with a low-dose antidepressant, may be all that is needed. However, when major depression occurs, consultation with a psychiatrist is strongly recommended for medical management. A major depressive episode implies a prominent and relatively persistent depressed or dysphoric mood that usually interferes with daily functioning (nearly every day for at least 2 weeks). At least four of the following eight symptoms should be demonstrated: change in appetite, change in sleep, psychomotor agitation or

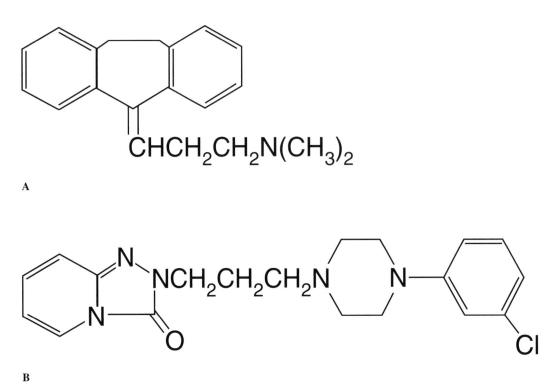

Figure 5-1. A. Chemical structure of amitriptyline. B. Chemical structure of trazodone, which is not a true tricyclic antidepressant.

retardation, loss of interest in usual activities or decrease in sexual drive, increased fatigue, feelings of guilt or worthlessness, slowed thinking or impaired concentration, and a suicide attempt or suicidal ideation [27]. Psychological counseling for depressed patients with chronic pain often requires special emphasis on and instruction in pain management strategies, pacing, relaxation techniques including biofeedback, and stress management. Involvement of other family members often is helpful.

Tricyclic Antidepressants

As previously mentioned, TCAs have several qualities that are useful for chronic pain patients. However, higher dosages often are required to achieve the antidepressant effects that are necessary for analgesia and sleep. Occasionally, TCA use is limited by anticholinergic effects (dry mouth, constipation, and urinary retention), daytime sedation, disturbed con-

centration, cardiac arrhythmias (heart block, tachycardia, and palpitations), and weight gain (particularly with Elavil).

TCAs inhibit the membrane pump mechanisms responsible for reuptake of norepinephrine and serotonin in adrenergic and serotoninergic neurons. The increased synaptic availability of these neurotransmitters is believed to underlie the antidepressant activity of the TCAs. Likewise, increased availability of norepinephrine and serotonin in the noradrenergic and serotoninergic descending pain pathways may explain the analgesic abilities of these neurotransmitters.

Selective Serotonin-Reuptake Inhibitor Antidepressants

Over the past decade, a new family of antidepressants has evolved that works by selectively inhibiting reuptake of the neurotransmitter serotonin. In general, this class of medication is better tolerated than the TCAs and has fewer side effects and sedative qualities. The medications available include fluoxetine hydrochloride (Prozac), sertraline hydrochloride (Zoloft), and paroxetine hydrochloride (Paxil).

These drugs all are orally administered antidepressants chemically unrelated to TCAs or other available antidepressants. Their mechanism of action is believed to be via selective inhibition of neuronal serotonin reuptake. As opposed to the TCAs, the selective serotonin-reuptake inhibitor antidepressants (SSRIs) have little affinity for muscarinic, histaminergic, and adrenergic receptors; antagonism of such receptors has been hypothesized to be associated with various anticholinergic, sedative, and cardiovascular effects seen with the TCAs.

The SSRIs are metabolized in the liver and excreted in the kidneys. Consequently, dosages must be adjusted appropriately in patients with liver and kidney disease. Serious and possibly fatal reactions can occur if SSRIs are used in conjunction with monoamine oxidase inhibitors (MAOIs). Therefore, SSRIs should not be used in combination with, or within 14 days of discontinuation of, an MAOI. The most commonly observed adverse reactions to SSRIs are listed in Table 5-6.

The usual dose ranges are 20–80 mg per day for Prozac, 50–200 mg per day for Zoloft, and 20–50 mg per day for Paxil. As with other antidepressants, the full antidepressant effect of SSRIs may be delayed until 4 weeks or more after treatment begins [28–34].

Venlafaxine Hydrochloride

Venlafaxine hydrochloride (Effexor) is chemically unrelated to the TCAs and SSRIs. The antidepressant action of Effexor is believed to be due to potent inhibition of norepinephrine and serotonin neuronal reuptake [35]. However, as opposed to the TCAs (which also inhibit norepinephrine and serotonin), Effexor has no significant affinity for muscarinic, histaminergic, and adrenergic receptors, thereby avoiding the anticholinergic, sedative, and cardiovascular effects of TCAs [35–37].

Effexor is metabolized extensively in the liver and excreted in the kidney. Like SSRIs, it should not be administered to patients on MAOIs or for 2 weeks after discontinuation of these drugs, and there is a similar side effect profile. The dose can

Table 5-6. Commonly Observed Adverse Reactions for the Selective Serotonin-Reuptake Inhibitors

Nervous system
  Anxiety
  Nervousness
  Insomnia
  Somnolence
  Tremor
  Dizziness
Gastrointestinal system
  Nausea
  Diarrhea
  Dyspepsia
  Anorexia
  Dry mouth
Other reactions
  Increased sweating
  Male sexual dysfunction (ejaculatory delay)

range from 75 to 225 mg per day for mild to moderate depression and up to 350 mg per day for severely depressed patients.

Bupropion Hydrochloride

Bupropion hydrochloride (Wellbutrin) is chemically unrelated to TCAs, SSRIs, and Effexor. The neurochemical mechanism of its antidepressant effect is not known, but it appears to be a stimulant for the central nervous system. There is a fourfold increased incidence of seizure activity in patients on Wellbutrin as compared with other marketed antidepressants. Therefore, Wellbutrin is contraindicated in patients with a seizure disorder and in patients with anorexia and bulimia, because of a higher incidence of seizures in such patients. Common side effects of this drug include agitation, dry mouth, insomnia, headaches, nausea, vomiting, constipation, and tremor. The usual adult dose is 300 mg per day in divided doses [38,39].

Myofascial Pain Syndrome

The myofascial pain associated with CTDs may persist as long as there is peripheral noxious input, or it may continue indefinitely. MPS must be

Table 5-7. Common Muscle Relaxants

Trade Name	Generic Name
Flexeril	Cyclobenzaprine
Lioresal	Baclofen
Norflex	Orphenadrine citrate
Norgesic	Orphenadrine citrate 25 mg + aspirin 385 mg + caffeine 30 mg
Norgesic Forte	Orphenadrine citrate 50 mg + aspirin 770 mg + caffeine 60 mg
Parafon Forte DSC	Chlorzoxazone
Robaxin	Methocarbamol
Robaxin-750	Methocarbamol
Skelaxin	Metaxalone
Soma	Carisoprodol 350 mg
Soma Compound	Carisoprodol 200 mg + aspirin 325 mg
Valium	Diazepam

addressed to decrease overall pain levels and to prevent migration of the myofascial pain over time.

Physical and occupational therapy play an important role in the management of MPS. Therapeutic modalities including hot packs, cold packs, ultrasound, massage, electrical stimulation, daily stretching, and therapeutic exercise can be applied to loosen up tight painful muscles, break myofascial adhesions, and improve blood flow to tissues. A goal of treatment is to decrease afferent nociceptive input from these tissues, thereby lessening or breaking the vicious cycle of pain and reactive spasm that perpetuates the condition.

Other treatments available for the management of chronic MPS include trigger-point injection therapy, transcutaneous electrical nerve stimulation (TENS), and medications such as nonsteroidal anti-inflammatory drugs and muscle relaxants. Nonsteroidal anti-inflammatory drugs may or may not be effective analgesics for patients with MPS or fibromyalgia. However, a component of low-grade inflammation may present that might respond favorably to this class of medication.

Muscle relaxants are generally indicated for short-term use in treatment of acute muscle spasm. Flexeril, which is structurally similar to the TCAs, might be appropriate for long-term use in patients with fibromyalgia. It can be sedating and might be appropriate for treatment of sleep disturbances associated with MPS. Around-the-clock usage (40

mg/day) has been described as being effective in some fibromyalgia patients [40–42]. Although many other muscle relaxants are available (Table 5-7), none is recommended for long-term treatment of MPS. The chronic use of diazepam (Valium) should be avoided as it is sedating, may worsen depression, and is potentially habit forming. Carisoprodol (Soma) is a commonly prescribed, uncontrolled, skeletal muscle relaxant whose active metabolite is meprobamate. Patients for whom carisoprodol is prescribed are at risk for meprobamate dependency, toxicity, and withdrawal. Therefore, carisoprodol should be used with caution [43].

Neurogenic Pain

The pain of CTD is usually multifactorial and includes chronic musculoskeletal, myofascial, and neurogenic components. Neurogenic pain may be due to nerve irritation by tight forearm or thoracic outlet muscles (i.e., scalene and pectoralis muscles) or to damaged nerve fibers (with positive electrodiagnostic studies). Clinical features of neurogenic pain include pain out of proportion to what would be expected given the clinical examination, burning or shooting pain, and physical findings consistent with nerve irritation (positive Tinel's sign, allodynia, hyperalgesia).

If neurogenic pain is believed to be contributing to the symptom complex, the following treatment modalities may prove helpful: TENS, capsaicin (Zostrix) cream, TCAs (discussed earlier), Tegretol and other anticonvulsants, mexiletine, and clonidine.

Transcutaneous Electrical Nerve Stimulation

TENS is a therapeutic modality that may prove helpful for one or more of the chronic pain problems associated with CTDs (neurogenic pain, chronic tendinitis, myofascial pain, and headaches). Its pathophysiologic efficacy is believed to be explained by Melzack and Wall's gate-control hypothesis [44,45]. Melzack and Wall proposed that large-diameter, myelinated, primary afferents exert an inhibitory effect on dorsal horn pain-transmission neurons and that selective stimulation of such afferent fibers would alleviate pain. The large-diameter afferents are easy to activate with externally applied, low-threshold electrical stimuli. In contrast, unmyelinated nociceptive afferent fibers are less sensitive and will not be activated by low-level electrical stimulation.

TENS offers a number of advantages: It is a relatively inexpensive form of pain control if used in the long term. Also, it might help decrease oral analgesic requirements. TENS puts the patient in a position of control over his or her pain. Finally, the onset of pain relief is almost immediate. Occasionally, a few minutes of stimulation will provide for several hours of sustained analgesia [46,47].

Among the disadvantages of TENS is the fact that wire electrodes may prove awkward in the treatment of upper-extremity conditions. Also, skin irritation can be caused by the electrode adhesive. Finally, the effectiveness of TENS may wear off over time [48].

A variety of commercial stimulators are available [49]. On each unit, one can adjust the stimulation frequency and intensity. There are no standard settings or electrode locations that work best. A patient must experiment with different electrode locations and different unit parameters to achieve optimal success with the unit. There is general agreement that the most effective placements are close to the area of pain. In the case of distal peripheral nerve injury, placement of electrodes over a proximal portion of the involved nerve is recommended (Figure 5-2) [46].

It is critical that patients receive thorough instruction on the use of TENS (the various parameters and potential electrode locations) if optimal effectiveness is to be attained. Experienced professionals—whether physicians, nurses, therapists, or TENS vendors—should invest the time required to instruct patients on TENS use.

Capsaicin Preparations

Capsaicin (Zostrix 0.025%, or Zostrix High-Potency 0.075%) is a naturally occurring substance derived from plants of the Solanaceae (chili pepper) family. It is indicated for the temporary relief of pain from rheumatoid arthritis, osteoarthritis, and various neuralgias. Although the precise mechanism of action of capsaicin is not understood entirely, it is believed that this agent relieves pain by depleting and pre-

venting reaccumulation of substance P in peripheral sensory neurons. As noted in Chapter 4, substance P can activate or sensitize peripheral nociceptors, and it is a mediator of inflammation. The medication should be applied three to four times daily; the maximal effect can be expected within several weeks of the drug's use [50–53].

Tegretol and the Anticonvulsants

The usefulness of anticonvulsants has been established for the treatment only of neuropathic pains that have a paroxysmal component. Trigeminal neuralgia is the most common painful condition for which anticonvulsants are effective. Other conditions that respond to anticonvulsants include glossopharyngeal neuralgia, paroxysmal pains of multiple sclerosis, postlaminectomy pain, postamputation pain, postherpetic neuralgia, and diabetic neuropathy. In all these conditions, nerve damage is a prominent feature and a lancinating or shooting component is present. The efficacy of anticonvulsants for treating other types of pain is questionable, although there is evidence that nonlancinating neuropathic pain also may respond [54–60].

Patients with upper-extremity CTD whose clinical examination is consistent with persistent neural irritation of one or multiple nerves may benefit from a trial of Tegretol or one of the other anticonvulsants. This is especially true if there is a shooting paroxysmal quality to the pain.

The precise mechanism of anticonvulsant pain relief is incompletely understood. It is believed that damaged nerves bear demyelinated patches of primary afferent axons that become ectopic sites of impulse generation. The demyelinated regions are sites of ephaptic spread, and pain triggered from the periphery is due to the short-circuiting of impulses from non-nociceptive to nociceptive afferents at the site of damage (Figure 5-3). The anticonvulsants are specifically valuable for neuropathic pains because these agents have been shown to reduce discharge from sites of ectopic impulse generation in damaged peripheral nerve [26,61–63].

Some patients with CTD seem to have irritated nerves that respond to anticonvulsant therapy even though electrodiagnostic studies consistently fail to reveal nerve damage. In the upper extremities, there are many potential sites for nerve compression

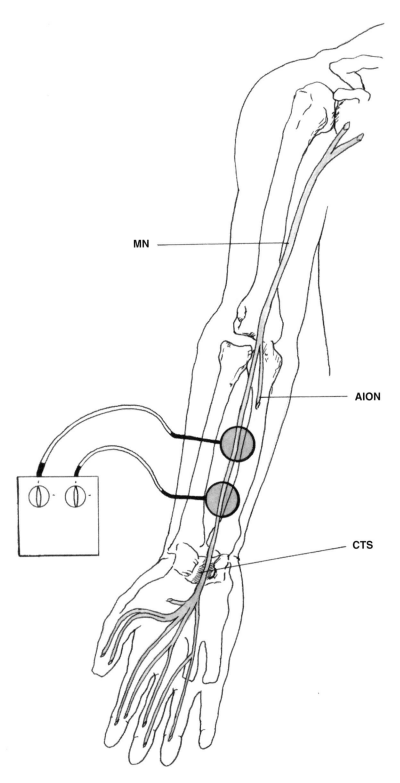

Figure 5-2. Transcutaneous electrical nerve stimulation electrode application. In the case of distal peripheral nerve injury (e.g., carpal tunnel syndrome [CTS]), placement of electrodes over a proximal portion of the involved nerve is recommended. (MN = median nerve; AION = anterior interosseous nerve.)

MN

AION

CTS

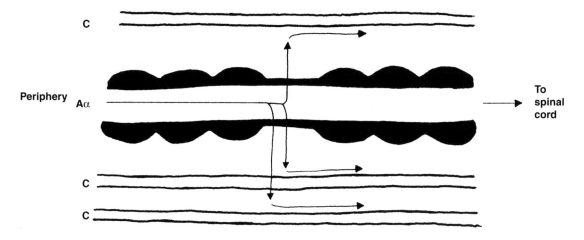

Figure 5-3. Ephaptic transmission. The demyelinated regions are sites of ephaptic spread. Pain is triggered from the periphery by a short-circuiting of impulses from non-nociceptive to nociceptive afferents at the site of damage. (C = unmyelinated C-nociceptive afferent fiber; Aα = myelinated non-nociceptive A alpha fiber.)

under ligaments (e.g., median nerve under the carpal tunnel), under taut myofascial bands (e.g., ulnar nerve under the flexor carpi ulnaris, radial nerve under the arcade of Frohse), and under tight muscles (e.g., pronator muscle and median nerve, pectoralis minor muscle and scalenes and brachial plexus). Persistent compression at these sites could theoretically lead to tiny regions of demyelinization and the development of ephaptic transmission or ectopic impulse generation and, in turn, to ultimate response to anticonvulsants, even in the face of unrevealing electrodiagnostic studies.

Currently, Tegretol is the first-line drug for the treatment of lancinating neuropathic pain. This medication needs to be started at the lowest possible dose and titrated appropriately until there is a therapeutic effect. Therapy is begun with a dose of as little as 100 mg per day, which can be increased progressively until pain relief is obtained or signs of toxicity appear. For most patients, relief is obtained at plasma concentrations between 5 and 10 µg/ml [64]. In any given patient, there is a very sharp Tegretol plasma level threshold required to obtain relief. Therefore, when a trial is being conducted with Tegretol, the dose should be titrated upward until there is a positive response or until side effects develop, to determine fully whether the drug will be effective. The most common dose-related side effects are sedation, ataxia, vertigo, blurry vision, nausea, and vomiting.

A mild leukopenia occurs in approximately 10% of patients, and in rare cases, there can be irreversible aplastic anemia. Regular monitoring of hematologic and liver functions is recommended.

Other anticonvulsants available include Dilantin, Depakote, and Klonopin. These drugs should also be titrated upward slowly until they prove effective or until the patient develops significant side effects. Dilantin should be started at 100 mg per day and can be increased to 400 mg per day. Therapeutic blood levels usually are between 10 and 20 µg/ml. Common adverse reactions include nystagmus, ataxia, slurred speech, decreased coordination, mental confusion, dizziness, insomnia, nervousness, and headache. It is recommended that serum drug levels, liver functions, and hematologic profiles be checked regularly.

Klonopin can be started at a dose of 0.5 mg two to three times per day, which can be titrated upward on the basis of clinical response. A principal side effect of Klonopin, as with other benzodiazepines, is sedation, which could be a problem during the day. However, with a half-life of 18–30 hours, it is possible that the majority of the dose can be administered at night, which also will promote better-quality sleep. The maximum recommended dose for seizure patients is 20 mg, although much lower doses are usually required to manage neurogenic pain. Klonopin can be tried in combination with other anticonvulsants.

Depakote should be started at a dose of 125–250 mg three to four times daily. The dose should be increased gradually to a maximum of 1–2 g per day. Optimum effectiveness may occur with serum levels between 50 and 100 µg/ml. Major untoward reactions include nausea and gastrointestinal upset, sedation, platelet dysfunction, hair loss, tremor, and hepatotoxicity. In children, hepatic dysfunction with fatal outcome has been reported. The drug is also potentially teratogenic. Depakote is relatively contraindicated in childhood and is contraindicated in pregnancy and significant hepatic disease. Hematologic and liver function studies should be checked before and during treatment. Blood level monitoring of the drug should be carried out periodically. It bears repeating that Depakote is teratogenic and should be used cautiously in fertile women [26,55,65].

Mexiletine Hydrochloride

Mexiletine hydrochloride (Mexitil) is an orally active antiarrhythmic agent that is structurally similar to lidocaine. It may prove helpful in the treatment of neurogenic pain when more traditional modalities and medications fail to provide symptom relief [66]. Mexitil, like lidocaine, inhibits the inward sodium current of neural membranes, thus reducing the rate of rise of the action potential and interfering with neural impulse transmission. It may prove useful in patients who appear clinically to have irritated peripheral nerves, damaged nerves, or neuromas.

Mexitil is well absorbed from the gastrointestinal tract. Peak blood levels are reached in 2–3 hours, and the half-life is 10–12 hours. The most common adverse reactions to Mexitil are reversible upper gastrointestinal distress and central nervous system effects (light-headedness, tremor, and coordination difficulties), which can often be avoided by administering the drug with food and by careful dose titration. The dose of Mexitil must be individualized on the basis of response and tolerance, which are dose related. Administration with food or an antacid is recommended. Early doses can be as low as 150 mg one to two times per day, with gradual titration every few days to a maximum dose of 1,200 mg per day. Mexitil is contraindicated in the presence of second- or third-degree atrioventricular block [67–69].

Clonidine

Clonidine (Catapres) is an antihypertensive agent with pain-relieving qualities. It is also sedating and, when given at night, may help promote better-quality sleep. In chronic painful conditions, clonidine has an antinociceptive action at the spinal cord level. As mentioned in Chapter 3, there are two descending pain modulatory pathways, a serotoninergic pathway from the rostroventral medulla and a noradrenergic pathway from the dorsolateral pons. Both pathways make up the dorsolateral funiculus. The noradrenergic inhibition of nociceptive transmission at the level of the spinal cord dorsal horn is mediated by an alpha$_2$-adrenergic receptor. Like norepinephrine, clonidine, a specific alpha$_2$ agonist, inhibits nociceptive dorsal horn neurons [70–76].

Because it often is sedating, clonidine can be initiated as a nighttime dose as low as 0.1 mg. If this is tolerated, the drug can be given two or three times daily or as a higher nighttime dose. Clonidine also is available in patch form (TTS-1, TTS-2, TTS-3); these patches can be changed weekly, providing for steady drug levels and greater convenience.

The most frequent adverse reactions, aside from sedation, are dry mouth, daytime drowsiness, dizziness, and constipation. Clonidine may be helpful in the treatment of neurogenic pain, myofascial pain, withdrawal from addictive substances, and sleep disturbances associated with chronic pain. It is nonaddictive and can enhance the potency of traditional analgesics, including opioids.

References

1. Saper JR, Silberstein S, Gordon CD, et al. Mechanisms and Theories of Head Pain. In JW Pine (ed), Handbook of Headache Management. Baltimore: Williams & Wilkins, 1993;16.
2. Andrasik F. Psychological and behavioral aspects of chronic headache. Neurol Clin 1990;8:961.
3. Holroyd KA, Andrasik F. A Cognitive-Behavioral Approach to Recurrent Tension and Migraine Headache. In PC Kendell (ed), Advances in Cognitive-Behavioral Research and Therapy. New York: Academic, 1982;275.
4. Lake AE III. Relaxation Therapy and Biofeedback in Headache Management. In JR Saper (ed), Help for Headaches. New York: Warner Books, 1987;163.
5. Shulman EA, Silberstein SD. Symptomatic and prophylactic treatment of migraine and tension-type headache. Neurology 1992;42(suppl 2):16.

6. Matthew RJ, Wilson WH. Caffeine-induced changes in cerebral circulation. Stroke 1985;16:814.

7. Ward N, Whitney C, Avery D, et al. The analgesic effects of caffeine in headache. Pain 1991;44:151.

8. Callaham MM, Raskin NH. A controlled study of dihydroergotamine in the treatment of acute migraine headache. Headache 1986;26:168.

9. Goldstein J. Ergot pharmacology in alternative delivery systems for ergotamine derivatives. Neurology 1992;42(suppl 2):45.

10. Peroutka SJ. The pharmacology of current antimigraine drugs. Headache 1990;30(suppl 1):5.

11. Silberstein SD, Shulman EA, Hopkins MM. Repetitive intravenous DHE in the treatment of refractory headache. Headache 1990;30:334.

12. Subcutaneous Sumatriptan International Study Group. Treatment of migraine attacks with sumatriptan. N Engl J Med 1991;5:316.

13. Couch JR, Hassanein RS. Amitriptyline in migraine prophylaxis. Arch Neurol 1979;21:263.

14. Gomersall JD, Stuart A. Amitriptyline in migraine prophylaxis. J Neurol Neurosurg Psychiatry 1973;36:684.

15. Diamond S, Baltes BJ. Chronic tension headache treated with amitriptyline—a double blind study. Headache 1971;11:110.

16. Lance JW, Curran DA. Treatment of chronic tension headache. Lancet 1964;1:1236.

17. Herring R, Kuritzky A. Sodium valproate in the prophylactic treatment of migraine: a double-blind study vs. placebo. Cephalgia 1992;12:81.

18. Mathew NT, Ali S. Valproate in the treatment of persistent chronic daily headache. An open-label study. Headache 1991;31:71.

19. Sorensen KV. Valproate: a new drug in migraine prophylaxis. Acta Neurol Scand 1988;78:346.

20. Watson CP, Evans RJ, Reed K, et al. Amitriptyline versus placebo in postherpetic neuralgia. Neurology 1982;32:671.

21. Gomez-Perez FJ, Rull JA, Dies H, et al. Nortriptyline and fluphenazine in the symptomatic treatment of diabetic neuropathy. A double-blind cross-over study. Pain 1985;23:395.

22. Kvinesdal B, Molin J, Froland A, et al. Imipramine treatment of painful diabetic neuropathy. JAMA 1984;251:1727.

23. Turkington RW. Depression masquerading as diabetic neuropathy. JAMA 1980;243:1147.

24. Gringas M. A clinical trial of Tofranil in rheumatic pain in general practice. J Int Med Res 1976;4:41.

25. Scott WAM. The relief of pain with an antidepressant in arthritis. Practitioner 1969;202:802.

26. Fields HL. Anticonvulsants, Psychotropics, and Antihistamine Drugs in Pain Management. In HL Fields (ed), Pain. New York: McGraw-Hill, 1987;285.

27. American Psychiatric Association. Diagnostic and Statistical Manual of Mental Disorders: DSM-IV (4th ed). Washington, DC: American Psychiatric Association, 1994.

28. Stokes PE. Fluoxetine: a five-year review. Clin Ther 1993;15:216.

29. Potter WZ, Rudorfer MV, Manji H. The pharmacologic treatment of depression. N Engl J Med 1991;325:633.

30. Tollefson GD. Antidepressant treatment and side effect consideration. J Clin Psychiatry 1991;52(suppl 6):4.

31. Thomas DR, Nelson DR, Johnson AM. Biochemical effects of the antidepressant paroxetine, a specific 5-hydroxytryptamine uptake inhibitor. Psychopharmacology 1987;93:193.

32. Bergstrom RF, Lemberger L, Farid NA, et al. Clinical pharmacology and pharmacokinetics of fluoxetine: a review. Br J Psychiatry 1988;153(suppl 3):47.

33. Physicians' Desk Reference (47th ed). Montvale, NJ: Medical Economics, 1993;2058.

34. Cooper GL. The safety of fluoxetine—an update. Br J Psychiatry 1988;153(suppl 3):77.

35. Effexor (venlafaxine HCl) prescribing information. Philadelphia: Wyeth-Ayerst Laboratories.

36. Richelson E. Synaptic pharmacology of antidepressants: an update. McLean Hosp J 1988;13:67.

37. Preskorn SH, Burke M. Somatic therapy for major depressive disorder: selection of an antidepressant. J Clin Psychiatry 1992;53(suppl 9):5.

38. Feinberg M. Bupropion: new therapy for depression. Am Fam Physician 1990;41:1787.

39. Bupropion for depression. Med Lett 1989;31:97.

40. Bennett RM, Gatter RA, Campbell SM, et al. A comparison of cyclobenzaprine and placebo in the management of fibrositis. A double-blind controlled study. Arthritis Rheum 1988;31:1535.

41. Hamaty D, Valentine JL, Howard R, et al. The plasma endorphin, prostaglandin and catecholamine profile of patients with fibrositis treated with cyclobenzaprine and placebo: a 5-month study. J Rheumatol 1989;19(suppl):164.

42. Reynolds W, Moldofsky H. The effects of cyclobenzaprine on sleep physiology and symptoms in FMS. J Rheumatol 1991;18:452.

43. Littrell RA, Hayes LR, Stillner V. Carisoprodol (Soma): a new and cautious perspective on an old agent. South Med J 1993;86:753.

44. Melzack R, Wall PD. Pain mechanisms: a new theory. Science 1965;150:971.

45. Melzack R, Wall PD. The Challenge of Pain. New York: Basic Books, 1982.

46. Fields HL. Nondrug Methods for Pain Control. In HL Fields (ed), Pain. New York: McGraw-Hill, 1987;307.

47. Meyer GA, Fields HL. Causalgia treated by selective large fibre stimulation of peripheral nerve. Brain 1972;95:163.

48. Woolf CJ. Transcutaneous and Implanted Nerve Stimulation. In PD Wall, R Melzack (eds), Textbook of Pain. Edinburgh: Churchill Livingstone, 1984.

49. Mannheimer JS, Lampe GN. Clinical Transcutaneous Electrical Nerve Stimulation. Philadelphia: Davis, 1984.

50. Buck SH, Burks TF. The neuropharmacology of capsaicin: review of some recent observations. Pharmacol Rev 1986;38:179.

51. Dickenson AH. Capsaicin: gaps in our knowledge start to be filled. Trends Neurosci 1991;14:265.

52. Dray A, Bettaney J, Forster P. Actions of capsaicin on peripheral nociceptors of the neonatal rat spinal cord-tail in vitro: dependence of extracellular ions and independence of second messengers. Br J Pharmacol 1990;101:727.

53. Lynn B. Capsaicin: actions on nociceptive C-fibres and therapeutic potential. Pain 1990;41:61.

54. Blom S. Tic douloureux treatment with new anticonvulsant. Arch Neurol 1963;9:285.

55. Maciewicz R, Bouckoms A, Martin JB. Drug therapy of neuropathic pain. Clin J Pain 1985;1:39.

56. Dunsker SB, Mayfield FH. Carbamazepine in the treatment of the flashing pain syndrome. J Neurosurg 1976;45:49.

57. Espir MLE, Millac P. Treatment of paroxysmal disorders in multiple sclerosis with carbamazepine (Tegretol). J Neurol Neurosurg Psychiatry 1970;33:528.

58. Fields HL, Raskin NH. Anticonvulsants and Pain. In HL Klawans (ed), Clinical Neuropharmacology. New York: Raven, 1976;173.

59. Shibasaki H, Kuroiwa Y. Painful tonic seizure in multiple sclerosis. Arch Neurol 1975;30:47.

60. Rull JA, Quibrera R, Gonzalez-Millan H, et al. Symptomatic treatment of peripheral diabetic neuropathy with carbamazepine (Tegretol): double blind crossover trial. Diabetologia 1969;5:215.

61. Wall PD. Changes in Damaged Nerve and Their Sensory Consequences. In JJ Bonica, JC Liebeskind, D Albe-Fessard (eds), Proceedings of the Second World Congress on Pain. New York: Raven, 1979;39.

62. Yaari Y, Devor M. Phenytoin suppresses spontaneous ectopic discharge in rat sciatic nerve neuromas. Neurosci Lett 1985;58:117.

63. Burchiel KJ. Carbamazepine inhibits spontaneous activity in experimental neuromas. Exp Neurol 1988;102:249.

64. Tomson T, Tybring G, Bertilsson L, et al. Carbamazepine therapy in trigeminal neuralgia: clinical effects in relation to plasma concentration. Arch Neurol 1980;37:699.

65. Rall TW, Schleifer LS. Drugs Effective in the Treatment of the Epilepsies. In AG Gilman, LS Goodman, A Gilman (eds), The Pharmacological Basis of Therapeutics. New York: Macmillan, 1985;446.

66. Davis RW. Phantom sensation, phantom pain, and stump pain. Arch Phys Med Rehabil 1993;74:79.

67. Chabal C, Russell LC, Burchiel KJ. The effect of intravenous lidocaine, tocainide, and mexiletine on spontaneously active fibers originating in rat sciatic neuromas. Pain 1989;38:333.

68. Dejgaard A, Petersen P, Kastrup J. Mexiletine for the treatment of chronic painful diabetic neuropathy. Lancet 1988;29:9.

69. Physicians' Desk Reference (48th ed). Montvale, NJ: Medical Economics, 1994;616.

70. Fleetwood-Walker S, Mitchell R, Hope PJ, et al. An α_2 receptor mediates the selective inhibition by noradrenaline of nociceptive responses of identified dorsal horn neurones. Brain Res 1985;334:243.

71. Yaksh TL, Reddy SVR. Studies in the primate on the analgesic effects associated with intrathecal actions of opiates, adrenergic agonists and baclofen. Anesthesiology 1981;54:451.

72. Wong KC, Franz DN, Tseng J. Clinical pharmacology of alpha$_2$-agonist and beta-adrenergic blocker. Anaesth Sinica 1989;27:357.

73. Spaulding TC, Fielding S, Venafro JJ, et al. Anti-nociceptive activity of clonidine and its potentiation of morphine analgesia. Eur J Pharmacol 1979;58:19.

74. Zemlan FP, Corrigan SA, Pfaff DW. Noradrenergic and serotonergic mediation of spinal analgesia mechanisms. Eur J Pharmacol 1980;61:111.

75. Reddy SVR, Maderdrut JL, Yaksh TL. Spinal cord pharmacology of adrenergic agonist-mediated antinociception. J Pharmacol Exp Ther 1980;213:525.

76. Fielding S, Spaulding T, Lal H. Antinociceptive Action of Clonidine. In S Fielding, T Spaulding, H Lal (eds), Psychopharmacology of Clonidine. New York: Alan R Liss, 1981;225.

Chapter 6

Occupation-Related Cumulative Trauma Disorders

Lyn Denise Weiss

Although the condition of cumulative trauma disorders (CTDs) is emerging as the by-product of modern technology, it should be noted that CTDs are not a new phenomenon. Ramazzini [1], in the seventeenth century, was one of the first to recognize work as a potential cause of chronic musculoskeletal disorders. He described "a harvest of diseases [ascribed to] certain violent and irregular motions of the body" [1]. References to occupation-related injury abound in the literature. In 1958, Sigerist [2] stated that "the development of industry has created many new sources of danger. Occupational diseases are socially different from other diseases, but not biologically." This astute physician raised an important point. Most of the conditions classified as CTDs are not unique to injured workers. However, the fact that such injuries occur in relation to a specific job task does separate these conditions not only socially but also economically, legally, and psychologically. In general, CTDs are considered tissue injuries caused by the cumulative effects of repetitive physical stress that exceeds physiologic limits [3].

The field of CTDs first became prominent in the mid-1980s in Australia. A rapid rise was reported in upper-limb pain largely among workers whose jobs involved repetitive hand movements. CTDs, then referred to as *repetitive strain injury*, became the focus of media attention and professional concern [4]. Some believe that the "epidemic" in Australia had to do with administrative bias, which favored the employee, and with the workers' compensation system, which facilitated recognition of the problem [5]. The incidence of new cases among keyboard workers in Australia peaked in 1985 and declined thereafter.

Many have debated whether this surge in the reporting of work-related injuries reflected an actual rise in such conditions as a result of new technologies (such as computers and improvements in automation) or whether the reporting merely appeared to increase as a result of extensive media coverage of the phenomenon of repetitive strain injury. More recent literature points to technologic advances as the cause of a true rise in the incidence of such injuries. The field of ergonomics (discussed later) grew out of this technologic expansion.

Impact of Cumulative Trauma Disorders

CTDs have physical, social, legal, psychological, and economic consequences. To refer only to the physical consequences of CTDs is to overlook the tremendous impact these disorders have on U.S. society. Consider the following statistics:

- The National Institute of Occupational Safety and Health (NIOSH) estimates that five million workers are currently susceptible to the development of CTDs [6].
- According to the National Council on Compensation Insurance, the average workers' compensation claim for a CTD injury in the United States costs $43,500 [7].

- The BLS reported that CTDs are the second most frequently reported category of occupational illness [8].
- According to the BLS, the number of cases of CTD was approximately 50,000 in 1986. By 1994, that number had increased to almost 350,000 cases [9].
- According to the BLS, CTDs accounted for one third of all workers' compensation costs in 1993 ($20 billion) [9].
- According to the Occupational Safety and Health Administration (OSHA) predictions for the year 2000, 50% of all injured worker's compensation cases will be related to CTDs [10].
- Twenty percent of workers in construction, food processing, manufacturing, mining industries, and office settings could be at risk for CTDs [8].
- According to the U.S. Department of Labor, CTDs accounted for 302,000 of 482,000 new cases of workplace illness in 1993 [11].
- According to the American Academy of Orthopedic Surgeons, CTDs cost the nation $27 billion annually in medical expenses and lost work [12].

The economic effects of CTDs are staggering and can be divided into direct and indirect costs. The direct costs include medical expenses and the cost of workers' compensation claims (wage replacements). Approximately 45% of the direct costs are medical expenses and 55% are wage replacements. The indirect costs, which frequently are not accounted for when the effects of CTDs are assessed, include lost productivity, the expense of employee retraining, and litigation expenses. When these costs are figured in, the economic effects of CTDs rise considerably.

The social and psychological stressors associated with CTDs should not be overlooked. In most societies, a person's social standing in the community is influenced by his or her occupation. The disabled worker often experiences psychological difficulties related to his or her new status in society in general (i.e., as a nonproducer) and in his or her family in particular (e.g., as one who is no longer able to provide). An individual's self-image is frequently tied to his or her body image; disability can have an extremely detrimental effect on a person's perception of self. It should be noted that the worker need not be totally disabled in order to suffer the emotional and social consequences of CTDs.

The development of CTDs has many legal ramifications as well. The determination of whether the disorder is occupation related may affect the type and amount of compensation the injured party receives. Often, it is not clear that a CTD is a direct result of occupational factors, as predisposing and concurrent factors can contribute to or be responsible for the development of CTDs. CTD sufferers who believe they have a legitimate claim of occupation-related injury may elect to bring suit against an employer. Such litigation is the topic of Chapter 15.

Although the cost of prevention of CTDs is almost always less than the cost of treatment, employees and insurance companies have been reluctant to pay for prevention. Nonetheless, prevention represents the most economical and humanitarian way to address the problem of CTDs.

Risk Factors for Cumulative Trauma Disorders in the Workplace

A number of risk factors have been associated with CTDs that are incurred in the workplace. Minimizing these factors is one way to reduce the number of occupation-related CTDs.

Repetition

Repetition has been regarded as the most important etiologic factor in CTDs. Repetition can be expressed as the number of exertions or movements per unit of time or as the length of time needed to complete a task or group of tasks (cycle time). Cycle times of less than 30 seconds or cycles in which the employee is involved in performing the same motion for more than 50% of the cycle are considered highly repetitive. In general, if the cumulative effect of repetitive stress exceeds the physiologic limits of any tissue, there is an increased likelihood that a CTD will develop.

Various ways exist to decrease the amount of repetition required for a task. One way is to combine jobs with short cycle times, thereby increasing the overall cycle time. This is known as job enlargement. In addition, automation can help to decrease the number of repetitions. However, when the number of repetitions is being decreased, care must be taken to avoid increasing the amount of force needed. Automation might actually increase the amount of repetition by decreasing the cycle time or by increasing the work load. Increased work load has been associated with increasing reports of CTDs [13,14].

Work pace has also been described as contributing to the development of CTDs [15,16]. In a study by Arndt [15], increased work pace was accompanied by an increased muscular effort, as identified by electromyographic data of flexor muscles of workers performing a highly repetitive task. It was suggested that work pace could have a dual effect on CTDs by increasing both the number of motions and the number of muscular activities associated with those motions. Increasing the work pace usually increases the number of repetitions performed in a given period of time.

There is a trend in industry to promote worker specialization. Although specializaiton may decrease training time and increase proficiency, it also increases the repetitiveness of the jobs. This is usually a result of decreased cycle time. Boredom and an increased risk for CTDs can ensue.

The human being is capable of millions of different movements, some very fine and some gross. The human machine is not, however, physiologically prepared for repetition. As Dobyns [17] aptly noted, "[T]he primate is a random action specialist, unique in the multiplicity of upper limb actions rather than the capacity for constant repetition."

Static Prolonged Positioning

Static prolonged positioning (also referred to as *static loading*) has been defined as the work that the muscles must perform in order to hold the body parts in certain positions. Static loading can increase the risk for CTDs. One example of static loading is the maintenance of isometric contractions. Muscles that remain contracted at more than 15–20% of maximal capacity may impair circulation. This positioning increases the risk for CTDs.

In a study by Larsson et al. [18], biopsies of the upper trapezius muscle were obtained from 17 patients with localized chronic myalgia related to static load during repetitive assembly work. Compared to each patient's nonpainful side, the affected trapezius muscle showed ragged fibers, indicating disturbed mitochondrial function in type 1 fibers. In addition, laser Doppler flowmeter recordings obtained on both sides revealed that myalgia correlated with reduced blood flow. This finding provides some pathologic evidence of the physical changes that occur with increased loading.

Increased muscular tension can occur in a person working at either too slow or too fast a pace. Assembly-line work with a conveyor belt restricts the work pace of the employee, whereas piecework usually increases a laborer's pace. With piecework, the employee can at least modify the pace to suit his or her individual comfort level. Permitting the worker to control and, in part, modify the work pace is likely to be beneficial in reducing the risk of CTDs.

Postures or Movements in a Non-Neutral Position

Humans have evolved into creatures that are best suited for postures in a neutral position. Many modern occupations require workers to assume positions or carry out movements that contribute to the development of CTDs. Among the movements commonly implicated in the development of CTDs are the following:

- Prolonged wrist dorsiflexion or extension
- Excessive wrist pronation or ulnar deviation
- Elbow flexion beyond 90 degrees (especially for tasks performed above elbow level)
- Internal rotation of the arms
- Elevation of the shoulder
- Excessive neck flexion
- Excessive hip flexion
- Excessive knee flexion
- Use of a pincer grip

Whereas limited unusual positioning may cause no ill effects, prolonged or repeated movements such as the ones listed here can stress physical structures and lead to the development of CTDs. For example, a pincer grip can produce up to fivefold greater positional stress than a power grip (Figure 6-1). Pincer grasps are especially detrimental to the metacarpophalangeal and carpometacarpal joints of

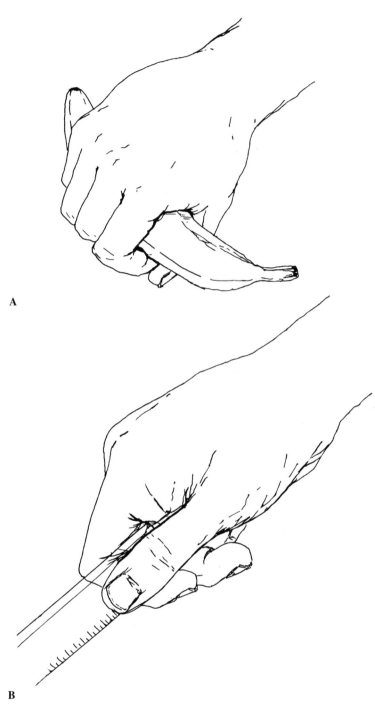

A

B

Figure 6-1. Power versus pincer grip. A. The power grip is performed by approximating digits 2–5 toward the thenar eminence. B. In the pincer grip, the thumb approximates the radial aspect of the index finger.

the thumb, as these joints are unsupported. A pincer grip can cause traumatic synovitis of the carpometacarpal joint. It also might aggravate an arthritic joint, as the movement can attenuate the action of the medial collateral ligament of the proximal joint of the thumb [19].

Long-Term Heavy Activity

Work that requires prolonged or repeated exertion of more than one-third of the patient's muscle strength (*force*) has been implicated in increasing the risk of CTDs. Efforts greater than 6 kg [8] or hand-force requirements of more than 40 N [4] have also been described as CTD-precipitating factors. The use of automation, mechanical tools, and power tools can help decrease the amount of force that the worker must apply. However, reducing force may increase repetition. Therefore, every task must be assessed individually.

NIOSH has established guidelines to assess job safety. The action limit (AL) can be calculated by the following formula [20]:

$$AL = 90 \ (6/H) \ (1 - 0.01 \ [V - 30])$$
$$(0.7 + 3/D) \ (1 - F/F_{max})$$

where H = horizontal distance from the hands at the origin of the lift to the center of the body; V = vertical distance measured from the hands to the floor at the origin of lift; D = the vertical travel distance from the origin to the destination of the lift; F = average number of lifts per minute; and F_{max} = duration of lifting in an 8-hour workday. More than 75% of women and 99% of men should be able to lift loads as calculated by the action limit.

The maximum permissible limit (MPL) can be found by multiplying the action limit by 3. Musculoskeletal injury rates and severity rates increase significantly when work is performed above the MPL. Only approximately 25% of male workers and fewer than 1% of female workers have the muscle strength to work above the MPL.

In general, the lifting requirements for tasks performed repeatedly should be limited to 30% of a worker's maximum isometric lifting capacity. Occasional lifting should be limited to 50% of a worker's maximum isometric lifting capacity [21].

Vibration

There is extensive evidence that vibration can cause CTDs [22–25]. Vibration-induced neuropathy has been described in the literature [23]. Both the vascular and nervous systems are involved in vibration-induced injury in workers. The neuritic component is usually characterized by numbness, tingling, perceptual decrement, and difficulty with fine hand control. *Vibration white finger* is the term frequently used to describe cold- or vibration-induced vascular spasm. Tools that produce high-frequency vibrations, such as industrial tools, have been known to cause these disorders.

NIOSH has estimated that 1.2 million Americans may have significant exposure to high-frequency vibration, and as many as 89% may be clinically affected in certain populations [22]. Riveters, pneumatic hammers, grinders, and rock drills have been implicated in the vibration syndrome [23,24,26–31]. Constant vibration has been associated with the development of low back pain in truck drivers.

Lundborg et al. [32] studied the pathologic effect of vibration in rats. Microscopic examination of involved nerves showed deranged axoplasmic structures or accumulation of smooth endoplasmic reticulum in unmyelinated fibers. Damage to these fibers is of interest because of their partial sympathetic composition, which may be responsible, in part, for the vasospasm observed in vibrational injuries [33].

Brammer et al. [22] have proposed a series of sensorineural stages of the hand-arm vibration syndrome (HAVS). At stage 0-SN are those workers exposed to vibration but displaying no symptoms. In stage 1-SN, the patient has intermittent numbness, with or without tingling. Stage 2-SN refers to those workers with intermittent or persistent numbness as well as reduced sensory perception. Stage 3-SN refers to those patients with intermittent or persistent numbness and reduced tactile discrimination or reduced manipulative dexterity.

The differential diagnosis of the vibration syndrome is extensive. Neurologic symptoms must be differentiated from other entities such as peripheral nerve entrapment (especially ulnar nerve entrapment), thoracic outlet syndrome (TOS), carpal tunnel syndrome (CTS), cervical radiculopathy, and peripheral neuropathy. Also included in the differential diagnosis are Raynaud's phenomenon, peripheral obstructive arterial disease, progressive systemic sclerosis, and rheumatoid arthritis.

For the most part, three methodologies have been used to diagnose the sensorineural complaints associated with HAVS: traditional clinical evaluations, electrodiagnosis via nerve conduction studies, and noninvasive quantitative tests of sensory performance [22]. Clinical tests such as pinprick, light touch, and two-point discrimination can be used in the office without elaborate equipment, but they are fairly insensitive and less objective relative to other measures. Nerve conduction studies have been useful in the evaluation of peripheral nerve slowing and peripheral nerve blocks. Measures of cutaneous vibrotactile performance and thermal sensitivity have been shown to be sensitive, reproducible, and quantifiable [23].

The vascular component of HAVS has been compared with primary Raynaud's phenomenon. Because primary Raynaud's phenomenon occurs in 8–10% of young females, it is important to establish whether there is a previous history of symptoms when evaluating such a patient for work-acquired causes. Different methods have been used to assess the vascular component, including measurement of the normalization time of fingertip temperature after cold challenge [34] and visual observation. The pathophysiologic change has been noted to be mostly reversible through pharmacologic sympathetic blockade [35,36]. Localized atherosclerosis has been noted in chronically affected patients [37,38].

The circulatory effects of acute vibration vary from those of chronic vibration. Whereas acute vibration exposure with cold tends to increase blood flow and decrease resistance, with chronic vibration exposure, cold will reduce blood flow and increase resistance [39]. Using a vibrational tool for an average of 1–2 hours per day may be sufficient to produce symptoms of HAVS.

A history of the frequency of vibrational tool use is essential. Documentation of the tool type is important also. Smaller tools such as metal burring wheels are especially damaging and may induce clinical changes with even limited use.

In addition to the vascular and neurologic complications of vibration, a diffuse syndrome of upper-extremity pain and muscle fatigue occurs in people exposed to vibration. Frequencies in excess of 70 Hz essentially decouple the wrist from the upper arm. Upper-arm transmission occurs at lower frequencies as well and is capable of producing resonances in the shoulder and arm [40].

Several methods have successfully decreased the effects of vibration on workers [23]. These include wearing antivibration gloves, using coated tool handles, replacing power tool operations with automated ultrasound welding, using a collar, and decreasing the amount of grip required to operate equipment. Although decreasing vibration exposure is important, in severe cases it might be necessary to eliminate any exposure to vibration.

Mechanical Stress

Tools or work equipment can exert pressure on muscles, tendons, nerves, or blood vessels. Prolonged exposure to such pressure can increase the risk of CTDs in the workplace. Tool usage is perhaps the most common culprit producing mechanical stress on body tissues. A very important way to reduce pressure is to ensure that the tools are appropriate for the task *and* fit the worker [41].

Tools should be designed for use with either hand. Use of right-handed tools by left-handed persons will put that 10% of the population at risk for CTDs. Orientation of the body to the work fixture will differ by as much as 140 degrees for a right-handed as compared to a left-handed individual.

If pathologic changes in the hand and wrist are to be avoided, weight, ease of operation, shock absorption, size, shape, texture, positioning, and purpose all must be taken into consideration when a tool is being designed [19]. In general, the lighter the tool, the less the hand becomes fatigued. Tools for women generally should be lighter than those for men, although this depends on the individual worker. The type of grip required may be more important than the weight of the tool. Oval handles usually fit a worker's hand better than do round handles. Handles should be designed for a power grip rather than a pincer grip. As stated previously, a pincer grip can produce up to fivefold greater positional stress than a power grip. The tool should be easy to operate. Spring loading will tend to minimize energy expenditure. However, a problem retaining the tool in the hand can be created by spring-loaded tools, by forcing the fingers of a small-handed worker toward full extension; this must be avoided.

Tools should be well within reach of the worker, so that he or she does not need to strain to acquire a tool. Overhead reaching is especially detrimental over prolonged periods.

Padding the tool for shock absorption is essential for reducing the risk of CTDs. Wos et al. [42] studied the effects of a bolt-gun support stand on impact loading of the hand-arm system while firing spiked bolts into a steel beam. The peak values of acceleration decreased more than eightfold during firing with the bolt-gun support. The shock-absorbing effect was noted at the thumb (metacarpal level) and the elbow. These investigators reported that the support stand improved working posture and helped to relieve the hand-arm system by distributing some of the shock to the legs, thereby permitting the legs to function as shock absorbers. The larger hip and knee joints are more stress-resistant than is the shoulder joint, and so, in most cases, it is beneficial to transfer some of the stress from the hand-arm system to the lower extremity. However, the worker must remember to maintain the legs in a slightly bent position if he or she is to maximize use of the legs for shock absorption.

The size of the tool is also important and, again, should be individualized for the worker. A tool that is too large for a hand requires that increased energy be expended to hold the tool, which can be a mechanism for intrinsic muscle strain. Because a partially stretched muscle contracts more forcefully than when it is unstretched at the time of activation [43], it is important that the tool fit the worker in such a way that the small joints of the hand are held in midflexion.

The shape of tools is also extremely important. Hand-held tools should fit the curve of the transverse palmar arch, thereby permitting an even application of force during instrumentation. The thenar and hypothenar eminences should be used on the proximal sides of any handles to prevent compression of the intrinsic neurovascular structures. Wrist flexors and extensors should be balanced whenever possible, and ulnar deviation should be avoided.

Texture, too, is important. A smooth finish sometimes increases the energy expenditure required for tool retention, whereas an overly coarse texture can lead to skin irritation, discomfort, and diminished efficiency. The texture should be adequate to allow the proper amount of friction between the tool handle and the skin surface. Various factors (e.g., environmental temperature, skin temperature, or individual physiology) may alter the amount of friction present [19].

Proper maintenance of tools is essential and may help decrease the risk of CTDs. This is especially true in such industries as meat packing (e.g., a dull knife usually requires increased force). In general, poorly maintained tools will require either increased force or poor biomechanical positioning on the part of the worker.

Positioning of the tool can affect the development of CTDs. Using a tool with the wrist acutely palmar flexed for prolonged periods can contribute to the development of CTS. de Quervain's disease can be caused by extreme ulnar deviation of the wrist during tool use or by excessive pinching, lateral striking of the thumb, or direct pressure on the tendons [19]. The hand and tool should be considered as a unit in task performance. Tools should be used only for the purpose for which they were devised. Educating workers in the proper use of tools and proper positioning during their use has been shown to help reduce the risk of CTDs [44].

Emotional Stress

Many studies relate high levels of work stress to CTDs in the upper extremities [15,45–49]. The stressors may include lack of control over the job, isolation, and decreased task diversity. In a study by Westgaard et al. [50], psychosocial problems at work were a risk factor for complaints in the shoulder and neck region. Work-related risk factors associated with symptoms of musculoskeletal complaints were correlated with psychosocial stress, either professional or personal. In a work by Bernard et al. [51], the most important predictors of CTDs were lack of social support and job variance.

One study of video display terminals (VDTs) [52] showed a highly significant association between occupational stress levels and some physical complaints. The presence of these associations has been interpreted as an indication that management of both physical and stress complaints should be tackled simultaneously.

In addition to job-related stress, frequently a CTD sufferer also experiences the stress of having to prove that his or her physical complaint is real. The symptoms of CTDs are often vague. In addition, many CTD sufferers are women, and the general notion that women tend to exaggerate or are emotionally labile diminishes their credibility. Reid et al. [53] suggested that the need to be believed and to establish his or her integrity dominates the plight of the worker who suffers from CTDs. These authors theorized that the chronicity of CTDs is connected to the failure of the predominant explanations of CTD to accommodate the psychosocial and political dimensions of the illness.

Temperature

Decreased temperatures can affect a worker's coordination as well as his or her manual dexterity. These effects could lead to a need for increased effort and additional manual force to perform the same task, or to maintain productivity levels. Hot or humid conditions also can affect a worker by causing excessive fatigue or decreased work capacity. Abnormal temperatures, whether hot or cold, can increase the ergonomic stress to which an individual is subjected.

Assessment of the Injured Worker

The worker with a possible CTD presents a potential challenge to the health care provider. Although the history and physical findings are often similar among CTD sufferers and patients with musculoskeletal maladies, attention must be paid to specific factors related to CTDs. Perhaps the most important fact that the health care provider must remember when evaluating the worker is that each worker is unique. Factors such as height, weight, medical history, previous injuries, social situation, strength, endurance, age, gender, and especially motivation must be assessed.

Most occupational tasks affect more than one joint, muscle, or tendon. Therefore, CTDs often occur in several body parts simultaneously [54]. The physician must not undertake a physical examination that concentrates solely on the area of pain. As with any other physical assessment, the structures proximal and distal to the area involved must be carefully examined.

A thorough history is part of any good clinical examination, and the evaluation of the injured worker is no exception. Only those aspects of the history specific to an evaluation for CTDs are addressed here. It is assumed that the health care provider will also obtain a thorough general history.

History of Previous Injury

A history of any previous injury should be documented. Some pre-existing conditions will enable the worker to be eligible for state aid (depending on the state). In addition, whether the patient is eligible for workers' compensation benefits may depend on a history of previous injury. An accurate assessment of the patient includes diagnosis, treatment, names and specialties of previous providers of treatment, previous medications and responses to these medications, diagnostic tests performed, any operations performed, and any physical or occupational therapy undergone (including modalities and treatment responses).

Other Medical Conditions

Certain systemic diseases, including rheumatoid arthritis, acromegaly, gout, diabetes, Paget's disease, myxedema, systemic lupus erythematosus, neoplasms, amyloidosis, scleroderma, and thyroid disease, may predispose a worker to CTDs. In female patients, pregnancy, use of oral contraceptives, menopause, and gynecologic surgery may affect the development of CTDs.

The employee's physical status must be considered in the evaluation of a worker with a CTD. In an article by Alund et al. [55], steel-industry transverse crane operators on long-term sick leave were analyzed in terms of case history, physical status, and active neck motion. In comparison with a reference group, the sick-listed crane operators had shorter necks. The authors noted that the somewhat shorter neck stature could be due to increased muscular tenseness. Although it usually is not possible to change the physical traits of a worker, it is possible to train or condition a worker effectively so that injuries can be minimized.

A thorough history must be obtained to assess for factors that might compound the diagnosis of CTD injury or might limit the patient's work capacity. Such factors might include poor cardiovascular fitness, congenital disorders, and chronic obstructive pulmonary disease.

History of Substance Abuse

It is important to obtain an accurate history of substance abuse in the injured worker. This includes use and abuse of prescription medications.

Psychosocial Issues

It is incumbent on the health care provider to note the social situation of the patient, including any support systems. In chronic cases of CTD, support systems may prove vital. Although sometimes difficult to obtain, information regarding the financial status of the injured worker, as well as financial incentives to continue in a disability status at work, should be sought, as these considerations may factor into the patient's motivation to comply with treatment plans. Perceptions of the patient's work ethic and feelings about returning to work should also be elicited.

There often is an adversarial relationship between the employer and the employee. An adversarial relationship may also exist between the health care provider who controls most of the decisions about return to work, continuation of sick leave, or designation of light duties, and the employee. Assessments by an insurance specialist are usually the most threatening for the worker. These consultations can elicit anxiety and fears about future financial security from the worker.

Job organization and psychosocial variables were found to be predictors of CTDs of the hand and wrist in departments composed of a large number of clerical and data-entry operators [51]. It is interesting to note that there were no psychosocial predictors of CTDs in an editorial department consisting of jobs that Bernard et al. [51] assumed were characterized by higher decision-making responsibilities, more latitude, and varied job tasks, despite a high work load.

Psychological Assessment and Testing

Psychological assessment and testing of the injured worker can contribute significantly to an evaluation, especially if the response to treatment is less than expected, if there is a suspicion of depression, or if the pain has been ongoing for more than 6 months (i.e., chronic pain). The visual analog scale can provide a nonverbal evaluation of a patient's perceived pain level and is relatively easy to use. A rating higher than seven on a visual analog scale in the setting of chronic pain can be predictive of a long-term disability [56].

Other psychological tests that may help in assessing the patient suffering from CTDs include the McGill Pain Questionnaire, behavior questionnaire, Word Descriptor Scale for Pain, Multidimensional Pain Inventory, profile of mood states, multidimensional health focus of control, and the Minnesota Multiphasic Personality Inventory (MMPI). Bird and Hill [57] suggest that a finding

of early loss of grip strength, as measured by a sphygmomanometer cuff, that improves with rest can be valuable in excluding compensation neurosis from the differential diagnosis.

Bigos et al. [58], in a retrospective evaluation, found that the strongest predictor of acute back-injury claims and chronic disability was an unsatisfactory employee appraisal rating by a supervisor within the 6 months prior to a back-injury claim. In a prospective study on work perceptions and psychosocial factors affecting the reporting of back injury, Bigos et al. [59] found that other than a previous history of back pain, factors most predictive of subsequent injury reports were work perceptions and certain psychosocial responses on the MMPI. Patients who stated that they "hardly ever" enjoyed their job tasks were two and a half times more likely to report a back injury. Obviously, the need to evaluate the worker in the context of the work environment cannot be overlooked.

Psychiatric Model of Cumulative Trauma Disorder Occurrence

One review of perspectives on the occurrence of CTDs included a psychiatric model [43], in which it was suggested that sufferers experience pain in the absence of organic disease. This report theorized that workers are afflicted with a conversion or somatization disorder. However, most of the literature refutes this theory and instead suggests that psychological issues arise as a result of CTDs [53,60] or can modify the severity of CTDs [61].

Psychological Issues: Precursor or Outcome of Cumulative Trauma Disorders?

It has been debated in the literature whether the psychological issues predate or are a result of a given injury. In a study by Helliwell et al. [61], subjects who expressed widespread somatic symptoms also reported experiencing more pain that they attributed to their jobs. Scores for anxiety, depression, and the Bradford Somatic Inventory (an inventory of somatic symptoms associated with anxiety and depression) were highly correlated. The investigators were unable to distinguish whether the subjects with pain had higher scores for psychological variables because they had pain or whether the psychological traits predisposed the subjects to symptoms.

A study by Helme et al. [60] provides objective evidence that patients with chronic CTDs have altered nociceptive mechanisms. The capsaicin-induced flare response, which has been noted to be diminished over a site of clinical pain, was reduced in patients with CTDs. The authors believed that this was consistent with the view that CTDs involved somatic pathophysiology. Psychological tests given to these patients revealed a denial of the presence of psychosocial pressures and low scores on hypochondriasis or phobic somatic assessment.

Psychosocial Issues and Chronic Illness

It has been suggested that the current concepts concerning CTDs fail to address the psychosocial and political concerns of workers with CTDs, contributing to the chronicity of the illness [53]. Many undertreated or untreated patients with CTDs eventually develop chronic pain syndromes. Associated anxiety and depression may be related to disruption of employment, financial difficulties, disturbed family relationships, and legal matters, and do not necessarily precede the development of symptoms. Cognitive behavior therapy has been shown to be helpful in chronic cases [62]. As Spaans [63] eloquently points out, "[T]hat neurotic symptoms are found in people confronted with the impossibility of continuing their vocations is not surprising and does not signify that neurotic factors determine the nature of the handicap."

Recreational History

Because recreational activities may play a part in the genesis of symptoms [64], the health care provider should obtain a history of a worker's leisure activities.

If compensation is allowed for work-related CTDs but not for play-related CTDs, more injuries might be attributed to one's job. As discussed in previous chapters, many recreational activities can contribute to the development of CTDs, and often the factors responsible for CTD development are not clear. For example, a VDT operator who is an avid tennis player and who presents with elbow pain might as easily have incurred injury on the tennis court as in the workplace. It can sometimes be extremely difficult to determine the offending behavior but, when compensation issues are involved, the worker might focus on occupational factors and ignore recreational factors that might be causative or contributory.

Occupational History

Time Off From Work

The amount of time that an employee is out of work has been documented as the most significant factor contributing to delayed recovery [52]. If the injured worker has been off for 6 months, there is a 50% likelihood that the patient will return to work. After a year, the likelihood that the patient will return to work drops to 25% and, after 2 years, this number plummets to 5%.

The amount of time that a worker has been employed is also an important part of the history of any worker with CTDs. A study by Buckle [65] showed that workers who had been at their jobs longer suffered from musculoskeletal disorders of the upper extremities more frequently than did those who had not been at their jobs as long.

Job Satisfaction and Stressors

Evidence in the literature supports the contention that job satisfaction is inversely related to injury risk, time loss, and delayed recovery [52]. In a study by Muffly-Elsey and Flinn-Wagner [66], a relationship was discovered between workers with CTDs and reported stress at work. The majority of workers who described their jobs as stressful had CTD symptoms. In addition, the authors found that a high percentage of workers who described their jobs as stressful and had symptoms of CTDs engaged in no leisure activities.

Job Evaluation

It is important that the health care provider obtain an accurate description of the type of movements performed, positions maintained, and tools used in a particular occupation. It may be helpful to obtain this information both from the employee and from the employer, as there are often discrepancies. Particular attention should be paid to risk factors such as repetition, long-term heavy activity or force, static prolonged positioning, loading or holding, vibration, mechanical stresses, pressure from tools on body tissues, and cold. Also important is the patient's perception of the amount of heavy work involved as compared to the employer's perception.

The job description is important in assessing the impact of CTDs on the ability of the worker to carry out his or her job. In one study by Viikari-Juntura et al. [67], it was noted that the prevalence of clinical epicondylitis in people in the sausage-making industry did not differ between workers in strenuous and nonstrenuous jobs. Sick leave, however, was much more common among workers in the strenuous jobs. The authors concluded that the most probable reason is that a meat cutter, sausage maker, or packer with epicondylitis is more disabled in his or her work than is a supervisor.

A *handicap* is a perceived mental or physical disability that reflects societal bias as experienced by the individual trying to fulfill a role. The presence or absence of a handicap depends on both the job and the employer [68]. If an employer will not accommodate a particular worker's perceived disability, then the worker might be considered handicapped for that position.

Job Availability

The health care provider should determine whether the patient's position is being held while the patient is out of work and, if so, for how long. In addition, it is important to note whether light or modified duty is allowed by the employer. If no light duty is permitted, the health care provider might be inclined to use more aggressive methods to return the patient to work quickly. These factors can influence the motivation of a worker to comply with a treatment regimen or to continue to report symptoms.

Workplace Evaluation

It usually is extremely helpful to observe the workplace and specific job requirements of the injured worker. Video recordings or serial photography have been used to analyze individual workstations. There is no substitute for a visit to the work site by the health care provider to assess job demands and conditions as well as worker movements.

Physical Examination

Because of legal or economic factors, the health care provider evaluating a patient for a CTD might question the validity of a patient's complaints. It is important to try to differentiate physiologic from nonphysiologic pain behavior. An excellent indicator of nonphysiologic pain is the Waddell's score on physical examination [69,70]. The Waddell's score was designed to evaluate patients with low-back complaints. The signs it seeks to elicit include superficial or nonanatomic tenderness, pain with axial rotation in block, differential response to straight-leg raising in the seated versus supine positions, nonanatomic weakness, nonanatomic sensory loss, and over-reaction to examination. A positive response to any one of these six tests should be reported. Although a positive test does not necessarily signify symptom magnification, a positive score on four of the six tests should be cause for suspicion.

The physical examination should include inspection for signs of inflammation, deformities, or ganglion cysts. Palpation of the extremity is important to identify areas of discomfort, signs of inflammation, swelling, or bony abnormalities. Range of motion (ROM)—active, passive, and active assisted—must be accurately documented, and areas and ranges of discomfort should be described. The strength of each limb must be documented.

Use of the 0-to-5 scale for documenting strength is widely accepted. On this scale, a score of 5 documents full strength against resistance; 4 denotes ability to move against some resistance but not full resistance; 3 indicates the ability to move the joint against gravity but not resistance; 2 indicates the ability to move the joint only if gravity is eliminated (accomplished by moving the joint so its plane of rotation is parallel to the ground); 1 signifies no functional movement, although muscular twitching may be present; and 0 indicates no movement.

Reflexes must also be tested. Other maneuvers may include a Tinel's, Phalen's, or Finkelstein's test. The speed of movements as well as tenderness on palpation must be assessed. The physical examination should include an evaluation of the patient's gait; whether the patient is able to dress and undress independently should also be noted. A useful tool for assessing workers in whom malingering is suspected is an evaluation of the patient's gait and activities in the waiting room, on the way into the health care provider's office, and on the way out.

Questions to Be Asked

In all suspected work-related injuries, an attempt must be made to answer the following questions [8]:

1. Is this injury work related?
2. What is the type of injury?
3. What is the extent of the injury?
4. What is the percentage loss of function?
5. When can the patient return to work and at what capacity?
6. When can the patient return to the job at full capacity?
7. Is this person physically capable of performing his or her job?
8. Are there structural or physiologic factors that predispose this person to developing CTDs?
9. Are improper body mechanics involved in the way this person performs his or her job?
10. Are the physiologic demands of that job excessive for this patient?

Treatment and Prevention of Occupation-Related Cumulative Trauma Disorders

Treatment

Therapy for the injured worker must focus on rest, alleviation of pain, elimination of provocative stressors (both occupational and nonoccupational) [8], treatment of any underlying disorder, limitation of scar formation, stress management, relaxation, and the preservation of elasticity, contractility, and strength [71]. Work-site analysis, with the goal of reducing the impact of any suspected precipitant, is helpful. Modification of the work site and alternative job placements [72], education, and ergonomic intervention are primary concerns. Preventive techniques, including stretching and exercise breaks, job rotation, task

rotation, work modification, early intervention, and early treatment should be included in any treatment program.

The most important aspect of CTD treatment is elimination of provocative stressors, which might necessitate modifying the workstation, the job description (i.e., light duty), or the work pace. Whether light duty is beneficial is the subject of controversy. Some argue that light duty encourages workers to report a disability because they may continue to work at an easier job, while others (including this author) believe that any modification that allows a worker to continue to perform a socially or economically useful function is beneficial.

Rest followed by reconditioning is the mainstay of treatment of CTDs. Splints are frequently used to rest an extremity. Although splints and braces can allow for repair of injured structures by resting the injured area, the practitioner must be careful not to divert the stress and strains to other parts of the body, such as the neck and shoulders [20]. In addition, prolonged splinting may lead to decreased ROM and, possibly, increased muscular strain.

Alleviation of Pain

Alleviation of pain is an essential component in the treatment of CTDs. Patients with mild symptoms may be treated with acetaminophen or over-the-counter nonsteroidal anti-inflammatory drugs (NSAIDs). In more severe cases, patients may require prescription medications (see Chapter 5). Therapy for patients with CTDs who go on to develop chronic pain syndromes is more complicated.

Treatment of the underlying disorder will depend on the specific condition involved. All CTDs cannot be treated by the same regimen. However, most disorders, if discovered early enough, will respond to rest, anti-inflammatory medications, and physical modalities. Occasionally, injection therapy is needed. Rarely is surgery indicated in CTD cases; in resistant cases, surgery should be considered.

Limiting scar formation and preserving elasticity, contractility, and strength are important aspects of any treatment program. Physical therapy usually helps in this regard, and should include stretching, ROM, and strengthening activities. Superficial heat prior to initiating therapy and icing after activity are also recommended for nonacute injuries.

Stress management and relaxation techniques may play a part in the treatment of CTDs if the health care provider believes that stress is a contributing factor. Stress may predispose the worker to, or might be a consequence of, CTDs.

Modification of the work site is a critical component of any treatment plan. The work site must accommodate the worker; it should not be designed merely for an average worker. There must be enough room to permit the employee to accomplish his or her task. For example, a secretarial worker should be able to turn in his or her chair (a chair on wheels is preferable) instead of straining to reach or see something. There should be ample leg room for the employee to sit comfortably while permitting frequent changes in position. Adequate space to allow the worker to stand and move about periodically also helps to reduce the incidence of CTDs.

Injections

Because injections are a treatment option in many of the disorders associated with CTDs, it is appropriate to discuss indications and contraindications at this time. It should be understood that injections (usually of a mixture of lidocaine and steroid preparation) treat only the initial inflammatory symptoms of any underlying injury. A proper therapeutic program must be initiated in conjunction with an injection. Controversies remain regarding the ability of corticosteroids to promote healing of damaged tissue. Response to injection is greater the earlier this modality is initiated in the treatment program. Chronic pain patients do not respond as well as acutely injured workers. At the chronic stage, the inflammatory reaction plays only a minor role in the pain mechanism.

An injection should be attempted only if there is discreet evidence of a tendon, bursal, or tenosynovial problem. Up to three injections per year may be given in any one area. These should be spaced several weeks apart. Relative rest of the involved extremity (to avoid the possibility of tendon rupture) should occur for the first week after injection. Passive ROM should be encouraged to increase mobility.

Injections should never be performed if there is evidence of acute trauma or infection. The tendon sheath, not the tendon itself, should be injected.

Injection immediately before competition is contraindicated [73].

The choice of anesthetic has been argued by many. One study suggests that long-acting bupivacaine has a better effect with overuse sports injuries than does a short-acting anesthetic (e.g., lidocaine) in local injections [74]. As with other treatment modalities, the success of an injection usually depends on the experience and skill of the physician administering treatment.

Education

Education can be considered both in the prevention and treatment of CTDs. In informing employees about the ergonomic hazards to which they might be exposed, workers will be better able to participate in both a prevention and a treatment program.

In one study of the effects of education on hand use among industrial workers in repetitive jobs [44], either handouts alone as an educational tool (group 1) or handouts in conjunction with hands-on demonstrations of the concepts in the handouts (group 2) were significantly effective (compared to a control group) in reducing the number of at-risk movements after only 1 week ($p = 0.02$ for group 1; $p = 0.04$ for group 2). No significant difference was found between the two study groups. It appears that a low-cost means of educating workers (i.e., a handout) can be effective in helping to decrease the incidence of CTDs.

Prevention

Prevention of CTDs involves a holistic approach and requires that the health care provider be able to assess the body as a whole, the individual worker, and multiple risk factors [75]. The practitioner must remember that no joint moves independently and that any change propagated by the action of one joint will affect most of the joints in that extremity.

Pre-Employment and Post-Hiring Testing

There is speculation that pre-employment testing can help prevent CTDs. Such testing might include physical examination, x-rays, or psychological inventories. However, these tests often cannot predict the subsequent development of CTDs, and their use may expose an employer to discrimination suits [21]. A more suitable solution is to provide on-the-job training, rotation of workers and workstations, use of correct ergonomic principles, and employee as well as employer education. Pre-employment testing of maximum isometric lifting capacity and a careful history to determine the presence of pre-existing or predisposing conditions might be useful. Assessment of a potential worker's ability to perform job-specific functions does not violate the Americans with Disabilities Act. An employer may require a post-hiring examination (with employment contingent on the results of the examination) only if the following conditions exist [68]: (1) All entering employees are required to take the same examination, (2) confidentiality is established, and (3) acceptable performance is related to pertinent job functions.

Functional capacity evaluations may help identify workers at risk for certain injuries due to physical limitations. Such evaluations cannot, however, predict the development of CTDs as a result of work conditions.

Job or Task Rotation

Job rotation is an effective means of preventing CTDs. It has also been found to be a positive motivating factor for employees, and productivity often is enhanced because overall fatigue is reduced [54]. Although additional cross-training is required, job rotation has been found to reduce body stressors significantly.

Task rotation is another method to help decrease the risk of CTDs. Heavy manual activities can be alternated with lighter activities. Alternating tasks that require sitting with tasks that require standing is also beneficial. Any change in task structure that increases cycle time will help decrease the risk of CTD.

Work-Site Modification

Work-site modification is often an effective way to prevent CTDs. The work site should be modified to decrease repetition, vibration, force, static loading, poor positioning, or poor body mechanics. Modifying tools, as described previously, is an important mechanism in prevention. Aids such as power assists, ergonomic chairs, proper seating, and redesign of workstations all are factors that can help prevent the incidence of CTDs. Moving the part to be manufactured closer to the worker can reduce extreme joint movements. It is possible to decrease work injuries by limiting the lifting required for repeated performed tasks to 30% below a worker's maximum isometric lifting capacity. For occasional lifting, the amount lifted should be less than 50% of a worker's maximum isometric lifting capacity [21].

Minimizing Repetitive Movement

Any job for which the cycle time is less than 30 seconds should be carefully evaluated. Automation or enlarging the worker's task to include other steps decreases the time spent on any one individual motion and can therefore help prevent CTDs.

Repetitive movements can be diminished by job rotation, task rotation, and work modification. The ergonomic placement of work site and tools within the work site might reduce the need for repetitive neck movements. Repetition involving bending, twisting, and lifting can sometimes be minimized by ergonomic design, attention to body mechanics, education, frequent rest or stretch breaks, use of back stabilizers, and job modifications [54].

Decreasing Force

The force that a worker is required to produce may be decreased by using proper tools, lowering the load to maintain an ergonomically advantageous position, and using mechanical assists. Educating the worker about proper biomechanics can be extremely helpful in decreasing force.

Modifying Static Loading, Body Positioning, and Biomechanics

Static loading, another risk factor for CTDs, can be prevented by proper training, rest breaks, task rotation, and lowering the force required for holding tools or equipment.

Postures that require the body to be maintained in a position other than neutral frequently lead to CTDs. Here, ergonomic design is extremely important. Proper positioning of the back and neck in the chair can make a tremendous difference.

The body position that a worker must maintain should be analyzed in an attempt to decrease the risk of CTDs. Workers are frequently required to work in an antigravity situation (with the arm elevated above 90 degrees). Lowering the work, raising the worker, and rotating tasks are methods that might avoid an antigravity situation. An ergonomic assessment of the task is extremely important to avoid deviation of physiologic structures from the neutral position. Adjustable workstations, worker education, and worker training are also effective measures.

Reducing Vibration

Vibration has also been implicated in the development of CTDs. Limiting the use of vibrating tools is obviously an important aspect of prevention. If this is not possible, use of a gel or other shock-absorbing materials as a cushion to absorb the impact of vibration can help. Vibration has been implicated in back disorders in truck drivers and others who must frequently ride in a surface vehicle. Suspension seats have proved helpful in such situations.

Rests or Breaks

Rests or breaks appropriately placed in the workday are probably the easiest and most effective way to prevent CTDs. Rests may mean physical time away from the job, a change in the type of work, or a change in work pace. Equally important is a break-in period for new workers or workers who are returning after an injury. Workers should gradually be introduced to the normal work pace. To rush this process is to put the worker at risk for developing or redeveloping a CTD.

Stretching

Stretching exercises performed two to three times daily have been suggested as a means of preventing CTDs in asymptomatic employees [75]. However, a controlled study by Silverstein et al. [76] found these stretching programs ineffective. Whether or not the stretching is effective, it affords the benefit of an enforced work break.

Stretching for CTS has been suggested [54] and includes wrist and finger extension, forearm pronation, overhead elbow stretches, and elbow retraction [77]. Again, the efficacy of stretching has yet to be proved.

Education

Education is perhaps the most important aspect of prevention. It is essential that employees, supervisors, and management personnel be educated about the causes, early signs, symptoms, and prevention of CTDs. A program in which all personnel are working toward the same goal is much more likely to succeed than one in which the participants are at odds with one another.

Role of the Health Care Provider in Treatment and Prevention

Many factors—including the variability of workers' compensation laws and practices, disincentives to return to work, confusion regarding treatment options, harassment of the injured worker, social and financial secondary gains, and administrative blockade to efficient management—complicate the treatment of CTDs [17].

The health care provider must become astute in areas other than the diagnosis and treatment of physical conditions. His or her role in treating CTDs often involves a continuum of care and may include (1) pre-employment examination, (2) post-injury assessment and treatment, (3) recovery assessment, (4) impairment rating, (5) Social Security disability evaluation, (6) independent medical evaluation, (7) compliance with regulations of the Americans with Disabilities Act, (8) prevention of CTDs, and (9) control of the return-to-work agenda [68,78].

The health care provider should be properly trained and available to the employees within a reasonable time frame. It is important that the health care provider be a part of the ergonomics team and be knowledgeable in the prevention, early recognition, evaluation, treatment, and rehabilitation of CTDs. Knowledge of the principles of ergonomics, physical assessment of the employees, and OSHA record-keeping requirements is also essential. The health care provider should conduct periodic walk-throughs of the workplace, if possible, to identify potential light-duty jobs, maintain contact with employees, and understand work practices. It is important to maintain a list of jobs with lower ergonomic risks so that he or she can recommend assignment for light or modified duty. The health care provider should try to identify jobs that are associated with an excessively high rate of CTDs and institute programs for CTD prevention.

The health care provider should obtain a baseline health assessment of each employee, to be used as a comparison in the event that a CTD develops. The health care provider should also set up a conditioning period for new employees and employees who have been on leave. The usual recommended break-in period is 4–6 weeks. It is helpful to perform follow-up assessments after the break-in period to determine whether the conditioning has been successful.

Employees should be encouraged to report any symptoms of CTDs to the health care provider as early as possible. Early in the course of a CTD, treatment, employee education, and any necessary ergonomic modifications are usually successful. Most importantly, objective measures of musculoskeletal outcomes must be developed, validated, and applied [79].

Common Cumulative Trauma Disorder Injuries

Many factors enter into whether an individual worker will develop a CTD and, if so, which physiologic structures will be involved. Some of the more common injuries that can occur as manifestations of a CTD are discussed in this section. It should be understood that these injuries frequently occur in individuals who are not at risk for CTDs. For example, it is not unusual for CTS to develop during pregnancy; this is usually attributable to increased fluid retention, which decreases the space available in the carpal tunnel. One should not assume that a diagnosis of one of these conditions is indicative of the presence of a CTD. A careful history may or may not reveal an underlying cause for the disorder.

Carpal Tunnel Syndrome

CTS results from compression of the median nerve in the carpal tunnel of the wrist. Other names commonly given to this syndrome include *writer's cramp* and *median neuritis*. Whereas most of the tendon sheaths as well as the ulnar and radial nerves usually pass through the wrist unimpeded, the median nerve and the finger flexor tendons must pass between the carpal bones and the transverse carpal ligament (Figure 6-2). A decrease in the size of the tunnel or swelling of the tendon sheath can lead to compression of the median nerve. In addition, wrist extension or flexion and ulnar or radial deviation can decrease the available space in the carpal tunnel.

Any activities that involve repetitive or prolonged wrist flexion, extension, or deviation can increase the risk of CTS. Such activities may be occupation or recreation related. The intracanal pressure increases 40- to 120-fold with wrist hyperflexion or extension [52]. Occupational factors that have been reported to contribute to CTS include force, repetition, awkward posture, vibration, and mechanical stress. Activities that might increase the risk of CTS include typing, keying, cashiering, knitting, sewing, polishing, sanding, packing, cooking, butchering, scrubbing, hammering, buffing, or grinding.

The symptoms of CTS include tingling or numbness in the distribution of the median nerve (Figure 6-3). In most individuals, the median nerve provides sensation to the first, second, third, and radial half of the fourth finger. Sensation is supplied to the palmar aspect of the hand as well as to the distal dorsal aspect of the corresponding digits. In the hand, the median nerve supplies the abductor pollicis brevis, opponens pollicis, flexor pollicis brevis (superficial head), and lumbricales I and II. Therefore, disorders involving the median nerve at the carpal tunnel usually lead to numbness in the sensory distribution and/or weakness of the thumb. The sensory alterations are much more commonly seen than are motor disturbances. Occasionally, the pain from CTS may radiate up the arm to the shoulder, and the patient may complain of a dull aching in the forearm.

The diagnosis is usually made clinically, with confirmation by electrodiagnostic testing. A history usually reveals tingling or numbness in the median distribution and, occasionally, weakness in the thumb. Wasting may be seen in the abductor pollicis brevis muscle. Tinel's, Phalen's, or the median compression test usually is positive. Tinel's test involves tapping over the median nerve at the wrist, which elicits reproduction of the symptoms. Phalen's test involves hyperflexion of the wrist for approximately a minute, thereby reproducing the symptoms. Occasionally, a reverse Phalen's test, in which hyperextension of the wrist leads to reproduction of the

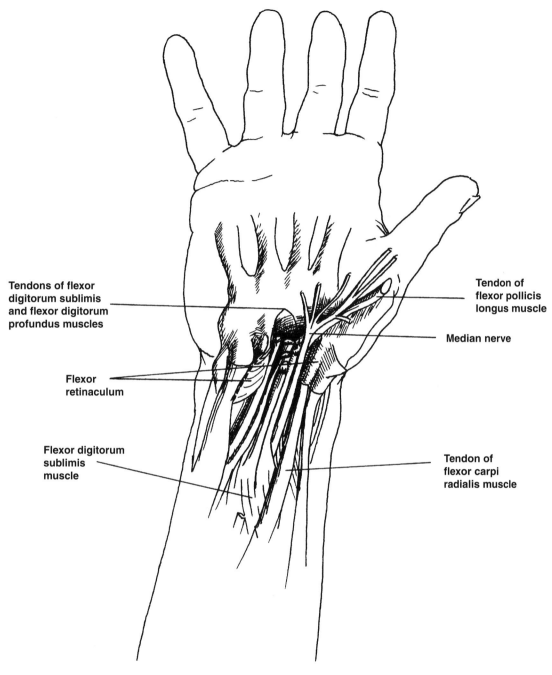

Figure 6-2. Anatomy of the carpal tunnel.

symptoms, is positive. Electrodiagnostic testing reveals slowing of the conduction velocity of the median nerve across the carpal tunnel.

Muffly-Elsey and Flinn-Wagner [66] contend that a diagnosis of CTS must be based on three or more of the following findings: (1) a positive Tinel's sign over the carpal tunnel, (2) a positive Phalen's sign for median nerve distribution, (3) a subjective report of morning swelling in the hands, (4) a reduced three-jaw chuck pinch as compared to

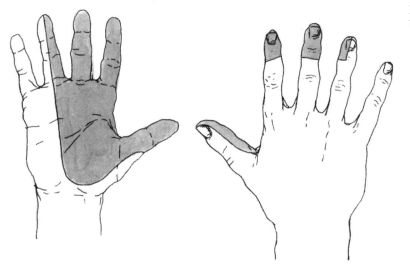

Figure 6-3. The sensory distribution of the median nerve.

published norms, (5) a square wrist dimension, and (6) elevated vibrometer readings as compared with the contralateral side in the median nerve distribution. Most authors consider electrodiagnostic testing the gold standard for diagnosis.

Prevention of CTS involves attempting to maintain the wrist in a neutral position and decreasing the amount of force if the wrist must be held in a flexed or extended position. Of course, it is also advantageous to decrease any predisposing factors that would lessen the available space in the carpal tunnel (e.g., reduce any swelling).

Interestingly, one study correlated systemic blood pressure with the functional response of nerve to local compression [80]. The authors studied the response of the median nerve to varied compression within the carpal tunnel and suggested that patients with either increased or reduced blood pressure might respond differently to a given level of mechanical compression of peripheral nerves. In patients with CTS, carpal tunnel pressures are elevated. These pressures are affected by wrist position and are perhaps modified, the authors suggest, by systemic factors.

Treatment of CTS is usually conservative unless the symptoms persist in interfering with the patient's occupation or activities of daily living or if evidence of denervation is noted on electrodiagnostic testing. Avoiding non-neutral wrist positions and repetitive wrist movement should be the first line of treatment. Splints, which maintain the wrist in a neutral position, can usually be worn at night

to help alleviate many of the symptoms. Injection of a combination of lidocaine and a steroid preparation into the carpal tunnel has been used successfully, but the effects are sometimes short lived. Physical therapy has also been used, though, again, the effects are usually short lived. Medications such as NSAIDs might provide relief. Treatment options include a short course of oral steroids. If increased swelling is believed to be contributing to the CTS, diuretics may be indicated, especially in women whose symptoms appear premenstrually. Surgery to release the carpal tunnel is usually successful, especially in the hands of a skilled surgeon.

de Quervain's Disease

de Quervain's disease is a name given to stenosing tenosynovitis of the first extensor compartment. This condition affects the tendons of the abductor pollicis longus and extensor pollicis brevis as they pass through the first extensor osteoligamentous compartments. The tendons of the thumb share a common sheath in this area. The patient will complain of pain over the radial styloid, which is usually aggravated by thumb motion. There may also be swelling and radiating pain into the thumb and forearm.

de Quervain's disease involves inflammation of the tenosynovium, the tissue that lines the tendon and provides a gliding surface at sites of friction. Either direct trauma or repetitive sheer forces can lead to

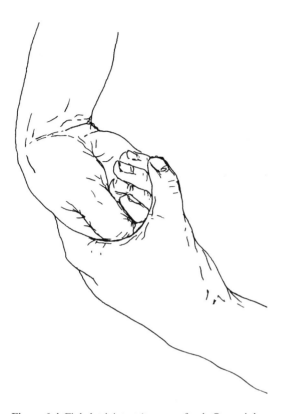

Figure 6-4. Finkelstein's test (to assess for de Quervain's disease). The affected wrist is forced into ulnar deviation with the thumb flexed and abducted. The test is positive if pain is elicited.

inflammation, pain, and swelling of the tenosynovium. The frictional component will increase as the tenosynovium thickens.

de Quervain's disease often results from forceful gripping and hand twisting. In addition, repetitive wrist extension with radial deviation may contribute to its development. Typical job activities that can contribute to the development of de Quervain's disease are sewing, cutting, butchering, grinding, polishing, sanding, buffing, and hammering.

The diagnosis of de Quervain's disease is usually made clinically by Finkelstein's test (Figure 6-4). In this test, the thumb is held to the palm and a fist is made over the thumb. The wrist is forced into ulnar deviation. If such a movement causes an exacerbation of the pain, the test is positive. Tenderness may also be found over the first extensor compartment. An x-ray is usually negative in de Quervain's disease, although it may be needed to rule out first

carpometacarpal joint osteoarthritis or an occult scaphoid fracture.

de Quervain's disease is usually managed conservatively. A thumb spica splint will provide rest for the tendon sheath, which may allow the inflammation to subside. Physical therapy, including ultrasonography, phonophoresis, and iontophoresis, has been used as treatment. Steroid injection into the sheaths is often successful. One must be cautious, however, to avoid injection into the radial nerve. The injection is a difficult one, as the tendon sheath is a very small area. A 62% long-term effectiveness rate has been reported with injection [81]. Surgery is used in recalcitrant cases. In one study by Witt et al. [81], of 30 wrists operated on for resistant de Quervain's tenosynovitis, 22 had a separate compartment for the extensor pollicis brevis.

Cubital Tunnel Syndrome

Cubital tunnel syndrome involves compression of the ulnar nerve at the medial aspect of the elbow. Symptoms include paresthesias in the fifth and ulnar aspect of the fourth digits. These may be accompanied by medial elbow pain or weakness of the ulnarly innervated hand muscles. The cubital tunnel syndrome is usually a result of activities that require flexion or extension of the elbow against resistance or activities that involve extended periods of resting the elbow on a hard surface (e.g., in hammering, carpet laying, or driving).

The diagnosis is made clinically by a combination of history, radiating pain, and presence of a Tinel's sign over the ulnar nerve at its entrance to the flexor fascia of the forearm. Nerve conduction studies are the definitive diagnostic test and will show a slowing of conduction velocity of the ulnar nerve across the elbow. A decrease in amplitude of more than 50% from the proximal to the distal segment is evidence of a conduction block. Evidence of denervation in the ulnarly innervated muscles portends an axonal lesion as opposed to a demyelinating lesion.

Treatment includes rest, elbow padding, and cessation of any exacerbating movements. Anti-inflammatory medications may be used, and local steroid injection may be beneficial. Surgery, usually involving transposition of the ulnar nerve, is used in cases resistant to conservative treatment.

Lateral Epicondylitis

Lateral epicondylitis, also known as *tennis elbow* (for its predilection among tennis players) affects 1–3% of the population. It is caused by repetitive mechanical overload of the tendinous origins of the extensor muscles on the lateral epicondyle of the humerus. Such overload results in reactive inflammation, which prompts the development of granulation tissue, usually within the tendinous origin of the extensor carpi radialis brevis muscle.

The symptoms include severe pain and tenderness over the lateral epicondyle, which is usually increased with resisted wrist extension. Passive wrist flexion may aggravate the symptoms. The patient may complain of a weakened hand grip. Usually, there is tenderness to palpation over the lateral epicondyle and a lack of tenderness near the radial head (where the posterior interosseous nerve penetrates the supinator muscle). According to Muffly-Elsey and Flinn-Wagner [66], the diagnosis of lateral epicondylitis should include the presence of three or more of the following symptoms: (1) pain with combined resistive wrist extension and elbow extension, (2) pain with combined resistive supination and elbow extension, (3) symptoms with resistive finger extension, and (4) point tenderness over the lateral epicondyle.

Although probably most well known for its occurrence among tennis players, lateral epicondylitis is also common among workers in occupational conditions that require unaccustomed forceful movements, wrist repetition, forceful grip, or repeated supination and pronation. Epicondylitis is an occupational hazard for politicians who must shake hands frequently. Other activities that can predispose to this disorder include hammering, small-parts assembly, screwing, woodworking, window cleaning, floor scrubbing, tree pruning, and yard raking.

Treatment for epicondylitis is usually conservative and includes rest, NSAIDs, and physical therapy. Splinting of the wrist in the neutral position is also beneficial. A strap worn just below the elbow (below the lateral epicondyle) may be used to help dissipate forces over a more distal area. Local corticosteroid injection has been used for cases unresponsive to more conservative methods. Such injections display a 48% long-term effectiveness [83], although there is debate about whether the relief provided is by the local anti-inflammatory

action or by acceleration of the microdegeneration of tendon fibers, which in turn reduces the tension. Epicondylitis may take months to resolve and frequently recurs. If conservative methods fail, surgery may be performed for debridement or release of the tendinous origins. Surgery is indicated in only 5–10% of refractory cases [83].

Prevention of lateral epicondylitis includes adequate rest periods and reduction of repetitive movements, especially wrist extension against resistance. Strengthening of the wrist extensors has been advocated once the initial symptoms have resolved.

In cases of resistant lateral epicondylitis, the diagnosis of posterior interosseous nerve entrapment should be entertained. The posterior interosseous nerve is a motor branch of the radial nerve that innervates the supinator, abductor pollicis longus, and all of the radially innervated forearm extensor muscles.

Medial Epicondylitis

Medial epicondylitis is similar to lateral epicondylitis, except that in the former the tendon irritation occurs over the medial epicondyle of the humerus where the wrist flexor muscles insert. The pain occurs over the medial epicondyle and is increased with resisted wrist flexion or pronation. This condition is also known as *golfer's elbow* because of its predilection among golfers. The treatment is similar to that discussed for lateral epicondylitis.

Ganglion Cyst

A ganglion cyst is a fluid-filled cavity that arises from a joint or tendon sheath. These cysts are usually found in the upper extremity along the digital flexor sheath, the dorsal capsule of the wrist, or the volar radial capsule of the wrist. However, ganglion cysts can arise from any joint or tendon sheath. It is suggested that repeated trauma may lead to a breakdown in the sheath's structure so that the normal lubricating fluid found within a tendon sheath or joint is released externally. The patient usually complains of a bump under the skin. The cyst might also produce discomfort and limit the ROM. Although many sources associate ganglion cysts with occupational overuse injuries [8,84,85], other authors [86] believe that ganglions are not caused by occupational activity but can worsen in people who perform repetitive movements. Movements that can increase the likelihood of developing a ganglion cyst include grinding, pressing, sawing, polishing, cutting, and pushing.

Treatment includes aspiration with or without injection of local steroids. Historically, treatment of ganglion cysts consisted of smashing with a heavy book; because a Bible was often used, these cysts came to be known as *Bible bumps.* Occasionally, taping may be useful. In recalcitrant cases in which the patient is in severe pain or the cyst limits mobility, surgery may be indicated.

Trigger Finger

Trigger finger is a type of tenosynovitis of the flexor tendons in the fingers or thumb. Constriction occurs within the fibrous annular pulleys such that movement of the tendon becomes restricted. Whereas normally movement of the finger is smooth, movement of a trigger finger exhibits snapping or jerking of the digit. There may be pain and tenderness over the involved area, and locking occurs in flexion. Trigger finger is seen in workers whose jobs require frequent grasping of hard objects (such as in the case of a machinist or a barber). It is also found in workers who must finger a trigger.

Occasionally, extension splinting of the affected finger at night will prevent painful flexion during sleep. Injection of local anesthetics and corticosteroids into the flexor tendon sheath usually provides some relief. Local corticosteroid injections have been reported to be effective in the long term in 90% of flexor tenosynovitis patients [87]. Of patients who responded positively for trigger finger, 61% received a single injection; 27% of those patients who received a second injection were reported to have had good results [87]. After any injection with corticosteroid, the patient should be advised to rest the joint to decrease the risk of tendon rupture. Activity should be modified for 3–4 weeks. Occasionally, surgical release of the fibrous annular pulleys of the finger or the flexor tendon is required. Some have advocated padding the palmar aspect of the hand in patients at risk for developing trigger finger.

Thoracic Outlet Syndrome

TOS is a vague entity that has been used to classify a number of varied complaints. TOS is alternately referred to as *neurovascular compression syndrome, cervicobrachial disorder, brachial plexus neuritis, costoclavicular syndrome,* and *hyperabduction syndrome.* True TOS is considered to be compression of the brachial plexus by an anatomically abnormal structure. Its incidence has been estimated by Cuetter and Bartoszek [88] to be one in 1 million. True TOS may result from compression of the brachial plexus and the brachial artery between the clavicle and first and second ribs by the pectoralis minor muscle or a hypertrophic anterior scalene muscle. Compression of the neurovascular bundle results in numbness, ischemia, and pain in the distal upper extremity. An increase in pain and a diminution of the radial pulse may be noted with hyperextension and retraction of the shoulder (Adson's maneuver) or by the abduction external rotation test, in which, with the shoulder in 90-degree abduction and externally rotated and the elbow flexed, the hand is opened and closed every other second for 3 minutes.

There is debate about whether this condition can be considered a CTD because it is usually considered an anatomic abnormality [86]. Some authors note that occupations that require frequent reaching above the shoulder level, prolonged carrying of heavy loads at the side of the body, the wearing of straps around the shoulder, or carrying of heavy loads with the arms extended may contribute to this condition [85,89]. Activities that have been purported to increase the incidence of TOS include buffing, grinding, overhead assembly, cashiering, automobile repair, sanding, typing, keying, stacking, work done by operating room personnel, truck driving, and letter carrying.

Before a definitive diagnosis of TOS is made, electrodiagnostic testing should be performed to confirm nerve involvement at the brachial plexus level. Such nerve involvement usually affects the lower trunk and leads to symptoms in an ulnar distribution. X-rays should be obtained to evaluate for a cervical rib or other anatomic abnormalities.

In patients with distal upper-extremity pain, it is important not to use TOS as a "wastebasket diagnosis," as the incidence is extremely low. True TOS

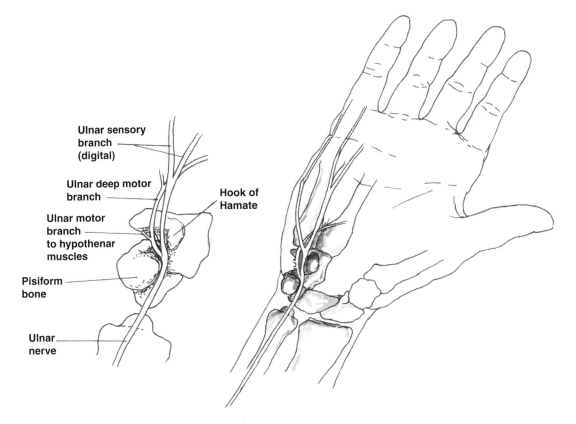

Figure 6-5. Anatomy of Guyon's canal.

has been treated conservatively, using physical therapy, diathermy, and transcutaneous electrical nerve stimulation. Often, avoidance of shoulder hyperextension will reduce the incidence of pain. In severe cases that are resistant to conservative methods, surgery might be required [90].

Ulnar Nerve Entrapment at Guyon's Tunnel

Guyon's tunnel syndrome (GTS) results from entrapment of the ulnar nerve as it passes within or distal to Guyon's canal in the wrist (Figure 6-5). Entrapment of the nerve can be caused by trauma, prolonged pressure, masses, anomalies, or inflammation. In the case of occupation-related GTS, prolonged flexion and extension of the wrist or repeated pressure on the hypothenar eminence of the palm could precipitate symptoms, which include paresthesias in an ulnar distribution and weakness of the ulnarly innervated

hand muscles. Diagnosis is made by electrodiagnostic testing, which may show slowing of ulnar nerve conduction across the wrist, loss of compound muscle action potential amplitude, and possibly denervation of the ulnarly innervated hand muscles.

GTS may be noted with prolonged bicycling, brick laying, hammering, carpentering, or playing of musical instruments. Treatment is usually conservative, involving avoidance of wrist flexion or extension. Splinting might be useful in certain cases. In cases that do not respond to conservative management, surgical exploration and decompression should be performed.

Reflex Sympathetic Dystrophy

Reflex sympathetic dystrophy can be caused by cumulative trauma. This entity is discussed in detail in Chapter 11.

Vibration White Finger

Vibration white finger (also referred to as *dead finger*, *Raynaud's phenomenon*, and *vibration syndrome*) is a condition that results from vasospasm of the digital arteries, which is usually triggered by vibration. The symptoms include decreased sensation and decreased control of finger movements. Blanching may occur, with the fingers turning cold and numb.

Vibration white-finger syndrome is seen frequently in workers whose occupations require the use of vibrating tools. There has been speculation as to the extent to which force influences the development of this syndrome. Because most vibrating power tools require high hand forces, it is difficult to separate which of the two effects—vibration or force—is the major contributor. However, the literature suggests that vibration is the etiologic agent [23]. Vibration affects both the neural and vascular elements in the hand. The resulting symptoms include vasospasm and a diffuse distal neuropathy.

Among the activities that can lead to the development of vibration white-finger syndrome are the use of such vibrating tools as chain saws, grinders, jackhammers, and sanders. Cold may exacerbate the condition.

Electrodiagnostic testing may reveal a diffuse distal neuropathy and is necessary to differentiate this condition from CTS. Treatment involves cessation of the activity that caused the disorder. Decreasing the force required to use vibrating tools has been advocated, as has been the use of padded gloves to decrease the transmission of the vibration [23].

Pronator Teres Syndrome

The pronator teres syndrome is a neuropathy resulting from compression of the median nerve in the proximal third of the forearm where it passes through the two heads (superficial and deep) of the pronator teres muscle. Pain, which usually worsens with activity, is noted in the proximal volar forearm. Paresthesias and dysesthesias occur in a median nerve distribution. There may also be weakness of median innervated muscles. Clinically, weakness of thumb and index finger flexion may be noted.

This condition is seen most commonly in workers whose occupations require strenuous pronation, flexion of the wrist and elbow, or repetitive rotation. It can occur in switchboard operators and bookbinders and in those who perform activities such as soldering, buffing, grinding, polishing, or sanding.

Diagnosis is made clinically and confirmed by electrodiagnostic studies. Electrodiagnostic testing will reveal a decrease in the amplitude of the median sensory action potentials on the affected side. Denervation might also be noted in median innervated muscles, usually with sparing of the pronator teres.

Conservative treatment involves the use of anti-inflammatory medications and splints for the elbow (to avoid excessive elbow flexion) and wrist (to avoid excessive pronation). Avoidance of exacerbating activities is especially beneficial. Surgical measures might be required and involve decompression of the median nerve in the proximal forearm, with release of anatomic structures that contribute to nerve entrapment (i.e., the fascia of the superficial and deep head of the pronator teres).

Anterior Interosseus Syndrome

The anterior interosseus syndrome is a compressive neuropathy of the anterior interosseus branch of the median nerve in the forearm (Figure 6-6). As this is purely a motor branch, sensory symptoms are absent. Patients usually complain of vague pain in the volar proximal forearm. The anterior interosseus nerve innervates the flexor digitorum profundus to digits 2 and 3, the flexor pollicis longus, and the pronator quadratus. As a result, patients might complain of decreased ability to approximate the thumb and index finger together with flexion of the distal interphalangeal joints (this is referred to also as the *OK sign*). When the patient is asked to make the OK sign (Figure 6-7), the patient will approximate the distal interphalangeal joints of the index finger and thumb instead of the pulp of the digits. Pain is usually exacerbated by repetitive strenuous activities and relieved with rest.

Diagnosis is made clinically and confirmed by electrodiagnostic testing. Nerve conduction studies are normal. Denervation may be found in the flexor digitorum profundus to digits 2 and 3, the flexor pollicis longus, and the pronator quadratus.

Management involves avoiding any activity that exacerbates the symptoms, resting the affected limb,

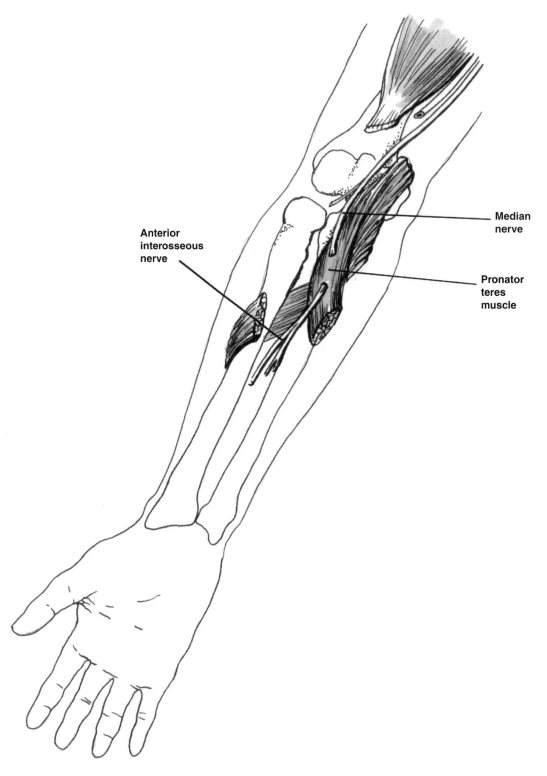

Figure 6-6. Anatomy of the anterior interosseus nerve.

and NSAIDs. Surgical exploration should be considered after 8–12 weeks if no improvement occurs.

Radial Tunnel Syndrome

Radial tunnel syndrome, also known as the *supinator syndrome*, is an entrapment neuropathy of the deep branch of the radial nerve (the posterior interosseus nerve). This entrapment occurs in the proximal forearm at the edge of the supinator muscle near the radial head (Figure 6-8). The patient presents with a deep, aching pain in the proximal forearm over the extensor muscles. The pain may radiate proximally along the lateral epicondyle or distally along the dorsal lateral aspect of the forearm. Motor weakness of the extensors of the wrist and fingers may be noted. There is, however, sparing of the extensor carpi radialis longus and brevis. If any of the fibers of the superficial sensory branch of the radial nerve are entrapped, paresthesias and dysesthesias in the radial distribution may be present.

This syndrome is seen frequently with repetitive wrist extension and forearm supination, especially with resisted movements. Radial tunnel syndrome may occur in assembly line workers or other workers whose jobs require repetitive motion.

This syndrome is frequently misdiagnosed as lateral epicondylitis. A careful examination will reveal tenderness within the extensor muscle mass in the proximal forearm in radial tunnel syndrome, whereas the tenderness is located over the lateral epicondyle in lateral epicondylitis. Electrodiagnostic testing may reveal a decrease in amplitude of the sensory nerve action potential of the radial nerve in the affected arm. Denervation in the radially innervated muscles of the posterior interosseus nerve may be seen if axonal damage is present. The radial nerve may be entrapped by one of several structures, including (1) the fibrous arcade of Frohse (the superior tendinous edge of the supinator muscle), (2) the fibrous origin of the extensor carpi radialis brevis, or (3) entrapment of the nerve between the muscular fibers of the supinator and the long axis of the radius. Symptoms are aggravated by resisted supination.

Treatment is directed at avoidance of any exacerbating activities as well as use of splinting and NSAIDs. Surgical decompression may be required in cases resistant to conservative management.

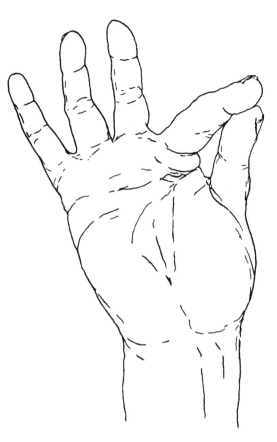

Figure 6-7. OK sign as a test for the anterior interosseus syndrome. Note weakness of flexion in the distal phalanx of the index finger and thumb.

Intersection Syndrome

The intersection syndrome, also known as *peritendinitis crepitans*, is characterized by pain, swelling, tenderness and, in some instances, crepitus in the region of the abductor pollicis longus and extensor pollicis brevis muscle bellies as they cross the radial wrist extensors (Figure 6-9). This occurs approximately 4–6 cm proximal to the wrist joint. It is unclear whether this syndrome is a result of friction produced by the abductor pollicis longus and extensor pollicis brevis muscle bellies rubbing on the radial wrist extensors or is a true tenosynovitis of the radial wrist extensors (extensor carpi radialis longus and extensor carpi radialis brevis). It has been suggested that this syndrome is a result of the development of an adventitious bursa [91] or an inflammatory peritendinitis [92]. It is seen frequently in workers

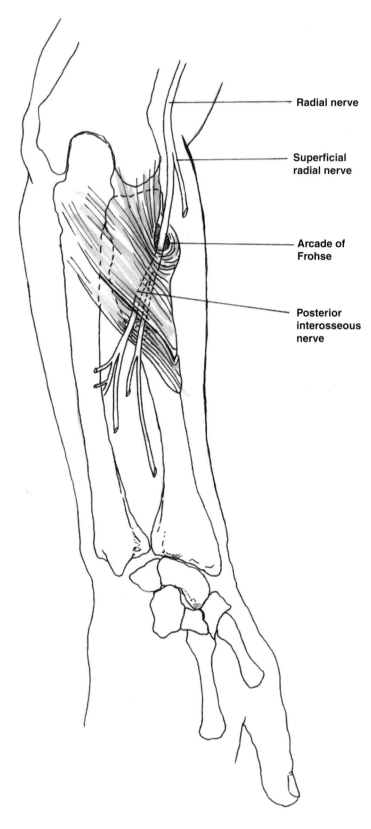

Figure 6-8. Radial and posterior interosseous nerves.

Radial nerve

Superficial radial nerve

Arcade of Frohse

Posterior interosseous nerve

Figure 6-9. Anatomy of the intersection syndrome.

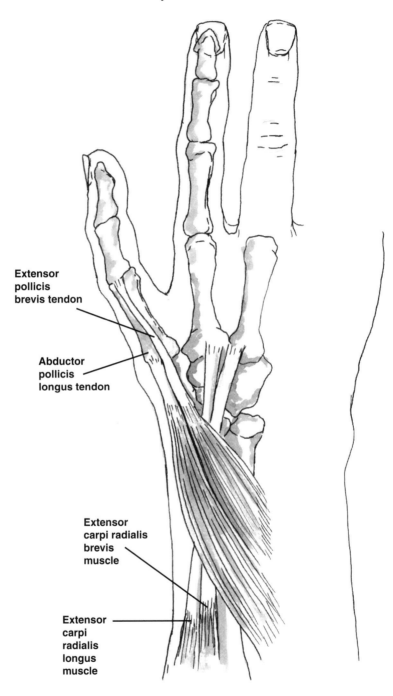

Extensor pollicis brevis tendon

Abductor pollicis longus tendon

Extensor carpi radialis brevis muscle

Extensor carpi radialis longus muscle

required to perform repetitive wrist extension against resistance—for example, painters, assembly-line workers, weight lifters, rowers, and canoeists.

The diagnosis is made clinically on the basis of pain, swelling, tenderness, or crepitation in the area of the abductor pollicis longus and extensor pollicis brevis muscle bellies as they cross the radial wrist extensors. de Quervain's disease must be ruled out as the symptoms may be similar.

Conservative treatment consists of modification of work activities to reduce repetitive wrist exten- sion, splinting of the wrist in 20 degrees of dorsi-

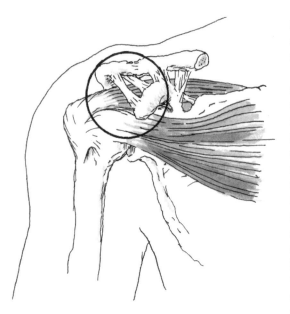

Figure 6-10. Area of impingement in the impingement syndrome. The tendons of the rotator cuff are compressed between the coracoacromial arch and the humeral head.

flexion, and administration of NSAIDs. Corticosteroid injections in the second extensor compartment have been beneficial. Cases that do not respond to conservative management may require surgical exploration of the intersection and decompression of the second dorsal compartment.

Tendinitis

Tendinitis refers to inflammation of the tendon and the tendon-muscle attachment. (Note that some authors refer to inflammation of the muscle-tendon junction and adjacent muscle tissues as *peritendinitis*.) The risk of hand and wrist tendinitis in patients who perform highly repetitive and forceful jobs is 29 times greater than in those who perform low-repetition and low-force jobs [4]. Some authors assert that there is a distinction between an overuse syndrome and a tendinitis or a tenosynovitis [93]. Stern [93] contends that the two conditions are differentiated histologically in that inflammation can be documented with tendinitis and tenosynovitis but not with overuse syndrome. It is the belief of this author, however, that overuse of an extremity can lead to a tendinitis or

tenosynovitis and, therefore, the differentiation is one of cause and effect rather than of two different entities.

The human body is capable of making extraordinary changes to adapt to various stressors. Muscles might undergo hypertrophy, alter contractile characteristics, or modify capillary density. The response of bone to stress is remodeling. The tendon units, however, are not as adaptable to changes in stress. Non-neutral positions might impair the mechanical advantage of the muscle tendon units and increase compressive forces at sites where tendons change direction [8]. Changes might be noted in the degree of cross-linkage, the amount of mucopolysaccharide content, or an increase in the cross-sectional area. However, when demands placed on a tendon exceed its adaptive limits, damage can occur. This may take the form of an acute traumatic injury (single supermaximal load) or repetitive microtrauma (frequent submaximal loads, as occur in CTDs), which might initiate a repair response in that tissue [17]. Repair occurs by noncontracting and inelastic scar formation, which decreases efficiency and increases the risk of future injury [72]. Injury can result in collagen damage, microvascular damage, and oxygen deprivation [94].

Whereas virtually any tendon in the body has the potential to become inflamed, certain tendons are more likely to become inflamed in cases of CTDs. Discussed here as examples are rotator cuff tendinitis and bicipital tendinitis. The diagnosis and treatment of other types of tendinitis can be extrapolated from these examples.

Rotator Cuff Tendinitis

Rotator cuff tendinitis has also been referred to as the *impingement syndrome* or *supraspinatus tendinitis*. The rotator cuff is composed of four muscles: the supraspinatus, infraspinatus, teres minor, and subscapularis. These muscles all originate from the scapula and insert onto the humerus. The supraspinatus, infraspinatus, and teres minor all insert on the greater tubercle, whereas the subscapularis inserts on the lesser tubercle (Figure 6-10).

The supraspinatus tendon in particular is at risk for impingement as it passes beneath the acromion. The tendon approximates the acromion with abduction of the arm from 70 to 100 degrees.

If the tendon is inflamed, movement within this range will produce the "painful arc" or impingement syndrome.

Supraspinatus tendinitis can occur among workers who maintain a position, under conditions of load, of shoulder abduction with the elbow extended. Persistent overhead work, buffing, welding, painting, riveting, construction work, grinding, polishing, sanding, or any job that requires constant elevation of the arm above 70 degrees increases the likelihood of occurrence of this disorder. Symptoms include pain at the shoulder that increases with abduction from 70 to 100 degrees. Frequently, a bursitis will precede, exacerbate, or result from a rotator cuff tendinitis. This is because the bursa acts as a cushion between the humerus and the acromion.

Diagnosis is usually made clinically on the basis of history and physical findings. An x-ray of the shoulder may reveal calcific deposits in the tendon. Magnetic resonance imaging usually identifies the lesion but is generally unnecessary and should be obtained only if the injury does not respond to conservative management. Treatment usually consists of rest. Physical therapies, including ultrasound, heat, and passive ROM exercises to prevent the development of frozen shoulder should be performed. NSAIDs are useful in patients for whom no contraindication exists. Local injections of corticosteroids are usually beneficial.

Bicipital Tendinitis

Bicipital tendinitis often occurs concurrently with rotator cuff tendinitis, or it may occur as a separate entity. The main complaint is usually pain in the area of the biceps tendon. Bicipital tendinitis is common among workers required to do overhead work, such as assembly workers, window washers, construction workers, and cleaners. Pain is usually elicited on resisted flexion of the elbow with supination of the forearm (Yergason's sign) (Figure 6-11) or resisted forward flexion of the shoulder with forearm supination and elbow extension (Speed's test) (Figure 6-12). Tenderness may also be noted on palpation of the biceps tendon as it passes over the bicipital groove and under the acromion. Management is similar to that of rotator cuff tendinitis.

Tension Myalgia

Tension myalgia, also referred to as *tension neck syndrome*, is a complex of symptoms including pain, tenderness, and stiffness in the neck muscles, which may be accompanied by headache. Spasm of the levator scapulae and trapezius muscle group is usually palpable. On physical examination, there is tenderness to palpation of the neck muscles, decreased ROM, and pain on ROM of the neck. Trigger points may be elicited. This condition results from static sustained muscle contraction and is common among secretaries, computer operators, cashiers, small-parts assemblers, and those whose work requires them to carry loads either in the hands or on the shoulders. It might also be seen after repeated or sustained overhead work, maintenance of a restricted posture with activities of the forearm, or bracing at the shoulder. Exacerbating conditions include awkward positions, prolonged positioning, and increased tension.

Treatment for tension myalgia is conservative and includes relaxation exercises, physical therapy, and local heat. A soft cervical collar may help to relieve symptoms temporarily. Stretching exercises are beneficial, especially if done consistently. Positioning is extremely important, and the author has found that a figure-eight harness to keep the shoulders retracted is usually effective. Relaxation and stress management techniques are also beneficial.

Types of Workers Commonly Affected with Cumulative Trauma Disorders

In this section, CTDs found in VDT operators, dental hygienists, sign-language interpreters, and workers in manufacturing industries are described. These four occupations can be viewed as models for evaluation of predisposing conditions contributing to CTDs. We study these four types of workers to understand the underlying factors that must be evaluated when treating a worker with a CTD. Several common stressors are characteristic of many occupations. These include repetition, forceful exertions, mechanical stressors, and posture. In any occupation, it is important to analyze the risk factors for CTDs, with the understanding that it is easier and less expensive to take preventive measures than to treat an established CTD.

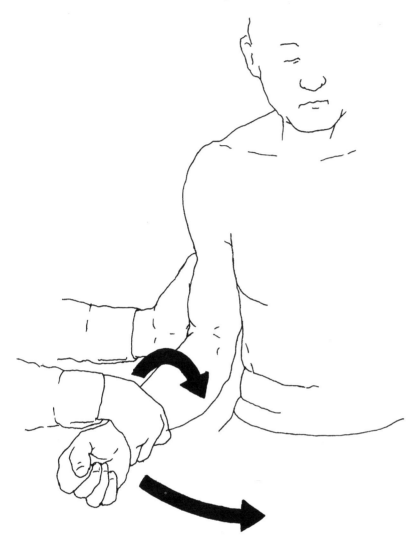

Figure 6-11. Yergason's sign for bicipital tendinitis. Pain is elicited in the area of the bicipital groove with resisted forearm supination.

Computer and Video Display Terminal Operators

Advances made possible through the use of computers have touched almost every industry in the United States today. More than 40 million people (approximately 40% of the work force) use a computer keyboard. The use of computers has allowed for technical breakthroughs of unimagined proportions. The downside has been a significant surge in the number of cumulative trauma injuries related to the use of VDTs. VDT operators have complained of headaches, neck problems, backaches, fatigue, moodiness, nausea, eye strain, burning and itching of the eyes, and a multitude of musculoskeletal pains and nerve entrapments.

The proliferation of high-speed computers has aided in the proliferation of CTDs such that CTDs now are tagged as "the industrial disease of the information age" [95]. The number of VDTs in the United States alone exceeds 70 million.

There is a plethora of literature linking computers and data entry with CTDs [96–98]. The equipment usually consists of a keyboard, a monitor, and a connection to the central processing unit of the computer. However, it is the interaction of the person with the machine that will determine whether musculoskeletal injuries occur. Most problems are short term and reversible. However, more serious problems develop if causes are not addressed.

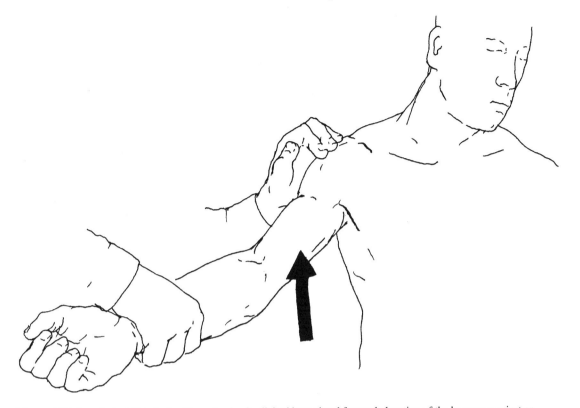

Figure 6-12. Speed's test. Pain in the biceps tendon is elicited by resisted forward elevation of the humerus against an extended elbow.

The World Health Organization [99] concluded that "musculoskeletal discomfort was commonplace during work with video display terminals" and that "injury from repeated stress is possible." The exact mechanism of injury and the best way to prevent injury have been intensely debated. Initial studies found a positive association between deviant work postures among keyboard or VDT operators and musculoskeletal signs and symptoms [100–103]. Subsequent studies, however, did not support these findings [104–108]. Various researchers have attempted to pinpoint solutions to the problem of CTDs in VDT workers [100,109,110]. Changes in both the worker and the workstation must be considered.

The statistics are convincing. *The New York Times* reported that 61% of 645 Associated Press News employees who took part in a survey said that they had neck and back pain. In another study, 17% of 2,100 *Los Angeles Times* employees complained of symptoms [111]. Considerable media attention

and litigation have ensued as a result of the high percentage of workers affected with CTDs.

It has been suggested that women are more susceptible to CTDs than are men. Pregnancy, use of oral contraceptives, menopause, and gynecologic surgery have been reported to contribute to the development of CTS. Because these conditions are unique to women, these factors may be responsible for the disproportionately high incidence of CTS in women [112]. Although it has been suggested that small wrist circumference also predisposed women to CTS, CTS has not been found to be related to wrist circumference [113]. There are at least two reasons that CTS is more likely to affect women than men: (1) More women are involved with typing and data-entry jobs, which carry a high incidence of CTDs, and (2) retention of fluids, as occurs during pregnancy or at certain times in the menstrual cycle, can increase the likelihood of CTDs.

One technologic advancement that may reduce significantly the incidence of CTDs in keyboard operators is the development of voice-recognition systems. Although this technology is not yet perfected, such systems could play an important role in the reduction of CTDs by reducing the amount of necessary keyboard work.

Repetitive Motion

As compared to traditional typewriters, computer keyboards have decreased the amount of energy exerted by the fingers of the operators. However, the number of activations per unit of time has increased. In many clerical jobs, tasks are defined by the number of keystrokes per hour. These can range from 8,000 to 15,000 or more keystrokes per hour, which translates to approximately two to five key hits per second. According to one author, a clerk who types 60 words per minute touches the keys 18,000 times per hour [77]. This equals 108,000 strokes in 6 hours. If the average keyboard typist uses 8 oz of force to depress each key, then the 60-words-per-minute typist presses 50,000 lbs (25 tons) through the fingertips in 1 day.

Repetitive motion puts the worker at risk for nerve entrapments (especially CTS), tendinitis, and muscular arm pain. CTS has been among the most widely reported nerve entrapments associated with CTDs. It is interesting to note that computer keyboards, which automatically scroll, actually increase the repetition factor. Typists used to have to stop keying in order to return to the next line. The fact that the typist working at a computer keyboard does not get that break may contribute to the increase in CTDs in the computer era.

Frequent rest breaks are an important component in preventing CTDs. It is recommended that VDT workers take at least a 10-minute break every hour. It should be noted that this means a break from keystroking. Another nonkeystroking job can be performed during this rest.

Hagberg and Sundelin [97] demonstrated that the introduction of 15-second pauses every 6 minutes gave a lower rating or perceived shoulder discomfort in VDT workers. Pauses of at least 2 seconds' duration resulted in decreased complaints of discomfort in the neck and shoulder [98]. A study by Waersted and Westgaard [16] suggested that frequent daily rotation between strenuous (repetitive) and less strenuous tasks only delayed the onset of musculoskeletal complaints in the neck

and shoulders. These authors suggested that reorganization of the work activities should be aimed at breaking up the muscular activity pattern over time.

Prolonged Sitting

An employee working at a VDT is frequently required to sit for prolonged periods performing a repetitive task. The job may require the worker to stay in the same position without moving for many hours. As noted earlier, frequent rest breaks are important in CTD prevention. Some software programs regularly remind the typist to stop typing and stretch. The prolonged static loading involved in VDT work subjects the individual to a variety of muscular disorders, especially fatigue.

Poor Posture

Fatigue and CTS often occur as a result of poor posture at the workstation. The individual might sit with shoulders hunched forward and neck flexed. Such individuals are at risk for neck and shoulder pain. These patients frequently suffer from myofascial pain syndrome. Pressure on the back increases almost 600% in the sitting position as compared to lying. Slouching increases the pressure by 740% [77].

Prevention depends on redesigning the workstation to fit the worker. Patients with myofascial pain frequently respond well to rest periods, physical therapy, and trigger-point injections. Although not yet described in the literature, the author has found that a figure-eight harness provides both a psychological and a physical reminder of good posturing.

Poor Positioning

A VDT worker is prone to CTDs secondary to poor positioning of the chair, the desk, the keyboard, the screen, or the manuscripts to be typed. The workstation is usually easily modifiable, although substantial expense may be incurred. However, the cost of a new desk or chair cannot be compared to the cost of even one workers' compensation claim. It is usually in the best interests of the employer to provide an adequate workstation, from both a financial and a personnel standpoint.

CTS may result from severe wrist flexion or extension that compromises the median nerve within the carpal tunnel. Users of VDTs may position the keyboard too high, thereby necessitating that they extend the wrist excessively, compromising the median nerve within the carpal tunnel. Ideally, the wrist should be held between neutral and 20 degrees of extension. Splints are frequently used to maintain the wrist in neutral during keystroking. However, it is much more advisable to redesign the workstation so that the wrist can be held in a neutral position.

Adjustability is probably the single most important feature of any desk or chair. If the worker is too high or too low relative to the desk and the keyboard, he or she is at risk for low-back pain, neck strain, peripheral nerve entrapments, tendinitis, myofascial pain, tenosynovitis, rotator cuff syndrome, and muscular strain. Each worker should be analyzed individually to assess height, leg length, arm length, and trunk length. The objectives of modifying the workstation are to minimize wrist flexion, wrist extension, and ulnar deviation; to avoid twisting or bending whenever possible; to maintain the keyboard below the elbow level and the neck and shoulders in a relaxed and neutral position; to keep the knees and hips flexed at 90 degrees; to maintain most objects (e.g., papers) within a 14- to 18-in. reach of the worker; and to position the screen where it can be seen comfortably, without twisting or turning the head (usually 20–28 in. away).

The chair is of utmost importance in preventing myofascial pain, including neck aches and backaches as well as maladies of the legs. Some type of lumbar support is recommended to accommodate lumbar lordosis. Here again, adjustability is important. The chair should be adjustable both vertically and from front to back. The feet should be able to rest flat on the floor with the legs perpendicular to the floor. The wrist and lower arms should be parallel to the floor. The chair should be padded to avoid uneven pressure on the buttocks. The average chair life span is 5 years. After this time, the chair becomes too soft to support the worker properly.

There has been a recent surge in the marketing of ergonomically designed products to assist in decreasing CTDs. These devices include wrist-support systems, modified keyboards, modifications in mouse pads, wrist pads, arm supports, forearm supports, workstations, chairs, footrests, and lumbar supports. Again, however, it must be emphasized that each worker should be analyzed for his or her particular job, work habits, and work risks. Before an employer spends a large amount of money, it is best to obtain a demonstration of the equipment and, if possible, to test the equipment for 1–2 weeks before buying it. The best equipment permits the worker to make adjustments throughout the day. Periodically, it may become necessary to modify the workstation to decrease the repetitiveness of motion.

The employer must be made aware that there are additional benefits of using proper equipment besides the obvious decrease in injury level (and, therefore, decreased workers' compensation payments). With the proper equipment, productivity and efficiency can also be increased. There are no scientific means by which to measure increased morale or the effect morale has on increased productivity.

Recommendations for Cumulative Trauma Disorder Prevention

In 1981, NIOSH [114] issued the following recommendations for VDT operators: a 15-minute rest break to be taken after 2 hours of continuous VDT work for operators under moderate visual demands or work load and a 15-minute rest break to be taken after 1 hour of continuous VDT work for operators under high visual demands or high work loads or for those engaged in repetitive work tasks.

In 1990, San Francisco enacted a law requiring workers who spend more than 50% of their time at VDTs be given a paid 15-minute break every 2 hours. Mandatory training sessions were regulated for employees who spent at least 20 hours per week at VDTs. In 1992, a California judge struck down the San Francisco law, stating that such measures should be regulated by the state. More and more states are now creating legislation to help decrease the incidence of CTDs [77].

Computers and VDTs have become an integral part of almost every industry. Currently, many people use computers daily; in the future, such interaction will be even more commonplace. Whereas computers have greatly increased the quality of life for many people, those who have suffered from CTDs associated with VDTs constitute a major exception.

Dental Hygienists

Many authors have evaluated why dental hygienists are at high risk for CTDs of the upper extremities [115–118]. Dental hygienists, as a rule, perform highly repetitive motions that frequently include an awkward posture, excessive force, mechanical stresses, vibration, and abnormally low temperatures. As such, they are subject to most of the risk factors for CTDs. MacDonald et al. [119] studied 2,400 California dental hygienists and noted statistically significant correlations between the incidence of CTS and the number of years practiced, number of days worked per week, and number of patients seen per day.

Repetitive Motion

A high degree of repetition is seen in hygienists' work. Repetition can be expressed as the number of exertions or movements per unit of time or as the length of time needed to complete a task or group of tasks (i.e., cycle time) [120]. Scaling and polishing activities both require a high degree of repetition. Dental hygienists can decrease the amount of repetition (and thereby decrease their risk of CTDs) by (1) using ultrasonic scalers, (2) interspersing non–hand-intensive activities (x-ray, patient care instructions, etc.) with hand-intensive activities, (3) allowing sufficient time to treat the patient and staggering the scheduling of patients who require hand-intensive motions, and (4) using very sharp instruments.

Poor Posture

Posture is another factor that puts a dental hygienist at occupational risk for CTDs. Frequently the hygienist is angled over the patient's mouth and the hygienist's elbows are elevated more than 30 degrees. The hygienist might hunch over the patient to improve his or her view of the mouth. This position is usually maintained for prolonged periods. Such positioning increases the risk of myofascial pain.

The force involved in such work places the hygienist at increased risk for CTDs. Smooth instrument handles tend to increase the amount of force that is needed. In addition, a constant pinching grasp is usually used. The element of force can be decreased by using minimum pressure in instrument grasp, selecting instrument handles that are serrated or textured, and using instruments of adequate weight.

Mechanical Factors

Mechanical forces factor into the development of CTDs as well. As in any other industry, evaluation of the tools that the hygienist uses in his or her daily routine is critical. Certain situations obviously increase the risk for CTDs. Ill-fitting gloves decrease manual dexterity and therefore require increased pressure. Larger-diameter rounded instrument handles avoid a pinching grasp and allow for a more equal distribution of forces throughout the hand and wrist. Electrically powered instruments whose cords are too short limit positioning and increase force in an awkward position. Retractable cords are perhaps one of the worst offenders, as they pull on the wrist while it is in a non-neutral position. Vibration might play a role in the development of CTDs in dental hygienists, depending on the type of tools used.

Temperature

As in other industries, temperature affects one's risk of developing a CTD. A cold environment can lead to decreased finger dexterity and decreased circulation in the digits. Hands should be washed in warm water with the goal of maintaining a temperature of 77°F in the distal phalanges. Instruments may be warmed before use. Temperature is particularly problematic with metal instruments, which tend to stay cooler.

Dental hygienists should be counseled to exercise their hands between patients. This serves both to warm up and to relax the muscles. Hand-exercising putty is especially beneficial as it is easily accessible and simple to use.

Recommendations for Cumulative Trauma Disorder Prevention

It is recommended that dental chairs be used that allow for the best possible access to the patient's mouth [121]. A good chair should have a comfortable seat that is adjustable. A footrest is advisable, as are armrests that can be adjusted; this will allow some elbow support when needed. A good chair also offers a backrest with up-and-down as well as forward-and-back adjustments.

It is recommended that the hygienist take rest breaks whenever possible, but especially if he or she is experiencing pain. Other suggestions include using the nondominant hand whenever possible, use of very sharp instruments, use of sonic and ultrasonic scalers, or changing to a less physically stressful procedure (e.g., patient education). Patient education is important, as is having the patient return more frequently for cleaning. This reduces the amount of forceful work required in patients who build up excessive calculus. Finally, dental hygienists should be aware of other causes of or factors that contribute to CTDs, including diabetes, rheumatoid arthritis, previous trauma, fluid retention, and pregnancy. Hobbies such as knitting, tennis, typing, or writing that put the patient at increased risk for repetitive forces of the hand and wrist should be avoided if symptoms of a CTD develop.

Sign-Language Interpreters

Sign-language interpretation is another field that has been investigated because of its high association with CTDs [122–124]. According to Podhorodecki and Spielholz [122], sign language is the fourth most common language in the United States. The types of CTDs encountered most often by sign-language interpreters include CTS, neuropathy, tendinitis, fasciitis, synovitis, and other nerve entrapments. Interestingly, deaf signers report that signing is less stressful, most likely because it was learned at an earlier age. This may imply a greater efficiency and more natural body mechanics for the deaf users, or it may reflect better-developed muscles that can better handle the stresses.

The common forces that increase the risk of CTDs—repetition, forceful exertions, and mechanical stress—come into play in sign-language interpreters as they do in other workers. Posture and vibration are not considered significant risk factors for sign-language interpreters.

Interpreters frequently complain of upper-extremity pain. This pain is believed to be more likely due to soft-tissue traumas attributable to repetitive use than to nerve entrapment. In one study, a higher proportion of nerve entrapments in sign-language inter-

preters compared to age-matched controls (i.e., non-signers) was not demonstrated [122]. It is believed that repetitive use of the hands may cause microtearing or friction that results in a local inflammatory reaction. In addition, fatigue with a local accumulation of metabolites has been suspected as a causative factor of pain after prolonged activity. Finally, pain could result from the abnormal positions that the signer is required to maintain for prolonged periods. Signing usually involves wrist dorsiflexion, ulnar deviation, and forearm pronation.

Although different methods of treatment have been tried, including NSAIDs, local steroid injections, splinting, bracing, icing, heat application, and physical therapy, the only treatment that appears to help consistently is rest. Studies involving interpreters for the deaf note that rest is the most effective way to relieve symptoms. An interpreter frequently has to perform his or her job for a prolonged period without rest. It was noted in one study that the average amount of time spent interpreting before the onset of symptoms was 1.8 hours [123]. Most patients experience symptoms within just less than 2 hours of signing. The study inferred that it is logical to take a break after signing continuously for 2 hours. It is also suggested that team interpreters be used. Job rotation is helpful. Progressive resistance exercises to increase both strength and endurance currently are being investigated to determine their effects. In addition, technique modification is being studied. Sebright [125] suggests that the wearing of gloves or restraints that limit movement but allow for adequate dexterity may be useful. Finger spelling, as opposed to the signing of entire words at one time, requires more speed and more finger movements and should be avoided whenever possible.

Manufacturing Industry Workers

CTDs have been studied in many of the major manufacturing industries, including meat processing [67,126], steel production [55], sewing (e.g., clothing manufacture) [16], chicken processing [65,66,127], automobile manufacture [128], manufactured housing production [129], painting [130], retail grocery sales [131,132], assembly-line work [18,44,133,134], chain sawing [22], manufacture of suture and wound-closure products [135], ski manufacture [136], and even baking [137]. The high incidence of CTDs in manufacturing industries is directly attributable to the major factors that predispose to CTDs: repetition, force, poor posture, and mechanical stressors.

Repetitive Motion

In some industries, pay based on piecework or a monitored number of completed cycles prompts workers to increase the amount of repetition. Increased automation has greatly enhanced the repetitiveness of most tasks. In many jobs, the worker is required to stand in one position and not move from the machinery as he or she is handed task after task to complete. Methods have been devised to help reduce job repetitiveness, some of which include worker rotation, more regular rest periods, enlargement of the job content to include a wider variety of motions, mechanical aids, automation, and a decreased work pace.

Excessive Force

More forceful and more frequent movements also put a worker at greater risk for CTDs. Work that requires prolonged or repeated exertion of more than approximately one-third of the worker's static muscular strength is an example of such forceful activity. Ergonomically designed tools might help to decrease forceful exertion. The weight of the objects held in the hand should be reduced. Tool handles that enhance the frictional quality of the object being held should be encouraged, as less forceful exertions might then be required. The use of mechanical aids can substitute for holding objects. Ill-fitting equipment (e.g., gloves) must be avoided. Hand force should not exceed 45 N.

Poor Posture

Maintained isometric contraction of muscles is often associated with CTDs. Muscles that remain contracted at more than 15–20% of their maximal capacity impair circulation [70]. Any positions of the hand that keep the wrist dorsiflexed increase the risk of CTS. In addition, prolonged wrist extension can contribute to this syndrome.

Several articles have described electromyographic recordings from neck and shoulder muscles to ascertain how much of an effect muscle activity and pos-

ture have on CTDs [138,139]. These studies failed to show a relationship between the level of muscle activity and complaints. However, it was noted that periods of shoulder rest lasting more than 2 seconds were negatively correlated with complaints. Veiersted et al. [138] suggested that pauses of a very short duration are beneficial for avoiding musculoskeletal complaints. A 50% reduction in total daily work hours resulted in only moderate delays in the development of musculoskeletal complaints. It therefore appears that short, frequent, well-placed rests are more beneficial than long, infrequent breaks.

The following postures should be avoided as much as possible: excessive wrist pronation, excessive ulnar deviation, excessive wrist flexion or extension, elbow flexion beyond 90 degrees (especially when the task heights are above elbow level), internal rotation of the arms and elevation of the shoulder, excessive neck flexion, and excessive hip and knee flexion.

Posture can be improved by relocating and redesigning tools as well as relocating and reorienting the workstation. Perhaps the most important constituent is the adjustability of the workstation.

Mechanical Stresses

Concentrated mechanical stress is another factor involved in the development of CTDs. Forces should be dissipated over as large an area of the body as possible. This could include rounding or padding surfaces that come in contact with the body, using tool handles that are long enough to extend beyond the palm, and avoiding the use of the hands for pounding [120]. Using belts is an excellent way to distribute force.

Lowering the work load, raising the worker's position, and rotating tasks are all methods used to alleviate an antigravity situation. An ergonomic assessment of the task is extremely important to avoid deviation of physiologic structures from the neutral position. Adjustable workstations, worker education, and worker training are other effective measures. Education is perhaps the most important aspect of prevention. It is essential that employees, supervisors, and management personnel be educated about the causes, early signs, symptoms, and consequences of CTDs. The reader is referred to the section on OSHA's Four-Step Program to Reduce Ergonomic Hazards.

Occupational Safety and Health Act

In 1970, owing to the tremendous impact that job-related injuries and illnesses had on the American work force, a bipartisan Congress passed the Occupational Safety and Health Act (hereinafter referred to simply as the *Act*). Its purpose was "to assure so far as possible every working man and woman in the nation safe and healthful working conditions and to preserve our human resources." The Act affected five million employers and 90 million employees. The goal was to keep the workplace free of hazards and to ensure safety of all workers [140].

Until 1970, there was no provision for protection against workplace injury and health hazards. The Act extends to all employers and their employees in the 50 states, the District of Columbia, Puerto Rico, and all other territories under U.S. federal government jurisdiction. The states may elect to adopt standards and enforce requirements that are at least as effective as federal requirements. To date, 25 states administer their own occupational safety and health programs through plans approved by the Act. Twenty-three of these plans cover the private and public sectors, while two cover the public sector only.

Establishment of the Occupational Safety and Health Administration

The Act was structured to emphasize employer responsibilities and rights as well as employee responsibilities and rights. Under the Act, each participant is a partner in the establishment of safe workplace practices. OSHA's general-duty clause requires employers to furnish each employee with a place of employment that is free from recognized hazards that are causing, or are likely to cause, death or serious physical harm [141]. OSHA authorizes enforcement and has the authority to initiate citations and penalties for any violations of the Act. Fines of up to $250,000 for an individual or $500,000 for a corporation may be imposed for a criminal conviction. OSHA also provides research, information, education, and training in the field of health and occupational safety. It develops and sets mandatory occupational safety and health standards for any business involved in interstate commerce [142]. The Act encompasses 20,000 rules

and regulations and is referable to industry and professional guidelines. OSHA issues voluntary guidelines for which it does not require compliance. However, it can use the general-duty clause to enforce certain regulations.

OSHA's goals include the following [143]:

- Encourage employers and employees to reduce workplace hazards and to implement new or improve existing safety and health programs.
- Provide for research in occupational safety and health to develop innovative ways of dealing with occupational safety and health problems.
- Establish "separate but dependent responsibilities and rights" for employers and employees for the achievement of better safety and health conditions.
- Maintain a reporting and recording system to monitor job-related injuries and illnesses.
- Establish training programs to increase the number and competence of occupational safety and health personnel.
- Develop mandatory job safety and health standards and enforce them effectively.
- Provide for the development, analysis, evaluation, and approval of state occupational safety and health programs.

Before the Act became effective, there was no centralized or systematic method by which to monitor occupational safety and health problems. According to the Act, employers of 11 or more employees must maintain records of occupational injuries and illnesses. An *occupational injury* is any injury that results from a work-related accident or from exposure involving a single incident in the work environment [143]. An *occupational illness* is any abnormal condition or disorder caused by exposure to environmental factors associated with employment. Included are acute and chronic illnesses. CTDs therefore fall into the category of an occupational illness.

Per OSHA regulations, record-keeping forms must be maintained for 5 years and include the OSHA 200 log and OSHA 101 supplementary record of occupational injuries and illnesses. All recordable occupational injuries and illnesses must be reported on the OSHA 200 log within 6 working days from the time the employer learns of the illness or injury. OSHA 101 is a form that contains details about each injury or illness and also must be completed within 6 working days from the time the employer learns of the work-related injury or illness.

Most CTDs are recorded on the OSHA 200 form as an occupational illness under the F7 column, Disorders Associated with Repeated Trauma. These disorders are caused, aggravated, or precipitated by repeated motion, vibration, or pressure [144]. Either physical findings or subjective symptoms and resulting actions must be documented. One of two requirements must be satisfied: (1) at least one physical finding (e.g., positive Tinel's, Phalen's, or Finkelstein's test; swelling, redness, or deformity; loss of motion); or (2) at least one subjective symptom (e.g., pain, tingling, numbness, aching, stiffness, or burning) accompanied by medical treatment including self-administered treatment when made available to employees by their employer, lost workdays including restricted work activity, or transfer or rotation to another job. Interestingly, unless the case was caused solely by a non–work-related event or off-premise exposure, the case is presumed to be work related [144].

"Disorders associated with repeated trauma" are the most frequently reported occupational illnesses [145]. This category includes noise-induced hearing loss and illnesses caused by ergonomic exposure. Hansen [146] defines the term *ergonomic illness* as "any diagnosis of gradual onset for which ergonomic exposure increases relative risk." According to OSHA 200 logs, the form companies are required to use to report occupational illnesses and injuries, disorders associated with repeated trauma rose 18% in 1981 and more than 50% in 1989.

A plethora of services, most funded by OSHA, are provided at no cost to the employer for those who require help in establishing and maintaining a safe and healthful workplace (see *All About OSHA*, for further details about individual programs [143]). Consultations can be scheduled to help employers identify and correct specific hazards, develop and implement effective workplace safety and health programs (with emphasis on the prevention of worker illness and injuries), and provide educational services [143].

The future of OSHA in the current political climate is cloudy. OSHA contends that imposing standards would save businesses $9.6 billion per year because of a decrease in time loss secondary to injuries and compensation claims. For example, a large manufacturer of microchips recently trained 18,000 of their 33,000 workers in ergonomics. The emphasis of the course was to reduce the risk of CTDs. The company noted a 30% decrease in the number of lost or restricted workdays attributable to CTDs. Other companies have reported similar or even larger savings. However, powerful lobbying groups that find OSHA's restrictiveness cumbersome seek to cut OSHA's budget. OSHA's future will probably depend on a number of variables, including political climate, employer and employee lobbying efforts, and bottom-line economic issues. It is interesting to note that although traumatically acquired injuries have been minimized, the number and causes of CTDs have risen.

OSHA's Four-Step Program to Reduce Ergonomic Hazards

OSHA attributes much of the recent increase in CTDs to "changes in the process and technology," which results in employee exposure to ergonomic risk factors such as high repetition [120]. However, determination of the overall incidence and prevalence of CTDs is difficult. Variations exist in diagnostic terminology and criteria. What one physician might classify as an occupational injury may simply be classified by another as CTS [147]. Reporting differences also complicate the issue as data collection is mandated differently by different states [148]. Compounding this, workers' compensation laws vary from state to state. It also is likely that, with the growing awareness of CTDs, many factors that were ignored or tolerated years ago are now being reported. Therefore, assessment of the precise incidence of CTDs is extremely difficult.

In 1990, OSHA began a nationwide program to help reduce or eliminate worker exposure to ergonomic hazards that lead to CTDs and related injuries and illnesses [143]. OSHA targeted the meat-packing industry because of its reported rate of CTDs, 75 times greater than that of industry as a whole. OSHA developed voluntary guidelines for this industry [144].

The ergonomics program developed for the meat-packing industry is composed of four major program elements, which can be generalized to most industries. These elements are work-site analysis, hazard prevention, medical management, and training and education.

Work-Site Analysis

Work-site analysis identifies existing hazards and conditions as well as potential hazards. Steps include analysis of safety logs and medical and insurance information, systematic analysis of the work site to identify work positions that might create potential hazards, the use of an ergonomist or other qualified person to analyze the data, and, finally, periodic surveys of the work site (to be done at least annually).

Hazard Prevention

Hazard prevention is achieved primarily through effective design of the workstation, tools, and job. The workstation should be designed to accommodate the person who performs the job and not a typical or average worker. Work methods should be designed to reduce static positioning, extreme and awkward postures, repetitive motions, and excessive force [144].

Tools and handles should be designed to reduce the risk of CTDs. Tools should be selected to minimize stressors, including chronic muscle contractions, steady force, extreme or awkward hand positions, repetitive forceful motions, vibrations, and excessive gripping, pinching, or force on the hands and fingers. Training and practice should be instituted to enforce proper work technique. New employees should undergo a conditioning or break-in period, which may last several weeks. Employees who are reassigned to new jobs should undergo a reconditioning period. At all levels, monitoring of proper work practices should be available.

Because repetition is such a prevalent factor in CTDs, it is necessary to include modifications of the work pace as well as the workplace. For example, in assembly-line work, the line speed should be adjustable, and staff should be rotated at different positions. Personal protective equipment should be selected with a concern for ergonomics. Proper fit is essential to facilitate grasping yet allow for tactile sensation. Insulation against extreme cold (less than 40°F) should be instituted

to minimize stress on joints and prevent peripheral vasospasm. Administrative controls to reduce exposures to ergonomic stressors must be a part of any program. These include limiting overtime work, decreasing production rates, building in rest pauses, decreasing cycle time, using job rotation, providing sufficient staff to avoid stress, and enlarging jobs.

Medical Management

Medical management must include proper record keeping of work-related illness or injury as well as early recognition, diagnosis, treatment, and reporting. Prompt evaluation and referral for conservative treatment is required if indicated. An appropriate return-to-work plan must be developed to decrease the likelihood of recurrence.

Training and Education

The fourth program element is training and education. This training must target all personnel—managers, supervisors, and employees. Training should include a description of potential illnesses and injuries, causes and early symptoms, and a means for prevention and treatment.

It is extremely important that workers be involved in the decision-making process. At UAW Ford, three ergonomic teams were developed to initiate projects and complete them within 1 year [149]. Two of those teams that included laborers initiated 28 projects and completed them within a year. The third team, which involved no laborers as team members, completed none of the 14 projects it began. Ethicon, Inc., also developed a successful ergonomics program by ensuring that the worker was involved in all phases of the program [135]. Two interesting aspects of their ergonomics program were the establishment of both an on-site physical therapy clinic and an on-site exercise program. Ethicon concluded that exercise used intermittently during the workday had both physiologic and psychological benefits, including improved posture and breathing, improved joint flexibility and muscle extensibility, improved balance and muscle tone, improved blood flow, reduced risk of inflammation, and reduced stress. Exercises were performed twice daily per shift for approximately 7 minutes at each session. Employees participated voluntarily.

The development of future programs to reduce ergonomic hazards—whether by OSHA, another regulating agency, or by industry itself—is sure to be beneficial in the future to a decrease in the rate of CTDs in the workplace.

Ergonomics

The term *ergonomics* has been defined as the study of work. Ergonomics addresses the need for human beings to interact compatibly with the work environment. This term implies an applied science that combines anthropology, biomechanics, physiology, biometrics, psychology, engineering, and occupational health. It studies the relationship between humans and machines [150].

Ergonomics seeks to adapt the job and workplace to the worker rather than trying to force the person to fit the job. It involves a proactive approach to improving safety, productivity, and quality [151]. This may be accomplished by designing or redesigning tasks, workstations, tools, and equipment that are within the worker's physical capabilities as well as limitations [152].

An ergonomic illness is defined as "any diagnosis of gradual onset for which ergonomic exposure increases relative risk" [146]. By this definition, many CTDs may be classified as an ergonomic illness.

Ergonomics has become big business. The office furniture industry, a $9 billion per year business, is releasing "ergonomically correct" products each year. There are, however, no official standards for what is ergonomically correct. Though there are accepted ergonomic principles, no standard yet defines what constitutes an ergonomically sound piece of equipment. It is therefore in the best interest of both the employer and the employee to try out any product before purchasing it. Each worker and work situation is different. Therefore, what is ergonomically correct for one worker in one job may be ergonomically incorrect for another.

Conclusion

According to Hadler [6], "[A CTD] is not a clinical event; it is a socio-political phenomenon." The treatment of CTDs is affected by legal, social, and compensation issues; treating the physical prob-lems of the individual without accounting for these other factors may be treating only a part of the problem. It is likely that questions will always remain regarding how much a disability is related to occupational factors versus individual predisposing factors.

Resolution of the CTD issue will require cooperation and communication from management, labor, government, academia, the insurance industry, medicine, and law [153]. The workers' compensation system in the United States is less effective in facilitating a worker's return to work than in other Western countries [68]. This issue must be addressed when searching for definitive treatments of CTDs. In the future, health maintenance organizations might be used to help control workers' compensation costs. Managed care has been projected to save 10–30% of medical costs. Whether this will result in better patient care has yet to be determined. It is hoped that, in the future, treatment "will be directed less at controlling pain and more at understanding and correcting underlying, intrinsic and extrinsic factors" [71].

References

1. Ramazzini B. Diseases of Workers (WC Wright, trans). New York: Hafner, 1964. (Original work published in 1700 and 1713.)
2. Sigerist HE. J Hist Med Allied Sci 1958;13:214.
3. Nakano K. Peripheral nerve entrapments, repetitive strain disorder, occupation-related syndromes, bursitis and tendinitis. Curr Opin Rheumatol 1991;3:226.
4. Armstrong T, Fine L, Goldstein S, et al. Ergonomics considerations in hand and wrist tendinitis. J Hand Surg [Am] 1987;12:830.
5. Hopkins A. The social recognition of repetitive strain injuries: an Australian/American comparison. Soc Sci Med 1990;30:365.
6. Hadler N. Cumulative trauma disorders. An iatrogenic concept. J Occup Med 1990;32:38.
7. Murphy K. What's correct ergonomically? Good question. The New York Times October 9, 1995;D3.
8. Idler R, Fischer T, Creighton J. Cumulative trauma disorders: current concepts in management. Indiana Med 1991;84:328.
9. Mason-Draffen C. High standards at work. Newsday March 9, 1997;F12.
10. Rempel DM, Harrison RJ, Barnhart S. Work-related cumulative trauma disorders of the upper extremity. JAMA 1992;267:838.
11. Mendels P. Gain from pain. Newsday March 5, 1995; p. 1 of Money and Careers.

12. Goldsmith WJ. Workplace ergonomics: a safety and health issue for the 90s. Employ Relat Law J 1989;Autumn.

13. Evans J. Women, men, VDU work and health. A questionnaire survey of British VDU operators. Work Stress 1987;1:271.

14. Sauter SL, Harding GE, Gottlieb MD. VDT-Computer Automation of Work Practices as a Stressor in Information-Processing Jobs: Some Methodological Considerations. In G Salvendy, MJ Smith (eds), Proceedings of the International Conference on Machine Pacing and Occupational Stress. London: Taylor & Frances, 1981;355.

15. Arndt R. Work pace, stress, and cumulative trauma disorder. J Hand Surg [Am] 1987;12:866.

16. Waersted M, Westgaard R. Working hours as a risk factor in the development of musculoskeletal complaints. Ergonomics 1991;34:265.

17. Dobyns J. Cumulative trauma disorders of the upper limb. Hand Clin 1991;7:587.

18. Larsson S, Bodegard L, Henriksson K, et al. Chronic trapezius myalgia morphology and blood flow studied in 17 patients. Acta Orthop Scand 1990;61:394.

19. Meagher S. Tool design for prevention of hand and wrist injuries. J Hand Surg [Am] 1987;12:855.

20. Aja D. Occupational therapy intervention for overuse syndrome. Am J Occup Ther 1991;45:746.

21. Taylor RS, Bonfiglio RP. Industrial rehabilitation medicine: 4. Assessment of the outcome of treatment in industrial medicine, program development, documentation, and testimony. Arch Phys Med Rehabil 1992;73(suppl 5):369.

22. Brammer A, Piercy J, Auger P, et al. Tactile perception in hands occupationally exposed to vibration. J Hand Surg [Am] 1987;12:870.

23. Cherniack MG. Raynaud's phenomenon of occupational origin. Arch Intern Med 1990;150:519.

24. Brubaker RL, MacKenzie CJG, Hutton SG. The study of vibration white finger disease among rock drillers. J Low Freq Noise Vibration 1985;4:66.

25. Toomingas A, Hagberg M, Jorulf L, et al. Outcome of the abduction external rotation test among manual and office workers. Am J Ind Med 1991;19:215.

26. National Institute for Occupational Safety and Health. Vibration White Finger Disease in US Workers Using Pneumatic Chipping and Grinding Hand Tools: I. Epidemiology (Vol 18). Washington, DC: US Department of Health and Human Services, 1982;118.

27. Lidstrom IM. Vibration Injury in Rock Drillers, Chiselers and Grinders: The International Occupational Hand and Arm Conference. US Department of Health, Education and Welfare Publication No. 77-170. Washington, DC: National Institute of Occupational Safety and Health, 1977.

28. Agate JN, Druett HA, Tombleson JBL. Raynaud's phenomenon in grinders of small metal casting. Br J Ind Med 1946;3:157.

29. Bovenzi M, Petronio L, DiMarino F. Epidemiological study of ship yard workers exposed to hand-arm vibration. Int Arch Occup Environ Health 1980;46:251.

30. Hunter D, McLaughlin AIC, Perry KMA. Effects of the use of pneumatic tools. Br J Ind Med 1945;2:10.

31. Suzuki H. Vibration syndrome of vibrating tool users in a factory of a steel foundry. Jpn J Ind Health 1978;20:261.

32. Lundborg G, Dahlin LB, Hansson, HA, et al. Vibration exposure and peripheral nerve fiber damage. J Hand Surg [Am] 1990;15:346.

33. Zimmerman N, Zimmerman S, Clark G. Neuropathy in the work place. Hand Clin 1992;8:255.

34. Kurumatani N, Iki M, Hirata K, et al. Usefulness of fingertip skin temperature for examining peripheral circulatory disturbances of vibrating tool operators. Scand J Work Environ Health 1986;12:245.

35. Bovenzi M. Vibration white finger, digital blood pressure, and some biochemical findings on workers operating vibrating tools in the engine manufacturing industry. Am J Ind Med 1988;14:575.

36. Olsen N, Nielsen SL. Diagnosis of Raynaud's phenomenon in quarry men's traumatic vasospastic disease. Scand J Work Environ Health 1979;5:249.

37. Takeuchi T, Imanishi H. Histolopathologic observations in finger biopsy from thirty patients with Raynaud's phenomenon of occupational origin. J Kumamoto Med Soc 1984;58:56.

38. Takeuchi T, Futatsuka M, Imanishi H, et al. Pathological changes observed in the finger biopsy of patients with vibration-induced white finger. Scand J Work Environ Health 1986;12:280.

39. Futatsuka M, Pyykko I, Farkkila M, et al. Blood pressure, flow and peripheral resistance of digital arteries in vibration syndrome. Br J Ind Med 1983;40:434.

40. Reynolds DD, Falkenberg RJ. Three and Four Degrees of Freedom: Models of the Vibration Response of the Human Hand. In Vibration Effects on the Hand and Arm in Industry. New York: Wiley, 1982;17.

41. Thiry S. Tools must fit the worker. Occup Health Saf 1990;59:79.

42. Wos H, Lindberg J, Jakus R. Evaluation of impact loading and overwork using a bolt piston support. Ergonomics 1992;35:1069.

43. Gowitz KE, Milnear M. Understanding the Scientific Basis of Human Movement (2nd ed). Baltimore: Williams & Wilkins, 1980;95.

44. Dortch H, Trombly C. The effects of education on hand use with industrial workers in repetitive jobs. Am J Occup Ther 1990;44:777.

45. Deves L, Spillane R. Occupational health, stress and work organization in Australia. Int J Health Serv 1989;19:351.

46. Stellman JJ, Klitzman S, Gordon G, et al. Comparison of Well Being Among Non-Machine Interactive Clerical Workers and Full Time and Part Time VDT Users and Typists. In B Knavel, P Wideback (eds), Proceed-

ings of the International Conference on Work with Display Units. Amsterdam: Elsevier, 1987;605.

47. Wallace M, Buckle P. Ergonomic Aspects of Neck and Upper Limb Disorders. In DJ Osborne (ed), International Review and Ergonomics: Current Trends in Human Factors Research and Practice (vol 1). London: Taylor & Frances, 1987;173.

48. Linton SJ, Kamwendo K. Risk factors in the psychosocial work environment for neck and shoulder pain in secretaries. J Occup Med 1989;31:609.

49. Gao CS, Lu D, She Q. The effects of VDT data entry work on operators. Ergonomics 1990;33:917.

50. Westgaard R, Jensen C, Hansen K. Individual and work-related risk factors associated with symptoms of musculoskeletal complaints. Int Arch Occup Environ Health 1993;64:405.

51. Bernard B, Sauter S, Fine L, et al. Psychosocial and work organization risk factors for cumulative trauma disorders in the hands and wrists of newspaper employees. Scand J Work Environ Health 1992;18(suppl 2):119.

52. Pickett CW, Lees RE. A cross-sectional study of health complaints among 79 data entry operators using video display terminals. J Soc Occup Med 1991;41:113.

53. Reid J, Ewan C, Lowy E. Pilgrimage of pain: the illness experiences of women with repetitive strain injury and the search for credibility. Soc Sci Med 1991;32:601.

54. Iserhagen S. Principles of prevention for cumulative trauma. Occup Med 1992;7:147.

55. Alund M, Larsson SE, Lewin T. Work-related chronic neck impairment. Neck motion analysis in female transverse crane operators. Scand J Rehabil Med 1992;24:133.

56. Weinstein S, Scheer S. Industrial rehabilitation medicine: 2. Assessment of the problem, pathology and risk factors for disability. Arch Phys Med Rehabil 1992;73(suppl 5):360.

57. Bird H, Hill J. Repetitive strain disorder: towards diagnostic criteria. Ann Rheum Dis 1992;51:974.

58. Bigos S, Battie M, Fisher L. Methodology for evaluating predictive factors for the report of back injury. Spine 1991;16:669.

59. Bigos S, Battie M, Spengler D, et al. A prospective study of work perceptions and psychosocial factors affecting the report of back injury. Spine 1991;16:688.

60. Helme R, LeVasseur S, Gibson S. RSI revisited: evidence for psychological and physiological differences from an age, sex and occupation matched control group. Aust N Z J Med 1992;22:23.

61. Helliwell P, Mumford D, Smeathers J, et al. Work related upper limb disorder: the relationship between pain, cumulative load, disability, and psychological factors. Ann Rheum Dis 1992;51:1325.

62. Spence S. Cognitive behavior therapy in the treatment of chronic, occupational pain of the upper limbs: a two year follow-up. Behav Res Ther 1991;29:503.

63. Spaans F. Occupational Nerve Lesions. In PJ Vinken, GW Bruyn (eds), Diseases of Nerves, Vol 7: Handbook of Clinical Neurology. Amsterdam: North-Holland, 1970;326.

64. Louis D. Cumulative trauma disorders. J Hand Surg [Am] 1987;12:823.

65. Buckle P. Musculoskeletal disorders of the upper extremities: the use of epidemiologic approaches in industrial settings. J Hand Surg [Am] 1987;12:885.

66. Muffly-Elsey D, Flinn-Wagner S. Proposed screening tool for the detection of cumulative trauma disorders of the upper extremity. J Hand Surg [Am] 1987;12:931.

67. Viikari-Juntura E, Kurppa K, Kuosma E, et al. Prevalence of epicondylitis and elbow pain in the meat-processing industry. Scand J Work Environ Health 1991;17:38.

68. Scheer S, Weinstein S. Industrial rehabilitation medicine: 1. An overview. Arch Phys Med Rehabil 1992;73(suppl 5):356.

69. Waddell G, McCulloch JA, Kummel E, et al. Non-organic physical signs in low back pain. Spine 1980;5:117.

70. Waddell G, Main CJ, Morris EW, et al. Chronic low back pain, psychologic distress and illness behavior. Spine 1984;9:209.

71. McKeag D. Overuse injuries: the concept in 1992. Prim Care 1991;18:851.

72. Clairmont A, Bonfiglio R, Taylor R, et al. Industrial rehabilitation medicine: 3. Treatment. Arch Phys Med Rehabil 1992:73(suppl 5):366.

73. Leadbetter W, Mooar P, Lane G, et al. The surgical treatment of tendinitis, clinical rationale and biologic basis. Clin Sports Med 1992;11:679.

74. Kannus P, Jarvinen M, Niittymaki S. Long or short acting anesthetic with corticosteroid in local injections of overuse injuries. A prospective randomized double-blind study. Int J Sports Med 1990;11:397.

75. Allers V. Work place prevention program cuts costs of illness and injury. Occup Health Saf 1989;58(8):26.

76. Silverstein BA, Armstrong TJ, Longmate A, et al. Can in-plant exercise control musculoskeletal symptoms? J Occup Med 1988;30:922.

77. Martinez M, Lamoglia J. Hands-on answers to hidden health costs. HR Magazine 1992;37(3):48.

78. Dobyns J. Role of the physician in workers-compensation injuries. J Hand Surg [Am] 1987;12:826.

79. Gerr F, Letz R, Landrigan P. Upper extremity musculoskeletal disorders of occupational origin. Annu Rev Public Health 1991;12:543.

80. Szabo R, Gelberman R. The pathophysiology of nerve entrapment syndromes. J Hand Surg [Am] 1987;12:880.

81. Witt J, Pess G, Gelberman RH. Treatment of de Quervain's tenosynovitis. A prospective study of the results of injection of steroids and immobilization in a splint. J Bone Joint Surg Am 1991;73:219.

82. Price R, Sinclair H, Heinrich I, et al. Local injection, treatment of tennis elbow—hydrocortisone, triamcinolone and lidocaine compared. Br J Rheumatol 1991;30:39.

83. Livengood L. Occupational soft tissue disorders of the hand and forearm. Wis Med J 1992;91:583.

84. Hales T, Bertsche P. Management of upper extremity cumulative trauma disorders. AAOHN J 1992;40(3):118.

85. Kroemer K. Avoiding cumulative trauma disorders in shops and offices. Am Ind Hyg Assoc J 1992;53:596.

86. Barton NJ, Hooper G, Noble J, et al. Occupational causes of disorders in the upper limb. BMJ 1992;304:309.

87. Anderson B, Kaye F. Treatment of flexor tenosynovitis of the hand ("trigger finger") with corticosteroids. A prospective study of the response to local injection. Arch Intern Med 1991;151:153.

88. Cuetter AC, Bartoszek DM. The thoracic outlet syndrome: controversies over diagnosis, over treatment and recommendations for management. Muscle Nerve 1989;12:410.

89. Guidotti T. Occupational repetitive strain injury. Am Fam Physician 1992;45:585.

90. Sheon R. Peripheral nerve entrapment, occupation-related syndromes, and sports injuries. Curr Opin Rheumatol 1992;4:219.

91. Wood MB, Linscheid RL. Abductor pollicis bursitis. Clin Orthop 1973;93:293.

92. Howard NJ. Peritendinitis crepitans: a muscle effort syndrome. J Bone Joint Surg 1937;19:447.

93. Stern P. Tendinitis, overuse syndromes, and tendon injuries. Hand Clin 1990;6:467.

94. Chu BM, Blatz PJ. Cumulative micro damage model to describe the hysteresis of living tissue. Ann Biomed Eng 1972;1:204.

95. Thompson J, Phelps T. Repetitive strain injuries: how to deal with the "epidemic of the 1990s." Postgrad Med 1990;8:143.

96. Bammer G. How technologic change can increase the risk of repetitive motion injuries. Semin Occup Med 1987;2:25.

97. Hagberg M, Sundelin G. Discomfort and load on the upper trapezius muscle when operating a word processor. Ergonomics 1986;29:1637.

98. Kilbom A, Persson J. Work technique and its consequences for musculoskeletal disorders. Ergonomics 1987;30:273.

99. World Health Organization. Visual Display Terminals in Workers' Health. WHO Offset Publication No. 99. Geneva: World Health Organization, 1987.

100. Sauter S, Schleifer L, Kuntson S. Work posture, workstation design, and musculoskeletal discomfort in a VDT data entry task. Hum Factors 1991;33:151.

101. Duncan J, Ferguson D. Keyboard operating posture and symptoms in operating. Ergonomics 1974;17:651.

102. Hunting W, Laubli T, Grandjean E. Postural and visual loads at VDT workplaces: I. Constrained postures. Ergonomics 1981;24:917.

103. Maeda K, Hunting W, Grandjean E. Localized fatigue in accounting machine operators. J Occup Med 1980;22:810.

104. Kemmlert K, Kilbom A, Milerad E, Wistedt C. Musculoskeletal Trouble in the Neck and Shoulder: Relationship and Clinical Findings in Workplace Design Effects. In Proceedings on Working with Display Units.

Stockholm: Swedish National Board of Occupational Safety and Health, 1986;174.

105. Pot F, Padmos P, Brouwers A. Determinants of the VDU Operator's Well Being. In B Knave, PG Widback (eds), Work with Display Units '86. Amsterdam: North-Holland, 1986;16.

106. Ryan GA, Bampton M. Comparison of data process operators with and without upper limb symptoms. Community Health Studies 1988;12:63.

107. Sauter SL, Gottlieb MS, Jones KC, et al. Job and health implications of VDT use: initial results of the Wisconsin–NIOSA study. Communications ACM 1983;26:284.

108. Starr SJ, Shute SJ, Thompson CR. Relating posture to discomfort in VDT use. J Occup Med 1985;27:269.

109. Loomis V, Church J. Video display terminals: potential health hazards and possible solutions. J Biocommun 1990;17(4):20.

110. Putz-Anderson V, Doyle G, Hales T. Ergonomic analysis to characterize task constraint and repetitiveness as risk factors for musculoskeletal disorders in telecommunication office workers. Scand J Work Environ Health 1992;18(suppl 2):123.

111. Polakoff P. Repetitive-motion, radiation and eye concerns mount at computer work sites. Occup Health Saf 1991;60:34.

112. Morgan S. Most factors contributing to CTS can be minimized, if not eliminated. Occup Health Saf 1991;60(10):47, 50.

113. Bleecker M. Medical surveillance for carpal tunnel syndrome in workers. J Hand Surg [Am] 1987;12:845.

114. National Institute for Occupational Safety and Health. Potential Health Hazards of Video Display Terminals. DHHS [NIOSH] Publication No. 81-129. Washington, DC: National Institute for Occupational Safety and Health, 1981.

115. Gerwatowski L, McFall D, Stach D. Carpal tunnel syndrome risk factors and preventive strategies for the dental hygienist. J Dent Hyg 1992;66:89.

116. Conrad J, Conrad K, Osborn J. Median nerve dysfunction evaluated during dental hygiene education and practice (1986–1989). J Dent Hyg 1991;65:283.

117. Conrad J, Osborn J, Conrad K, et al. Peripheral nerve dysfunction in practicing dental hygienists. J Dent Hyg 1990;64:382.

118. Randolph S. Ergonomic strategies in the work place. AAOHN J 1992;40(3):103.

119. MacDonald G, Robertson MM, Erickson JA. Carpal tunnel syndrome among California dental hygienists. Dent Hyg 1988;62:322.

120. Frederick L. Cumulative trauma disorders and overview. AAOHN J 1992;40(3):113.

121. Strong D, Lennartz F. Carpal tunnel syndrome. J Cal Dent Assoc 1992;20(4):27.

122. Podhorodecki A, Spielholz N. Electromyographic study of overuse syndromes in sign language interpreters. Arch Phys Med Rehabil 1993;74:261.

123. Cohn L, Lowry R, Hart S. Overuse syndromes of the upper extremities in interpreters for the deaf. Orthopedics 1990;13:207.

124. Stedt J. Interpreters' wrist repetitive stress injury and carpal tunnel syndrome in sign language interpreters. Am Ann Deaf 1992;137:40.

125. Sebright JA. Gloves, behavioral changes can reduce carpal tunnel syndrome. Occup Health Saf 1986;55(9):18.

126. Higgs P, Young V, Seaton M, et al. Upper extremity impairment in workers performing repetitive tasks. Plast Reconstr Surg 1992;90:614.

127. Schottland J, Kirschberg G, Fillingin R, et al. Median nerve latencies in poultry processing workers: an approach to resolving the role of industrial "cumulative trauma" in the development of carpal tunnel syndrome. J Occup Med 1991;33:627.

128. Nelson N, Park R, Silverstein M, et al. Cumulative trauma disorders of the hand and wrist in the auto industry. Am J Public Health 1992;82:1550.

129. Kellerman R. Manufactured housing plant injuries in a rural family practice. J Fam Pract 1990;31:273.

130. Takami H, Takahashi S, Ando M, et al. Rupture of the extensor digitorum communis tendon caused by occupational overuse. J Hand Surg [Br] 1991;16:70.

131. Harber P, Bloswick D, Pena L, et al. The ergonomic challenge of repetitive motion with varying ergonomic stresses characterizing supermarket checking work. J Occup Med 1992;34:518.

132. Harber P, Pena L, Bland G, et al. Upper extremity symptoms in supermarket workers. Am J Ind Med 1992;22:873.

133. Magnusson M, Granqvist N, Jonson R, et al. The loads on the lumbar spine during work at an assembly line: the risks for fatigue injury of the vertebral bodies. Spine 1990;15:774.

134. Chatterjee D. Workplace upper limb disorders: a prospective study with intervention. Occup Med 1992;42:129.

135. Lutz G, Hansford T. Cumulative trauma disorder controls: the ergonomics program at Ethicon, Inc. J Hand Surg [Am] 1987;12:863.

136. Barnhart S, Demers P, Miller M, et al. Carpal tunnel syndrome among ski manufacturing workers. Scand J Work Environ Health 1991;17:46.

137. McDonald E, Marino C. Manual labor metacarpophalangeal arthropathy in a baker. N Y State J Med 1990;90:268.

138. Veiersted K, Westgaard R, Andersen P. Pattern of muscle activity during stereotyped work and its relation to muscle pain. Int Arch Occup Environ Health 1990;62:31.

139. Hansson G, Stromberg U, Larsson B, et al. Electromyographic fatigue in neck/shoulder muscles and endurance in women with repetitive work. Ergonomics 1992;35:1341.

140. Occupational Safety and Health Act of 1970. Public Law 91-5/96. S.2193;1970.

141. O'Brien RF, Gallagher. OSHA and the general duty clause. Prof Safety 1991;31.

142. Haag AB. Ergonomic standards, guidelines and strategies for prevention of back injury. Occup Med 1992;7:155.

143. All About OSHA. OSHA Publication No. 3125. Washington, DC: US Department of Labor, Occupational Safety and Health Administration, 1991.

144. National Institute for Occupational Safety and Health. Ergonomics Program: Management Guidelines for Meat Packing Plants. DHHS Publication No. 3123. Washington, DC: National Institute for Occupational Safety and Health, 1990.

145. Bureau of Labor Statistics. Occupational Injuries and Illnesses in the United States by Industry, 1988. Washington, DC: US Department of Labor, 1990.

146. Hansen J. OSHA regulation of ergonomic health. J Occup Med 1993;35:42.

147. Jensen RC, Klein BP Sanderson LM. Motion related wrist disorders traced to industries, occupational groups. Monthly Labor Rev 1983;106:113.

148. Brown CD, Nolan BN, Faithfull DK. Occupational repetitive strain injuries: guidelines for diagnosis and management. Med J Aust 1984;140:329.

149. Brandon K. Ergonomics at UAW-Ford. Occup Health Saf 1992;61(6):44.

150. Blair S, Bear-Lehman J. Prevention of upper extremity occupational disorders [editorial comment]. J Hand Surg [Am] 1987;12:821.

151. Joyce M. Ergonomics will take center stage in the 90's and into the new century. Safety professionals and engineers must work together to address ergonomic issues. Occup Health Saf 1991;60(1):31.

152. National Institute for Occupational Safety and Health. Ergonomics: The Study of Work. DHHS Publication No. 3092. Washington, DC: National Institute for Occupational Safety and Health, 1991.

153. Thomas R. Report on the multi-disciplinary conference on control and prevention of cumulative trauma disorders (CTD) or repetitive motion trauma (RMT) in the textile, apparel, and fiber industries. Am Ind Hyg Assoc J 1991;52:A562.

Chapter 7
Entrapment Neuropathies

Jay Mitchell Weiss

Pathophysiologic Features of Nerve Compression

Entrapment neuropathies are generally insidious in nature. Frequently, the patient will note not a specific onset of a symptom but rather a gradual progression of symptoms. One exception is entrapment neuropathies due to cumulative trauma disorders (CTDs). Although entrapment neuropathies due to overuse can occur insidiously, they are often more acute in nature. Very frequently, a specific activity—for instance, the weekend building of a deck by a noncarpenter or the playing of a sport by someone unaccustomed to that sport—will cause the acute onset of a mononeuropathy.

In extreme cases, compression neuropathies can cause axon loss and wallerian degeneration, but most compression neuropathies tend to be demyelinating. The axons of motor nerves, as well as most of the sensory nerves, are covered with a myelin sheath, which permits a saltatory or jumping type of conductionat least 10 times faster than the conduction of unmyelinated fibers. Consequently, most myelinated motor and sensory fibers conduct in the range of 50 m per second or faster. Because of the excellent insulating properties of myelin, a depolarization at one node of Ranvier (the area of minimal myelin covering between one myelinated segment of nerve and the next) will cause enough current at the subsequent node of Ranvier to reach threshold potential. This causes the sodium channels to open, thus propagating the action potential [1].

Because the electric current traveling from one node of Ranvier to the next is essentially instantaneous, the conduction velocity of the nerve is limited by both the amount of time it takes the sodium channels at each node of Ranvier to open and the density of those nodes of Ranvier per unit of length. The depolarization of the nodes of Ranvier regenerates the potential and ensures its propagation. In a healthy myelinated nerve, the myelin is such a good insulator that it frequently depolarizes a second node simultaneously, further increasing the velocity of the action potential.

When a segment of myelinated nerve loses its myelin covering because of compression, that segment of myelinated nerve differs from an unmyelinated nerve. In unmyelinated nerves, sodium and potassium channels run the entire length of the nerve and can propagate action potentials across that entire length. A myelinated nerve that loses its covering is often unable to propagate an action potential owing to the scarcity of sodium channels along what was formerly an internodal region. In the absence of the insulating effects of the myelin, the depolarization current likely will not reach the next concentration of sodium channels (node of Ranvier) and, therefore, it will not regenerate the wave of depolarization [1]. This failure is referred to as a *conduction block*. The axon distal and proximal to the block can still conduct normally.

In addition to conduction blocks, slowing can occur due to a loss of the saltatory conduction or an increase in the internodal conduction time. This internodal conduction time is the amount of time it takes for action potential generation at the nodes of Ranvier [2].

In remyelination, several immature nodes of Ranvier might replace the previously healthy node. Damage and regeneration of the myelin sheath over a several-millimeter-long segment of axon can replace each mature node of Ranvier with several immature nodes of Ranvier. These immature nodes will have increased internodal conduction time. Hence, one would expect the velocity across that segment to decrease significantly. Fortunately, in most cases of demyelination secondary to nerve compression, the axon remains intact. If the offending activity is reduced, the nerve tends to remyelinate. A restoration of nerve function (be it in the form of normal strength or normal sensation) is highly likely.

These varying stages of myelin damage (demyelination and remyelination by immature myelin) can often be identified electrodiagnostically. Nerve conduction studies are important in determining the location and extent of nerve injury, which helps the clinician in determining a prognosis. In certain cases of recurrent injury, localization is very important because surgical release may be the definitive treatment.

Nerve conduction studies use an electrical impulse along the nerve to depolarize the nerve. The resulting depolarization or action potential propagates in both directions. Electrodes are placed over an area where the nerve is superficial or over muscles innervated by that nerve. An oscilloscope is synchronized to the shock so that a latency time between the stimulus and the recorded potential can be measured. The size of this response can be used to quantify the number of axons in the individual nerve that are functioning. By measuring the latency over a specific distance, the speed of the nerve can be calculated. The use of shorter segments can help to localize nerve injury precisely (the so-called inching technique).

Electromyography (EMG) involves the insertion of a thin needle, which is attached to an amplifier, into the muscle. The potentials are displayed on an oscilloscope or computer screen and are heard through a speaker. The muscle is examined for the presence of spontaneous activity (involuntary firing of the muscle fibers), as this is a common sign of denervation.

Voluntary muscle contractions are also analyzed. The strength of muscle contractions is augmented by increasing the frequency with which individual axons fire to stimulate muscle and by recruiting or adding axons. The recruitment pattern might indicate that part of the nerve is not functioning.

General Causes of Nerve Compression

Although technically not truly an entrapment, nerve compression due to external sources is occasionally noted in the ulnar, peroneal, and radial nerves. The peroneal nerve may be compressed at the fibular head, the ulnar nerve at the elbow, or the radial nerve at the spiral groove (Saturday night palsy). Any of these compressions can occur as a result of cumulative trauma, though each is more likely to occur as a single precipitating event.

Poor positioning and prolonged periods of unconsciousness that place pressure on these nerves frequently lead to significant conduction blocks and, at times, even to frank denervation. Most of these locally compressive neuropathies have in common a period of unconsciousness deeper than normal sleep. In a normal sleep, compression of any of these nerves will lead to dysesthesias that cause the patient to awaken and change position. Frequently, these position changes are effected subconsciously such that the patient does not realize he or she has awakened. Nonetheless, such alterations of position can be the cause of a restless sleep. When alcohol or anesthesia are introduced, these protective mechanisms (i.e., shifting positions to relieve paresthesias) are no longer present, and the compression can persist long enough to cause significant nerve damage [3–5].

Upper-Extremity Nerve Entrapments Due to Cumulative Trauma Disorders

Median Nerve

Carpal Tunnel Syndrome

Etiologic Features.   The carpal tunnel is a space located at the wrist. Its dorsal as well as medial and lateral boundaries are formed by the carpal bones, whereas its ventral border is formed by the palmar ligament. In this essentially nonyielding structure, the flexor tendons to all five digits (with the exception of the flexor pollicis brevis) pass through the carpal tunnel. In addition, the radial artery and median nerve pass through this tunnel.

Compression of the median nerve at the wrist was described as early as 1913 in an autopsy study by Marie and Foix [6]. Only recently has the general public become familiar with the term *carpal tunnel syndrome* (CTS). There is a danger that the amount of attention given to this disorder in the lay press will result in numerous nonspecific wrist complaints being classified as CTS.

Compression of the median nerve can occur by a narrowing of the carpal tunnel with extreme flexion or extension of the wrist or, more commonly, by a swelling of the other objects in this confined space. Frequently, tendons can become swollen due to repeated trauma or microtrauma that causes localized edema. Not surprisingly, CTS is frequently seen in pregnancy owing to fluid retention and peripheral swelling. In the early stages, the compression of the median nerve tends to be intermittent. As the condition progresses, electrodiagnostic signs of demyelination may develop. In extreme cases, denervation (axon loss) may be noted.

The clinical criteria for the diagnosis of CTS are well established. The history frequently includes complaints of numbness or tingling of the hand, which is generally much worse at night, in a median nerve distribution. Usually, this sensation has been ongoing for some time and will wake the patient from sleep. The patient commonly reports the need to shake or move his or her hand for several minutes until the paresthesias abate. On closer questioning, one can frequently confirm that these paresthesias and dysesthesias are limited to the median distribution. Additionally, on physical examination, there is usually decreased sensation in a median distribution, with normal sensation in the fifth digit and the ulnar half of the fourth digit. Abductor pollicis brevis weakness might be present, and Phalen's sign (hyperflexion of the wrists for a short period that brings on paresthesias or dysesthesias in a median distribution) or reverse Phalen's sign (symptoms with hyperextension of the wrist) is often positive [7]. In the author's experience, Tinel's sign is rarely helpful except in severe cases. Tinel's sign is elicited by tapping over the area of entrapment, which is 2–3 cm distal to the distal wrist crease (not at or proximal to the distal wrist crease). Symptoms of paresthesias or dysesthesias in a median nerve distribution should be elicited.

The contemporary reporting of CTS in epidemic numbers is attributed to the large amount of coverage this entity has achieved in the lay press. Certainly, there are psychosocial factors that encourage the reporting of complaints. Throughout most of the country, newspapers have highlighted the impact of CTS as well as other CTDs related to occupational exposures. Most health care workers who treat workers' compensation patients are very familiar with these complaints. Depending on the industrial makeup of a region, complaints of repetitive hand use occur with varying frequency. However, repetitive keyboard use among secretaries or transcriptionists is probably the most commonly reported precipitating factor in most locations. As mentioned elsewhere, factors that predispose one to CTDs are very prevalent in these workers. Such patients frequently spend long periods, even their entire day, performing the exact same activity, with little variation in movement. They also take infrequent breaks, and the activity in which they are engaged is repeated many times per second. Although this can lead to the development of CTS, in the author's opinion this diagnosis is somewhat over-reported. It would be inaccurate to classify all wrist pain as CTS. Certainly a highly significant number of these patients (especially the EMG-negative patients) are manifesting various tendinoses, sprains, or other overuse syndromes. de Quervain's disease (discussed in Chapter 6) and flexor tendinitis are commonly mistaken for CTS, especially by those who brand every wrist complaint in computer users as CTS.

Conditions associated with CTS include pregnancy, hypothyroidism, acromegaly, amyloidosis, multiple myeloma, and mucopolysaccharidoses. CTS is also more common in diabetic and dialysis patients (as are nerve entrapments in general) [5,8].

Electrodiagnostic Assessment.   CTS is probably the most common mononeuropathy seen in electrodiagnostic laboratories [9]. The definitive diagnosis of CTS is based on documenting a slowing of the motor or sensory fibers of the median nerve across the carpal tunnel. This slowing can be based on the distal latency (the amount of time it takes for an impulse to travel from a depolarization of the nerve at the wrist to the abductor pollicis brevis muscle of the thumb). The median latency can be compared with the distal latency measured from the ulnar nerve of the same hand or with the median nerve of the opposite hand. Other sensitive criteria include a loss of amplitude (corresponding to a block of motor nerve fibers) when comparing the results of a stimulus distal to the carpal tunnel and of one at the wrist.

Still other criteria include a comparison of the sensory latency from the median nerve with that from the radial nerve (which does not pass through the carpal tunnel and should therefore not be slowed). This sometimes is referred to as *Bactrian's sign* because of its characteristic two-humped appearance, which corresponds to the electrophysiologic representation of the median and radial fibers: The Bactrian camel has two humps.

Electromyography-Negative Carpal Tunnel Syndrome. In the vast majority of the cases meeting some or most of the previously cited clinical criteria, electrodiagnostic testing (particularly the nerve conduction velocity component) is positive for CTS. Rarely will patients with such specific clinical complaints as numbness in a median nerve distribution and hand pain that awakens them at night have a normal electrodiagnostic evaluation.

Nonetheless, there is debate among many electromyographers about the definitive electrodiagnosis of CTS: If EMG and nerve conduction velocities are the best tests we have for determining CTS, are they definitive or can there be false negatives? On the basis of some of the limitations of electrodiagnostic testing, it is this author's opinion that the possibility of EMG-negative CTS exists even though the vast majority of electrodiagnostic studies in a given patient might be normal because the CTS is not present or significant.

Generally, when performing electrodiagnostic tests, we are measuring the latency of the fastest-conducting fibers. If a very small portion of motor fibers is being compressed, a change in latency might not be apparent electrodiagnostically. If these fibers do show conduction block, the block will present as a small change in the amplitude of the evoked response. Depending on the number of fibers involved, this small change will frequently be ascribed to technical factors. Because of the limits of the testing, a change in amplitude of 10% or 20% cannot be said to be significant. Additionally, in intermittent compressions, if the compression itself is removed, there may be no change in the conduction of the nerve fiber.

Having presented this theoretic possibility, it is important to note that after a period of weeks or months of repetitive compressions, given the many parameters assessed electrodiagnostically in suspected cases of CTS, at least one or more parameters will show some subtle signs of involvement.

Treatment. As with most CTDs, modification of the offending activity and gradual building up of tolerance is usually the first line of treatment. Unfortunately, this frequently requires that a patient cease to work for a prolonged period. On his or her return to work, the patient often experiences a recurrence of the problem. Surgery is usually curative (when CTS has been documented according to the previously mentioned criteria) and permits resumption of normal activities. Such intervention allows the patient to continue vocational and avocational activities with minimal disruption and with minimal cost to the system and the individual.

Surgery should definitely be considered in cases for which there is electrodiagnostic evidence of axonal damage or in which symptoms interfere with an individual's activities of daily living. It is desirable to prevent permanent loss of sensation in the median nerve distribution of the hand (which is nearly the entire hand) and loss of significant grip strength (due to loss of a component of thumb opposition). In borderline cases, a resting hand splint worn during parts of the day or during sleep is often adequate to relieve symptoms sufficiently. Because of media attention to CTS, patients, their families, and physicians have improved knowledge of the signs of CTS and, therefore, a higher suspicion for this syndrome. Hence, the condition is more likely to be reported early and not to progress to a severe stage.

Frequently, an injection of corticosteroid into the carpal tunnel is sufficient to alleviate symptoms. Such an injection is considered both a diagnostic and a therapeutic procedure, because a positive response for even a short period helps to confirm the diagnosis of CTS.

Pronator Teres Syndrome

The somewhat controversial pronator teres syndrome is believed to occur owing to hypertrophy of the pronator teres muscle, which can compress the median nerve. Frequently, the median nerve will pierce the two heads of the pronator teres muscle before passing under it [9,10]. Very rarely does this produce significant weakness, but it might produce a diffuse pain in a median nerve distribution. Because of limitations of EMG and the fact that the nerve conduction studies tend to be performed over a larger area, minor nerve conduction slowing can easily be missed in cases of pronator teres syndrome. In patients who present with diffuse forearm pain, especially those who perform repetitive movements involving the pronator teres muscle (e.g., carpenters, mechanics), the pronator teres syndrome should be included in the differential diagnosis.

Anterior Interosseus Nerve

The anterior interosseous nerve is a motor branch of the median nerve that supplies the pronator quadratus muscle, flexor digitorum profundus muscles to digits 2 and 3, and flexor pollicis longus muscle. Entrapment of the anterior interosseous nerve can lead to weakness in the muscles it supplies.

Anterior interosseous neuropathy has been reported in association with excessive forearm exercises, but this is rare. Most often anterior interosseous neuropathies are caused by trauma.

Ulnar Nerve

Cubital Tunnel Syndrome

The most common site of ulnar nerve compression, especially compression due to CTDs, is in the region of the elbow. At the elbow, the nerve travels posterior to the medial epicondyle and below the aponeurotic arch formed by the bellies of the flexor carpi ulnaris muscles. This area is referred to as the *cubital tunnel*. Because of the location of the ulnar nerve in this region and the way that it winds around the medial epicondyle, the nerve is likely to be entrapped either under the aponeurosis of the flexor carpi ulnaris or in the ulnar groove behind the medial epicondyle.

Frequent hand use with the elbow in a flexed position has been reported to narrow the cubital tunnel and cause symptoms, generally paresthesias or dysesthesias in an ulnar distribution (fourth or

fifth digits of the affected hand) [11]. According to Stewart [5], repetitive elbow flexion can cause intermittent compression by the aponeurosis. As with most entrapments, the diagnosis of ulnar neuropathies is difficult when the complaints are relatively nonspecific. However, a detailed history may lead one to suspect cumulative trauma as a contributing or etiologic factor. Although electrodiagnostic testing should be performed in cases of suspected ulnar entrapment, the results often are not definitive. One exception is a conduction block or significant slowing of the ulnar nerve that can be documented across the elbow. Short segments (10–14 cm) are used in such testing to prevent the normal nerve (having a normal conduction velocity) from averaging out the relatively insignificant slowing we would see in the affected segment (Figure 7-1). However, the segment should be longer than 10 cm to decrease the likelihood of fictitious perceived slowing due to measurement error. Denervation may be present in ulnarly innervated muscles of the hand if there is significant ulnar neuropathy at the elbow. Usually, the flexor carpi ulnaris is spared, probably owing to the proximal branching of the nerve to the flexor carpi ulnaris.

Ulnar Neuropathy at the Wrist

Repetitive pressure in the hand can cause a neuropathy of the ulnar nerve. This disorder is seen frequently in bicycle riders after prolonged gripping of the handlebars. When the lesion occurs at the level of the hand, the motor branches to the abductor digiti minimi are usually spared. The interosseous and lumbrical muscles to digits 3 and 4 generally are involved. Similar types of repetitive trauma can occur with prolonged use of hand tools or repeated use of the hand as a hammer. The latter has been implicated also in many vascular injuries of the hand.

Radial Nerve

Crutch Palsy

When axillary crutches are used incorrectly, they can put a great deal of pressure on the axillae. Although the four major nerves of the arm—the median, ulnar, radial, and musculocutaneous—all

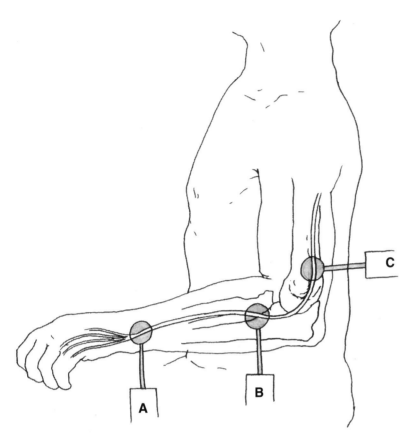

Figure 7-1. Common sites for stimulating the ulnar nerve to assess for entrapment: at wrist (A); below elbow (B); above elbow (C). An entrapment at the elbow may show up as a slowed conduction velocity between segments B and C at a small distance (approximately 10 cm). That same entrapment might yield a normal conduction velocity from A to C, as the larger normal area can raise the velocity over the entire segment to a normal range.

can be compressed to varying degrees at the axilla, the radial nerve is most likely to be affected. The diagnosis in this case may be suspected based on a history of arm pain, numbness, or weakness related to the use of axillary crutches. Reassessment of the patient's gait during crutch walking, to confirm that the crutches are not compressing the axillae significantly, may be helpful.

Supinator Syndrome

Among the most common upper-extremity compressive neuropathies resulting from overuse is the supinator syndrome. This syndrome usually is due to hypertrophy of the supinator muscle, which compresses the posterior interosseous nerve. The posterior interosseous nerve is considered purely a motor branch of the radial nerve. Like most motor nerves, however, it sends sensory branches to innervate the joints it crosses—in this case, the wrist.

The posterior interosseous nerve emerges in the proximal forearm where it penetrates the supinator muscle. The opening in the muscle is referred to as the *arcade of Frohse* and tends to have a fibrous border. Hypertrophy of this muscle, as commonly occurs with repetitive use of hand tools (e.g., screwdrivers, wrenches) can cause an acute posterior interosseous neuropathy. Posterior interosseous nerve injury or entrapment due to CTDs is also a common cause of refractory lateral epicondylitis (see Lateral Epicondylitis in Chapter 8). Indeed, posterior interosseous nerve entrapment should be considered in cases of lateral epicondylitis that do not respond to treatment.

The patient's history usually provides insight into the diagnosis. For example, a person not accustomed to performing intense manual labor who complains of weakness in the hand and a nonspecific or dull wrist pain and ache might be suffering an interosseous nerve entrapment. The clinician must assess the patient's neurologic status, including reflexes, strength, and sensation. Cessation of the offending activity generally provides some relief. Anti-inflammatory medications are commonly used unless contraindicated. After several weeks of relative rest, a gradually progressive strengthening program followed by progressive resumption of activity is usually all that is necessary.

In severe cases of the supinator syndrome, wrist drop and weakness of the finger extensors might be present. Forearm supination should not be involved, as the branch to the supinator muscle usually exits proximal to the entrapment.

As a general rule, in entrapments due to muscle hypertrophy, the muscle causing the entrapment is spared because the nerve supply to that muscle exits prior to the point of entrapment. In the author's experience, entrapments due to compression by muscle rarely lead to acute denervation. Unfortunately, in the absence of significant weakness, electrodiagnostic testing and EMG are of limited value both in supinator syndrome in particular and in posterior interosseous neuropathies in general. If significant axonotmesis is present, electrodiagnostic testing is usually positive.

Lower-Extremity Nerve Entrapments Due to Cumulative Trauma Disorders

Piriformis Syndrome

One of the most controversial nerve entrapments is the piriformis syndrome. Generally, the sciatic nerve travels beneath the piriformis muscle. However, in approximately 10% of people, the entire sciatic nerve or a portion of it pierces the piriformis muscle [12].

In those persons in whom all or part of the nerve pierces the piriformis muscle, it is conceivable that spasm or recurrent contractions of this muscle might cause an apparent sciatica. As is the case with most sciatic nerve injuries, the predominant picture is that of a peroneal nerve injury.

The piriformis muscle is predominantly a hip external rotator. Although on clinical examination numerous piriformis stressing maneuvers aggravate the symptoms, electrodiagnostic changes are relatively rare. More recent work by Fishman and Zieberg [13] suggests that electrodiagnostically, H-

reflex studies may be more sensitive than conventional EMG for localizing lesions of the sciatic nerve in the piriformis muscle. The H-reflex is tested with the patient's hip flexed, adducted, and internally rotated. An increase in the latency of the H-reflex in this position is indicative of the piriformis syndrome.

H-reflexes are analogous to the ankle-jerk reflex and probably use the same afferent and efferent nerve fibers. H-reflex testing is performed similarly to nerve conduction studies (described earlier).

In the H-reflex, the tibial nerve is stimulated in the popliteal fossa (instead of by tapping the Achilles tendon). As mentioned earlier, the wave of depolarization travels in both directions. A depolarization of the gastrocnemius muscle may be noted fairly early (<10 milliseconds) and corresponds with the depolarization of the nerve in a peripheral direction. The proximally traveling impulse along the sensory fibers will synapse in the spinal cord and send an impulse to the gastrocnemius muscle over the motor nerves. The H-reflex requires a stimulus that does not depolarize all the motor fibers, or these fibers will be refractory and the reflex will be lost. The response will occur at approximately 30 milliseconds, which corresponds to the amount of time it takes for the impulse to travel up the afferent sensory fibers, enter the spinal cord, synapse one or more times, leave the spinal cord, travel to the muscle, synapse, and depolarize the muscle (which is what is being recorded).

The treatment for piriformis syndrome most often consists of corticosteroid injections into the muscle, which theoretically relieves the muscle spasm. Gentle stretching of the piriformis muscle is also used. Avoidance of hip flexion, adduction, and internal rotation (i.e., crossing the legs) is advocated.

Common Peroneal Nerve Compression

Similar to ulnar nerve compression at the elbow, the common peroneal nerve is frequently compressed in the region of the fibular head. At this point, the nerve is superficial and very easily palpated. Compression from prolonged cross-legged sitting is well documented. EMG is helpful in determining the location of the lesion and in documenting a specific conduction block. Rarely, denervation is noted in the muscles supplied by the common peroneal nerve, except for the short head of the biceps femoris muscle, which is innervated proximally.

Cessation of the offending activity is often all that is necessary. In patients unable to move the legs or in anesthetized patients, protection of the peroneal nerve at the fibular head is essential.

Tarsal Tunnel Syndrome

Tarsal tunnel syndrome is a compression of the tibial nerve posterior to the medial malleolus. Because it is generally the result of anatomic factors and not overuse, it will not be discussed here.

Sural Nerve Compression

The sural nerve is a sensory nerve derived from the fibers of the tibial and peroneal nerves. It supplies sensation to the posterior lateral aspect of the distal leg. Sural nerve compression can occur from recurrent trauma or prolonged use of certain footwear (e.g., combat boots). It is conceivable to incur such injuries in very rigid boots such as ski boots or after frequent prolonged use of hard boots such as are worn in other activities (e.g., in-line skating). The location of the symptoms should lead the clinician to suspect a lesion of the sural nerve.

The sural nerve is very easily studied electrodiagnostically. However, given the limitations of sensory nerve conduction studies, a conduction block affecting 20% or fewer of the fibers may easily be missed, owing to the normal variability in sensory nerve action potential amplitudes obtained and the technical limitations of sensory studies. Sural nerve biopsies are rarely necessary in suspected cases, and a period of relative rest, including avoidance of the offending footwear, if applicable, should suffice.

Conclusion

Despite the great strides made in the past 20 or so years with regard to our knowledge of electrodiagnostic testing and computer technologies, our powers to diagnose many entrapment neuropathies remain limited. The one major exception to this is CTS; in fact, many electromyographers insist that CTS cannot exist in the absence of EMG evidence. As stated earlier, however, the existence of EMG-negative CTS is probable, although it occurs rarely. For most other entrapment neuropathies, in the absence of gross weakness or focal neurologic changes on examination, we are often unable to document the lesion definitively, because our best means of documenting subtle entrapments is through nerve conduction studies. Only in a few cases (e.g., the median nerve at the wrist and the ulnar nerve at the elbow) are we able to narrow the conduction studies to a short segment that is superficially located so we can detect accurately a small area of slowed conduction.

The median nerve at the wrist and the ulnar nerve at the elbow are also among the most commonly entrapped nerves. For these reasons, surgical releases for these two nerve entrapments (CTS to a greater degree and ulnar neuropathy at the elbow to a lesser degree) are the most commonly performed procedures of their kind. Surgical release in the carpal tunnel is exceptional because, in most patients, the operation is associated with very low morbidity and frequently returns the worker to work more quickly than a prolonged course of rest. In the case of definitively diagnosed CTS, it can be argued that surgical intervention is the most conservative form of treatment, as it can result in the least disruption of lifestyle and the most rapid resumption of normal activities. Nonetheless, current treatment often consists of immobilizing the worker. A temporary period of disability is observed while the patient waits for the symptoms to abate. Often, the original symptoms recur on resumption of work activities; meanwhile, months of employment and income have been lost.

Aside from these specific examples, the tenets of treating overuse injuries, specifically the period of relative rest and alteration of training schedules, is generally appropriate. We use the term *training* when referring to sports-related injuries. Similarly, alteration of the work requirements in occupational injuries frequently leads to resolution of symptoms. After symptoms resolve, activity can be resumed gradually in order to "work-harden" the tissues. This treatment method goes a long way toward restoring normal function without limitation.

References

1. Dumitru D. Electrodiagnostic Medicine. Philadelphia: Hanley & Belfus, 1995;119.
2. Rasminsky M, Seers TA. Internodal conduction in undissected demyelinated nerve fibers. J Physiol 1972;227:323.
3. Sunderland S. Traumatic injuries of peripheral nerves: simple compression injuries of the radial nerve. Brain 1945;68:56.
4. Parks BJ. Postoperative peripheral neuropathies. Surgery 1973;74:348.
5. Stewart JD. Focal Peripheral Neuropathies. New York: Elsevier Science, 1987;150.
6. Marie P, Foix C. Atrophie isolee de l'éminence thenar d'origine neuritique. Rôle du ligament annulare anterieur dans la localisation de la lesion. Rev Neural (Paris) 1913;26:647.
7. Magee DJ. Orthopedic Physical Assessment (2nd ed). Philadelphia: Saunders, 1987.
8. Potts F, Shahani BT, Young RR. A study on the coincidence of carpal tunnel syndrome and generalized peripheral neuropathy. Muscle Nerve 1980;3:440A.
9. Kimura J. Electrodiagnosis in Diseases of Nerve and Muscle: Principles and Practice (2nd ed). Philadelphia: Davis, 1989;500.
10. Ansen BJ. An Atlas of Human Anatomy (2nd ed). Philadelphia: Saunders, 1963.
11. Fendel W, Stratford J. The role of the cubital tunnel in tardy ulnar palsy. Can J Surg 1958;1:287.
12. Sunderland S. Nerve and Nerve Injuries. Edinburgh: Churchill Livingstone, 1978.
13. Fishman LM, Zieberg PA. Electrophysiologic evidence of piriformis syndrome. Arch Phys Med Rehab 1992;73:359.

Chapter 8
Cumulative Trauma Disorders in Sports

Jay Mitchell Weiss

Lower-Extremity Cumulative Trauma Disorders in Sports

Lower-extremity cumulative trauma disorders (CTDs) are frequently related to repetitive overloading. The fact that the lower extremities are usually called on to support the body's entire weight predisposes the lower extremities to certain types of injuries. It is difficult to conceive of a group of patients—with the exception of gymnasts and possibly paraplegics—who depend on the upper extremities to perform a significant amount of weight bearing.

Lower-extremity overuse injuries tend to be characterized by a common factor of recurrent lifting, especially of heavy loads. In the occupational setting, the incidence of such injuries is dwarfed by the incidence of back injuries. Many lower-extremity CTDs are athletically or recreationally induced. Errors in athletic training schedules or an intensive "weekend warrior" attitude on the part of some athletes commonly causes stressing of tissues that are not physiologically prepared for that level of strain. In this chapter, some of the more common sports-related CTDs of the lower extremities are discussed, as are the means of evaluating and treating them.

Leg pain should be adequately evaluated, and the tendency to "run through the pain" (i.e., exercise despite the pain) should be resisted. An adequate diagnosis must be sought. The healing period for a stress fracture varies from 1 month to more than 6 months, depending on the severity of the injury.

After an adequate healing period, activity should be resumed on a modified training schedule similar to that described in Table 8-1. Most lower-extremity overuse injuries respond to conservative treatment much more rapidly than do stress fractures, and therefore resumption of training can be initiated much earlier.

Stress Fractures

Stress fractures are due to repetitive strain that causes subtle tissue damage. This damage is compounded until it leads to tissue failure and clinical symptoms. In this case, the tissues are bone, and the microtrauma overwhelms the reparative capacity, causing stress fractures. Stress fractures are invariably attributable to CTDs.

Many of the best reports on stress fractures have come from military doctors. Because of the standard training regimen of military personnel, as well as the lack of individual freedom either to modify one's level of activity or to seek different treatment, military recruits are an ideal population for study. Data can be reliably obtained to document the specific training program. The group sample size is high, and patients are rarely lost to follow-up. Military recruits are discouraged from limiting activity owing to pain. This "no pain, no gain" philosophy is also found frequently among recreational and professional athletes. We must keep this lack of freedom in mind when evaluating studies. Nevertheless,

Table 8-1. Return to Running After Injury

Freedom from pain and tenderness during normal daily activities is essential before runners can return to training. On a scale of 0–10, where 0 is normal and 10 is severe pain, runners are asked to rate pain during normal activities; their rating must be 0 before training can resume.

I. If your pain score is 0: Run every other day for 2 weeks, then a maximum of 5 days per week for the next 4 weeks. If your previous training level was 4–6 miles per session, begin with 1 mile; if the previous level per session was less than 4 miles, begin with 0.5 mile per session. If you experience no pain while running, adhere to the following weekly mileage schedule (based on a previous training level of 4–6 miles per session):

	Miles per Day						
	Sunday	Monday	Tuesday	Wednesday	Thursday	Friday	Saturday
Week 1	1	0	1	0	1	0	2
Week 2	0	2	0	2	0	3	0
Week 3	3	2	0	3	3	0	4
Week 4	3	0	4	4	0	5	4
Week 5	0	5	5	0	6	5	0

II. If you experience short intervals of pain while running:
   A. Do not run for 2 weeks.
   B. Perform a 10-minute total workout, alternating a 4-minute run and a 1-minute walk. If no pain occurs, add 5 minutes every 3 days, working up to 30 minutes; then progress to the next step. If pain is experienced, cut back 5 minutes and work up.
   C. Perform a 15-minute total workout, alternating a 4.5-minute run and a 0.5-minute walk. If no pain occurs, add 5 minutes every 3 days, working up to 30 minutes; then progress to the next step. If pain is experienced, cut back 5 minutes and work up.
   D. Run steadily for 15 minutes, adding 5 minutes every 3 days. If pain is experienced, cut back 5 minutes and work up.

III. If you have pain after running:
   A. Decrease your mileage by 50% and progress by adding 10% a week.
   B. If you cut your workout 50% and still have pain, cut the workout again by 50% and progress by adding 10% per week.

IV. Running routine: Moist heat (5 minutes) → stretch → run as prescribed → ice massage (10 minutes). At night, moist heat (20 minutes) → stretch → weight lift → back exercises.

Source: Adapted with permission from DM Brody. Techniques in the evaluation and treatment of the injured runner. Orthop Clin North Am 1982;13:541.

the information obtained from large studies of military recruits can be extrapolated to nonmilitary personnel.

The prevalence of stress fractures (primarily of the lower extremities) in military recruits varies. Rates as low as 2% in the U.S. Army [1] and 5% in British paratroops recruits [2] have been reported. On the other end of the spectrum are reported rates of 30% in Israeli Army recruits [3] and up to 64% among Finnish soldiers [4].

Giladi et al. [3] followed a group of 312 recruits. In his study, soldiers were examined for stress fractures every 3 weeks during training. Soldiers with symptoms suggesting stress fractures were allowed 3 days of rest. If symptoms persisted, they were seen by an orthopedist. The diagnosis of stress fracture was made on the basis of a positive radiograph or scintigram (focal areas of increased uptake). Giladi et al. [3] found that 50% of the symptomatic recruits had stress fractures; 52% of these fractures were in the tibial diaphysis, 30% in the femoral diaphysis, and 9% in the metatarsals.

Anthropomorphic data indicate that women have relatively narrower bones than do men [5]. In one study of West Point cadets, women experienced 10 times the incidence of stress fractures compared to men [6], a finding that emphasizes the importance of body-part composition and tibial bone width to the propensity for stress fracture development. Other predisposing factors include osteoporosis (a factor with a female and Caucasian predominance) and excessive rotation of the hip [6]. As for most CTDs, a large increase in the frequency and duration of training in relatively unprepared individuals is cited as the primary cause of the injury.

The optimal treatment for stress fractures, as for most CTDs, is prevention. In addition to training errors, several mechanical factors may be modified. Compressive forces play a highly significant role in the development of stress fractures. Anything that minimizes the shock (primarily in the form of ground-reaction force) of activity involving the lower extremities is helpful. Viscoelastic shoe inserts or modification of the running surface (i.e., switching from artificial surfaces such as concrete or asphalt to a natural surface such as grass) are examples of means by which to minimize shock.

If localized tibial pain is believed to be due to a stress fracture, the period of rest will be considerably longer than for enthesitis or tendinitis. Generally, bracing is not required, and weight bearing can be permitted as long as high loads are avoided. During running, loads at impact can equal several times the weight of the body. Conventional radiographs are usually negative unless the stress fracture has progressed to an advanced stage. One of the dangers of overlooking a stress fracture is the potential for it to progress to a frank fracture from repeated insult.

Once a stress fracture has been diagnosed, treatment consists of relative rest, the cessation of training activities, and good nutrition. Obviously, after healing has occurred, care should be taken not to repeat the original training errors that caused the problem. Bone scan and radiographs should rule out a pathologic etiology for the fracture.

Achilles Tendinitis

Achilles tendinitis is one of the most common overuse injuries of the lower extremities. The Achilles tendon is the largest tendon in the body and must support nearly all the weight of the body. This tendon is the primary plantar flexor of the ankle. As

such, it is frequently called on to support the entire body weight. It is also rapidly stressed during ballistic movements such as jumping or landing.

Most Achilles tendon overuse injuries and frank disruptions occur within 6 cm of the calcaneal attachment, which corresponds with the watershed area, the area of the most tenuous blood supply [7]. This area is the histologic location of most disruptions of the internal tendon structures and of Achilles ruptures and is the clinical location of tenderness or pain.

The Achilles tendon gets most of its blood supply from the epitenon, the vascular connective tissue that coats the tendon. The epitenon is the continuation of the connective tissue covering the muscle.

Numerous mechanical factors predispose to Achilles tendinitis. Lack of stretching or frequent wearing of high-heeled shoes can lead to functional shortening of the tendon, which tends to decrease the tendon's elasticity. Shortening is usually accompanied by increased compensatory pronation of the foot, which tends to cause a twisting force on the tendon.

Like almost all other CTDs, training error, usually in the form of an increase in duration or frequency of exercise combined with a decrease in the resting interval, is often the precipitating factor in tendinitis. Changes in footwear are commonly reported by sufferers of Achilles tendinitis, even when no other specific alteration in training regimen can be observed.

Achilles tendinitis is common among women who take up running, especially when a significant part of the day is spent in high-heeled shoes. The combination of tightening of the Achilles tendon owing to the wearing of high-heeled shoes and the sudden demands made by running, especially if prior stretching is not done, places stress on the tendon.

Clinically, Achilles tendinitis patients most often complain of pain located in the distal aspect of the Achilles tendon several centimeters proximal to the calcaneus. The pain comes on after a period of exercise or strenuous walking. As the tendinitis progresses, the patient generally notes that the pain persists longer with each bout. The pain might even persist with rest or appear immediately on walking. Ankle dorsiflexion is frequently limited owing to pain.

On examination, the involved area of the tendon is often tender. Frequently, a swollen area can be palpated. A retrocalcaneal bursitis may manifest with symptoms similar to Achilles tendinitis. As with most overuse injuries, the early stages generally respond very well to a combination of anti-inflammatory agents and relative rest. Any training errors must be corrected before the patient reinitiates activity. If a recent change in athletic shoes predated the pain, the athletic shoes should be examined. If at all possible, the shoes should be changed. In those patients who do very well with a return to the type of athletic shoe originally worn, the importance of this factor should be stressed to the patient and he or she should be cautioned against switching again.

In more resistant Achilles tendon injuries, additional modalities are often necessary. As with any acute injury, cold should be used in the first 24–72 hours. Ultrasound is probably best used in the later stages of inflammation. When the symptoms have decreased, and before the patient's return to an activity, the patient should be started on a stretching program. If adequate stretching is not easily obtained with independent home exercises, then the patient should be given formal physical therapy to obtain an adequate stretch of the Achilles tendon. Stretching is one of the most important phases of therapy and is vital to preventing recurrence. Any return to activity should be done on a schedule that prevents overuse, for example, starting at less than 50% of the previous distance run and adding 1–2 minutes per mile. For a sample after-injury running program, see Table 8-1.

Shin Splints

The term *shin splint* is a nonspecific term that has various meanings, depending on who is using it. Generally, the term should be applied only to tibial pain, most often anteromedial pain on the midshaft of the tibia. Various etiologies have been proposed for shin splints. Undoubtedly, what are frequently categorized as shin splints usually constitute a combination of stress fractures, compartment syndromes, tendinitis, enthesitis, and muscle sprains or microtears.

Invariably, these are overuse injuries. The most commonly implicated activity is running. As with most running injuries, a detailed history, including the patient's running distance, frequency, rest intervals, and the type of surface and footwear, should

be examined in depth. Frequently, training errors in the form of a too-rapid increase in distance are implicated. Aside from compartment syndrome, all the etiologies of shin splints have in common the precipitating factor of overuse. Tissue failure occurs, owing either to an excessive load or to inability to heal in time for the next cycle of stress. Compartment syndrome can present in a similar manner. However, frequently there are associated paresthesias or hypoesthesias in the more distal parts of the extremity.

The etiology of an exertional compartment syndrome is hypertrophy of the muscle against a fixed, confining structure—in this case, the fascia. Intermittent claudication is due to the hypertrophy. In a chronic compartment syndrome, the symptoms frequently resolve with rest, which makes compartment syndrome difficult to distinguish from other causes of shin splints.

The chronic condition presents very differently from an acute compartment syndrome. In the acute form, compartment pressures are high, and immediate fasciotomy is required. In chronic exertional compartment syndrome, which is far more common than acute compartment syndrome, compartment pressures will likely be normal or high normal (but not specifically considered abnormal) during periods of rest. Peripheral pulses or Doppler ultrasonography might not be particularly helpful. Compartment pressure should be taken both at rest and after the patient has been running or exercising. Edwards and Myerson [8] do not recommend testing during exercise, because this is technically difficult and the movement makes readings less reliable. Pressures in excess of 10–15 mm Hg at rest and 15–25 mm Hg 5 minutes after exercise are considered diagnostic of compartment syndrome [9–13].

Enthesitis and Tendinitis

Enthesitis and tendinitis can occur from cumulative trauma to the insertion of the muscle or tendon with the bone or the tendon itself. These conditions are treated similarly in that a relative period of rest should be used to help promote early healing. Rest can be accomplished in conjunction with anti-inflammatory drugs and appropriate physical therapy. In mild cases, the healing should be relatively rapid, and the pain and tenderness should subside within a 1- to 2-week period. The goal is to resume training with a light schedule, which should enable the patient to progress gradually to the training level at which he or she was before the onset of symptoms. Enthesitis and tendinitis can be seen in all sports that involve running or repetition of lower-extremity movements.

Knee Disorders

Because of its mechanical structure, the knee, like most of the lower extremities, tends to develop overuse injuries owing to its weight-bearing characteristics. The upper extremities are rarely called on to support the entire body weight. The upper extremities, if used to support heavy loads, usually bear weight for a very limited time. For this reason, we see more skeletal abnormalities at the weight-bearing surfaces and their associated cartilage and apophyses than in the upper extremities. The soft-tissue symptoms, such as tendinitis and bursitis, are much less common in the knee than in the upper extremities. If such symptoms are a factor, frequently the cause is local irritation (e.g., housemaid's knee) or tendon overloading (e.g., patellar tendinitis).

Patellar Tendon Disorders

Pain in the patellar tendon is frequently referred to as *jumper's knee* because it is seen often in jumpers. Patellar tendon injuries are seen most commonly in sports, usually due to repetitive microtrauma. According to Nirschl [14], the histologic changes can be seen in the tendon itself and most often consist of mucoid degeneration and fibrinoid necrosis. Martens et al. [15] and King et al. [16] studied 18 patients with patellar tendon pain on activity who suffered persistent symptoms and failure to respond to lengthy conservative treatment. All patients were involved in sporting activities that required an explosive effort. The common finding on ultrasonography and computed tomography was expansion of the patellar ligament. Most injuries were treated conservatively in this series, and all patients were able to return to their original sport.

One commonly used staging system classifies patellar tendon injuries based on symptom charac-teristics [17–19]. In stage 1, pain appears after cessation of the activity and generally does not persist for a long time. In stage 2, pain occurs early in the course of the activity, disappears after warm-up, and recurs after activity. Stage 3 is characterized by pain that impairs function during and after activity, and stage 4 is complete tendon rupture.

Injuries in the first two stages are highly responsive to relatively conservative treatment, which consists of identifying and altering training errors, resting for a defined period, and increasing rest time between training sessions. Minimizing the explosive or ballistic forces placed on the tendon, combined with judicious use of ice and anti-inflammatory agents, generally allows the inflammation to subside. If decreased activity and increased rest intervals are not adequate, the patient should be prevented from participating in the offending activity for several weeks. Normal walking and other activities of daily living should be encouraged to prevent atrophy. It is relatively rare at stage 1 or 2 to require knee immobilization or other bracing, as cessation of the activity is usually adequate.

Stage 3 injuries can be handled conservatively on a trial basis. However, the activity restrictions should be much more stringent. It is important to realize that this is a continuum of symptoms, and the progression from one stage to another is somewhat arbitrary. Stage 4, tendon rupture, requires surgical repair.

Osgood-Schlatter Disease

The large mass of muscles that form the quadriceps group inserts on the patella. The patellar tendon then inserts on the relatively small tibial tubercle [20]. Osgood-Schlatter disease is epiphysitis or osteochondritis of the growth plate at the tibial tuberosity. Repeated contraction of the patellar tendon can lead to inflammation and partial avulsion at the secondary ossification center. Patellar tendon injuries should be separated from Osgood-Schlatter disease, which is a disorder of adolescence. The disease generally occurs during the rapid growth spurt of puberty, usually between years 10 and 12 in girls (although it can range from 8 to 13 and is often 1.0–1.5 years later in boys). In these patients, the area of greatest pain is at the tibial tuberosity. The pain is frequently aggravated by sports activities. In the early stages, plain radiographs are normal.

Later, radiographic changes include tuberosity fragmentation and soft-tissue changes.

On examination, an enlargement of the tibial tubercle is frequently present [21,22]. It is important to diagnose Osgood-Schlatter disease accurately to rule out other, more serious disorders, such as tumors or infection. Radiographs, along with routine blood work and a detailed examination, usually aid in diagnosis. Depending on the stage of the disease, enlarged or avulsed fragments may be visible on x-ray.

Treatment of Osgood-Schlatter disease does not generally extend beyond a period of cessation of heavy athletic activity. If he or she is on a sports team, the affected youth should be excused from that activity for a period of time. Generally, monthly checkups can be instituted. When the child is again asymptomatic during normal activities, including stair climbing and the normal running of childhood and adolescence, he or she can return to competitive sports on a limited basis. Progression of activities should be dictated by common sense, and the patient should be able to tolerate the activity at a certain frequency of play before gradually increasing the activity level. In more severe cases, it is not uncommon for a child to miss a season of play. However, with very few exceptions, these severely affected youths are almost all able to play the following season. Protracted symptoms or severe pain should be investigated to rule out tumor [21].

Patellofemoral Pain

Patellofemoral pain represents a group of disorders that have anterior knee pain in common. Most commonly, the pain is assumed to be due to compressive forces of the cartilage on the undersurface of the patella against the femoral condyles. Distal quadriceps tendinitis or enthesitis or proximal patellar tendon pain can be difficult to distinguish from patellofemoral pain. The factors aggravating both of these conditions are primarily contraction of the quadriceps against force, especially with the knee flexed. The term *chondromalacia* is frequently used, but this term refers to a specific pathologic process that is not always present. According to Reid [21], "Efforts to link what is obviously a constellation of etiologies and pathologies under one all encompassing term, *chondromalacia*, is not

likely to further the understanding of this difficult clinical problem."

Overloading of the joint, often in activities such as jumping or weight lifting, is a precipitating factor in patellofemoral pain. Milgrom et al. [23], in their prospective study of Israeli infantry recruits, found an approximate 15% incidence of patellofemoral pain among the subjects. "With only minimum periods of restriction of activity, all of the recruits who had patellofemoral pain due to overactivity were able to finish the training course." On follow-up 1 month later, these investigators found that approximately 60% of the knees still were symptomatic. According to Kujala et al. [24], increased height (which increased passive mediolateral range of motion) and unequal limb lengths were significant predisposing factors in exertional knee injuries in general. According to Milgrom et al. [23], increased medial tibial intercondylar distance and increased strength of the quadriceps are risk factors for patellofemoral pain caused by overactivity.

One of the mainstays of treatment is quadriceps-strengthening exercises, intended preferentially to strengthen the oblique musculi vastus medialis. Terminal extension exercises (from 15-degree knee flexion to neutral) help to strengthen the vastus medialis muscle. These exercises help to maintain the stability of the patella in the intercondylar groove between the femoral condyles. This is referred to as *patellar tracking*. This method of treatment is very effective when clinically the cause of the patellofemoral pain is patellofemoral laxity and an increased Q angle as opposed to a tight lateral retinaculum. The Q angle is the angle between a line from the center of the patella to the anterior superior iliac spine and a line from the center of the patella to the tibial tubercle—this angle is usually 15–20 degrees [25].

Treatment of patellofemoral pain by increasing the strength of the vastus medialis muscle might, at first glance, seem to be at odds with Milgrom's observation [23] that increased strength of the quadriceps muscle is a risk factor for this syndrome. Two arguments refute this theory, however. First, the patellofemoral pain that Milgrom et al. [23] described occurred in healthy young people who acutely increased their activities, including jumping and running. Generally, patellofemoral pain is encountered in a much older individual and is frequently brought on by normal daily activities such as ascending stairs. Second, Milgrom's group [23] was measuring maximum isometric strength of the quadriceps at 85-degree knee flexion. This is an overall measure of strength of the entire quadriceps group, of which the vastus medialis component is minor. In fact, a hypertrophied quadriceps would offer more lateral shear or stress to the patella and would therefore aggravate patellofemoral pain. Hence, this author believes that the rationale behind quadriceps-strengthening exercises (especially of the vastus medialis), even in the younger age group, is sound. As always, patients using these exercises should be monitored for any aggravation of symptoms.

A tight lateral retinaculum might cause a patient to fail to respond to terminal extension exercises. An inflexible lateral retinaculum would cause the quadriceps-strengthening exercises actually to put more strain on the patella rather than permitting the patella to stabilize by returning it to the anatomic groove. The inability of the patella to remain in the intercondylar groove between the femoral condyles is referred to as a *patellar tracking disorder*. A tight lateral retinaculum is one of the indicators for a lateral retinacular release, as quadriceps-strengthening exercises alone will not solve the underlying patellar tracking disorder.

Upper-Extremity Cumulative Trauma Disorders in Sports

Hand and Wrist Disorders

The hand is the part of the upper extremity that directly performs most repetitive actions. In most occupational or recreational activities, the function of the rest of the body, including the lower extremities, trunk, shoulder, elbow, and remainder of the upper extremity is to position the hand appropriately in space so that it can grasp, release, press, touch, or transport. With the exception of the hand's intrinsic muscles, most of the muscles involved in hand movement originate from the elbow region, which explains why repetitive hand movement often yields pathologic findings in the elbow and forearm.

Many hand injuries are due to acute as opposed to cumulative trauma. This is certainly predictable, given the role of the hand in most sports, especially

contact sports. In this chapter, however, we will concentrate only on those injuries related to cumulative trauma; evaluation and treatment of acute injuries are beyond the scope of this text.

Frequently, hand injuries due to cumulative trauma are not seriously attended to early in their course because the hand is not weight bearing and, in many instances, it can be immobilized relatively easily. A similar-level injury of the foot or lower extremity would render the injured individual incapable of walking and frequently bring him or her to medical attention relatively quickly. Left untreated, cumulative disorders of the hand can cause significant pain and disability.

de Quervain's Tenosynovitis

Probably the most common tendinous CTD of the wrist is de Quervain's tenosynovitis. In 1895, de Quervain described stenosing tenosynovitis of the abductor pollicis longus (APL) and extensor pollicis brevis (EPB) tendons (first dorsal compartment) [26], a disorder that still bears his name. de Quervain's disease is referred to as a stenosing tenosynovitis because the tendon sheaths become thick and restrictive. The patient's presenting symptom is pain just proximal to the radial styloid. The pain is reproduced or exacerbated by resisted ulnar deviation of the hand when the thumb is tucked into the fist (positive Finkelstein's sign) (Figure 8-1A). The tendons of the APL and EPB lie together in the most radial extreme of the wrist (Figure 8-1B). As such, they are active in radial deviation of the wrist and extension and radial deviation of the thumb. Whether the inflammation initiates within the tenosynovium or the tendon sheath itself is not clear [26,27].

As with most CTDs, a period of relative rest is usually indicated. However, because the hand is so involved in nearly every human activity, and because numerous wrist movements are performed without conscious effort, it is often not enough to use the relative rest principles that have been outlined elsewhere in this chapter. Specifically, cessation of the offending activity is not necessarily adequate because other injuries and stresses of the affected region will occur during the course of a day. A thumb spica splint usually is required for immobilization. A detailed history must be obtained to determine what specific changes in daily activi-

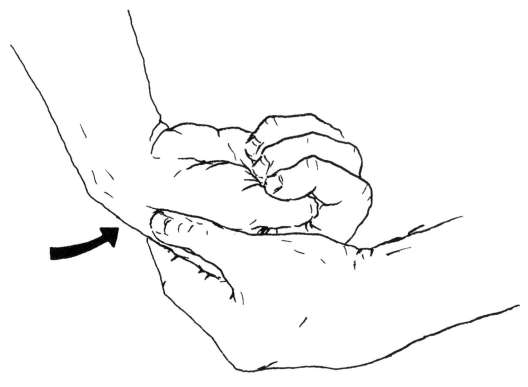

A

Figure 8-1. A. Finkelstein's test. The patient makes a fist and tucks in the thumb. The examiner then forces the hand into ulnar deviation. Pain over the abductor pollicis longus and extensor pollicis brevis tendons is consistent with de Quervain's tenosynovitis. B. Tendons involved in de Quervain's tenosynovitis. The abductor pollicis longus and extensor pollicis brevis tendons travel together in the first dorsal compartment. Tenderness occurs in the area of the radial styloid.

ties, occupational activities, or training activities corresponded with the onset of this injury.

Generally, enforced immobility is the mainstay of treatment, though anti-inflammatory medications are helpful adjuncts. Other physical therapeutic modalities, including underwater ultrasound, phonophoresis, iontophoresis, and ice, are helpful in some cases.

Refractory de Quervain's tenosynovitis frequently responds to injection with a corticosteroid in the region of the tendon sheath. Care must be taken to avoid the superficial branch of the radial nerve in such injections. As always, there is a likelihood that steroid injection might lead to weakening of the tendon and thereby increase the possibility of rupture.

Because the EPB tendon might occupy a separate compartment from the APL, steroid injection and immobilization might fail. In 20–30% of surgi-

cal cases, Froimson [28] found a septum dividing the first dorsal compartment into two separate tunnels. The incidence of separate tunnels is probably higher in refractory cases of de Quervain's tenosynovitis. Findings such as locking and clicking indicate significant stenosing of the tenosynovium and likely will require surgical release.

Intersection Syndrome

Intersection syndrome is much less common than de Quervain's tenosynovitis and therefore is diagnosed or considered infrequently. Intersection syndrome is presumed to be an inflammation at the point where the muscle bellies of the APL and EPB intersect as they travel medially and distally, crossing the radial wrist extensor, the extensor carpi radialis longus, and the extensor carpi radialis brevis. The area of tenderness is generally 4–6 cm

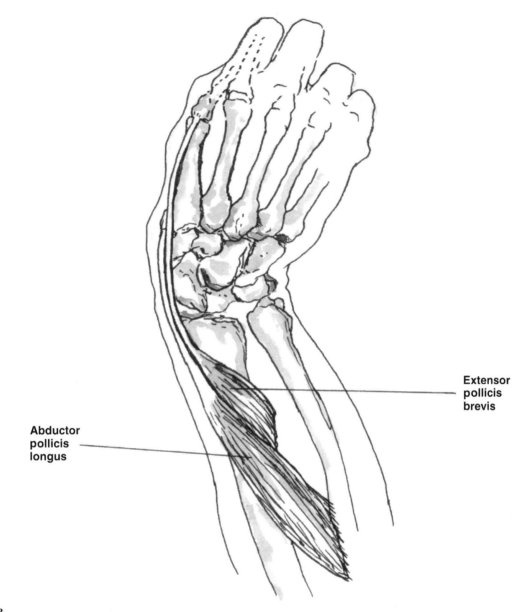

**Extensor
pollicis
brevis**

**Abductor
pollicis
longus**

B

proximal to the distal radius on the dorsal aspect of the arm.

As with other CTDs, relative rest along with splinting and anti-inflammatory medications are often adequate [29–31]. When given, corticosteroid injections are usually administered into the second dorsal compartment, as Grundberg and Regan [32] frequently found stenosing tenosynovitis of the second dorsal compartment.

Although less common, tenosynovitis has been variously diagnosed in the extensor pollicis longus, extensor digitorum communis, extensor digiti minimi, flexor carpi ulnaris, flexor carpi radialis, and flexor carpi ulnaris. This occurs relatively rarely, and the mainstay of treatment is the same as that for other CTDs. Although rare, tenosynovitis of the extensor pollicis longus can lead to rupture of the tendon and so must be considered. This condition was first reported approximately 100 hundred years ago by Dums [33], who observed it in Prussian drummers, which explains the origin of its alternative name, *drummer boy's palsy.*

Trigger Finger

Trigger finger results from a thickening of the proximal portion of the flexor tendon sheath around the metacarpophalangeal joint. Several reports have implicated direct pressure, such as prolonged forceful gripping of a racket or tool, as a causative factor [31,34]. Most cases, however, are idiopathic. It is postulated that prolonged mechanical irritation is sufficient to incite an inflammatory response that leads to trigger finger. Trigger finger frequently responds to corticosteroid injections in the region of the nodule. For a more detailed discussion of this condition, see Chapter 6.

Elbow and Wrist Joint Disorders

For several reasons, CTDs affecting the bones of the wrist area are a particular problem in gymnasts. Gymnastics, probably more than any other sport or activity, requires the wrist to accept primary weight-bearing responsibility for a significant amount of time. In addition, many of the movements, such as vaulting and floor handsprings, place a very large load on the wrist at impact. These factors alone would likely result in a great number of wrist injuries.

In addition, competitive women's gymnastics over the last several decades has come to be dominated by younger competitors, who are at greater risk for injuries owing to their skeletal immaturity. The prepubescent girl of short stature appears to have a significant advantage in many activities, notably the uneven parallel bars, for which height is an impediment. To compete at age 16, an athlete would have been required to undergo years of stressful training involving thousands of gymnastic movements during a skeletally immature age.

The fact that form is stressed in gymnastic maneuvers also places gymnasts at risk. Performance of a back handspring requires the maintenance of an extended elbow, without any flexion during the maneuver. Just as knee flexion during a landing acts as a shock absorber and dissipates some of the stress, elbow flexion during a back handspring would dissipate a significant amount of the compression force. However, elbow flexion during competition results in point deductions. Therefore, athletes are coached to perform these maneuvers in what is, biomechanically, a higher joint-loading situation [35]. Consequently, the stress is translated to the wrist.

These extremes of upper-extremity weight bearing and stress significantly affect both the elbow and wrist joints. We see valgus stresses in the elbow joint similar to those seen in pitchers, with lateral joint compression and medial joint distraction. Prolonged periods of wrist extension with weight bearing are grouped under the generic term *dorsiflexion jam syndrome.* Pain may be seen in different areas in the wrist, among these the wrist joint capsule, the carpal joints and bones, the distal radial epiphysis, and the triangular fibrocartilage complex. All probably play a part in various injuries.

Of note here is the distal radial epiphyseal stress syndrome, which appears to be effected by compressive forces. Wrist pain in this syndrome has been shown to increase with increased duration and intensity of workouts. This distal radial epiphyseal compression leads to radiographic abnormalities, such as widening and irregularity of the distal radial epiphysis. The compression has also been reported to lead to premature closure of the radial epiphysis [36]. After early radial epiphyseal closure with continual ulnar growth, the athlete might develop an acquired ulnar variance, which frequently leads to degenerative changes within the triangular fibrocartilage complex because of abnormal stress loads across this area [36].

Preventive therapy is infinitely preferable to surgical reconstruction, splinting, or any of the other interventions available. Training errors are the most common preventable problem among gymnasts. The pressure that coaches and parents put on these child athletes, and that the children impose on themselves, can be enormous. Any pain, especially wrist pain, must not be ignored.

Elbow Disorders

Anatomy of the Elbow

Before we look at specific elbow abnormalities and stresses, it is important to review the anatomy of the elbow. At first glance, the elbow appears to be one of the simpler joints of the body, acting essentially as a hinge. Whereas straight flexion and extension are the predominant motions of this joint, the elbow cannot be adequately examined or understood by defining it as just a single articulating hinge joint. In fact, the distal humerus has two articulating surfaces, the trochlear and capitellum. The trochlear articulates with the ulna; the capitellum articulates with the radial head.

In extension, the elbow joint is limited by the olecranon process of the ulna in the olecranon fossa of the humerus. Additionally, there is a radial ulnar articulation that permits pronation and supination.

In addition to bony stability and a joint capsule, medial and lateral collateral ligaments provide resistance against varus and valgus stresses, which are very common in the elbow. The distal end of the humerus becomes widened in a mediolateral direction just above the articulating surfaces, and these widened areas form the medial and lateral epicondyles. These bony protuberances are the origination point of most of the ventral and dorsal forearm muscles, respectively. The pronator teres, flexor carpi radialis, palmaris longus, flexor carpi ulnaris, and flexor digitorum superficialis originate totally or partially from the medial epicondyle. The extensor carpi radialis longus and brevis, extensor carpi ulnaris, and extensor digitorum communis originate from the lateral epicondyle. A great amount of stress from repetitive movement is transferred to these small bony areas.

The extended arm is in a slightly valgus position, averaging between 10 and 15 degrees, owing to an asymmetry of the trochlea posteriorly [37]. This valgus is referred to as the *carrying angle* of the elbow [38].

Lateral Epicondylitis

Probably the most common overuse injury of the elbow region and, in fact, one of the most common overuse injuries overall is lateral epicondylitis, often referred to as *tennis elbow*. Several authors cite both a medial and a lateral tennis elbow [20], but generally the term tennis elbow is reserved for lateral epicondylitis. Lateral epicondylitis was recognized more than 100 years ago [39]. Numerous anatomic locations and pathologies have been implicated in this disorder, but all agree that it is an injury of the

musculotendinous insertion of the wrist extensors at the region of the lateral epicondyle.

Nirschl and Petrone [40] reported the primary lesion to be pathologic alteration of the extensor carpi radialis brevis. Nirschl recommends the term *angiofibroblastic tendinosis*, referring to a degenerative process as opposed to an inflammatory process, because histologically inflammatory cells are not identified [41]. Other postulated primary lesions include a periostitis and enthesitis around the interdigitation of the common extensor tendon and the bone, a tendinitis of the common extensor tendon, and a tendinosis of the extensor digitorum communis [41].

Causes.   Although there is not complete agreement on the pathologic nature of lateral epicondylitis, most authors agree on its cause and treatment. The etiology is invariably one of cumulative trauma. As with most CTDs, epicondylitis is a function of the amount of strain placed on the common extensors combined with the duration and frequency with which those strains are applied and the rest interval between subsequent periods of use.

In most cases, the history is crucial in elucidating the specific characteristics of overuse. Lateral epicondylitis generally occurs in players older than 35 years [21,42]. Several factors tend to occur commonly in tennis players who complain of lateral epicondylitis. Among these are an acute increase in playing frequency and diminished rest time between periods of play. The body cannot compensate for the stresses imposed on it, which are frequently due to faulty mechanics.

Faulty mechanics, most often in the form of a poor backhand, often predispose a tennis player to lateral epicondylitis. Generally, a shot that leads with the elbow or a late swing requires a player to use excessive wrist extension to "save" the shot. Usually, these players use a single-handed backhand, which puts more stress on the lateral epicondyle. A new racquet or restringing of an old racquet at a higher level can transmit more pressure to the elbow. In the case of a new racquet, the grip should be checked to ensure that the racquet is the proper size for the playing hand. The easiest means of testing for this is to insert an index finger between the base of the thumb and the tips of the fingers of the playing hand while it grips the racquet normally. The index finger should fit snugly in that location (Figure 8-2A). An alternative method

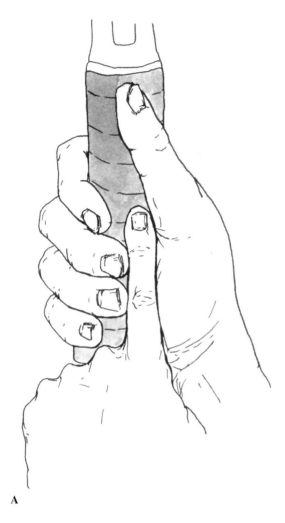

A

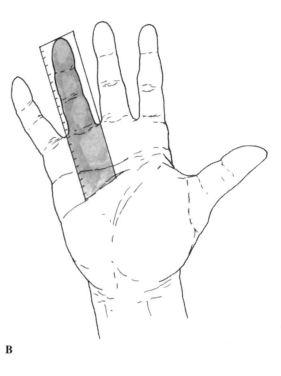

B

Figure 8-2. A. Method for properly sizing a grip on a tennis racquet. An index finger should fit snugly between the base of the thumb and the tips of the fingers. B. Alternative method for measuring a tennis racquet grip. The distance from the proximal palm crease to the tip of the fourth finger should equal the circumference of the grip.

is to measure the distance from the proximal palmar crease to the tip of the fourth finger. This measurement should equal the circumference of the racquet grip (Figure 8-2B).

The etiologic factors associated with lateral epicondylitis in tennis players are similar to the changes in intensity or specific demands that can be elicited in a comprehensive history of occupation-induced lateral epicondylitis. In the case of occupation-induced lateral epicondylitis, it is unlikely that the work frequency increased from once weekly to several times per week; more likely the proportion of time spent performing specific tasks has changed—for example, a typist who is working overtime during busy periods of the year or a person who is returning to work after a period away from

work. In either of these cases, as in the case of the tennis player, an increased demand was placed on tissues, and the regenerative and reparative capacity was overwhelmed.

The diagnosis of lateral epicondylitis depends to a large degree on the history. On physical examination, tenderness is commonly noted in the region of the lateral epicondyle. This tenderness is often aggravated by resisted extension of the wrist. There is also pain in this region on passive flexion of the wrist when the arm is fully extended.

Nirschl reports seven phases of pain in tendinitis [41]:

- Phase 1: Mild postexercise pain that resolves within 24 hours

- Phase 2: Postexercise pain that exceeds 48 hours and resolves with warm-up
- Phase 3: Exercise-induced pain that does not alter activity
- Phase 4: Exercise-induced pain that alters activity
- Phase 5: Pain caused by heavy activities of daily living
- Phase 6: Intermittent pain at rest that does not disturb sleep and is caused by activities of daily living
- Phase 7: Constant dull and aching rest pain and pain that disturbs sleep

The differential diagnosis of lateral epicondylitis, especially refractory lateral epicondylitis, should include posterior interosseous nerve syndrome. Therefore, a detailed neurologic examination of the strength of the more distally radial innervated muscles, particularly the extensor indicis proprius, should be performed. Diagnosis of posterior interosseus nerve syndrome is difficult on examination and, unfortunately, because of the nature of the entrapment, electrodiagnostic testing is often not helpful.

Treatment.   Lateral epicondylitis can generally be treated in phases. The first phase is a relative period of rest to minimize the cumulative trauma and to prevent the disorder from becoming chronic. This treatment rationale makes sense regardless of whether the fundamental abnormality is a degenerative one, as Nirschl proposes [41], or a truly inflammatory one.

In milder cases, rest alone will be adequate to promote healing. Ice after use of the affected area and anti-inflammatory medications are helpful adjuncts to treatment. In rare cases, corticosteroid injection may be beneficial or necessary. Physical therapy in the form of ultrasound, iontophoresis, or phonophoresis is helpful in resolving this disorder.

Later phases of treatment should be initiated after the area becomes asymptomatic. A flexibility and strengthening program for the lateral extensor group and an ergonomic assessment are features of this treatment phase. Any strengthening program should increase the load on the epicondyle gradually so as not to repeat the original injury or overwhelm the reparative capacity of the tissues. Usually, this is accomplished with wrist extension exercises, using manual resistance (by the therapist or the patient's

other hand), elastic bands, or other exercise equipment. The rationale behind the strengthening is that the extensor mechanism will build resistance to this repeated level of stress, thus allowing resumption of activities.

In tennis-induced lateral epicondylitis, abnormalities of mechanics that cause abnormal stresses of the region are seen. Several lessons with a teaching professional usually help the patient identify and correct certain mistakes, such as starting or swinging late and meeting the ball behind the body. The aforementioned racquet-grip or string abnormalities should be examined. Many patients find that wearing a tennis-elbow brace just distal to the elbow tends to dissipate the forces from the lateral epicondyle to surrounding tissues. Such a brace can also be used in lateral epicondylitis of occupational or industrial origin.

In refractory cases, local corticosteroid injection is frequently helpful. As is the case in most areas of the body, corticosteroid use should not be considered a first-line treatment as there is significant evidence that corticosteroid injection predisposes to tendon rupture. It does appear to be a reasonable treatment option, particularly for refractory lateral epicondylitis that is keeping a patient from work.

Surgical therapy for tennis elbow is nearly always successful, with positive results ranging from a low of 73% in the study by Goldberg et al. [43] to a high of 100% in Conrad and Hopper's group [44]. Most authors report a 90% or better success rate, regardless of the specific technique used. A significant component of the success of surgical intervention is probably subsequent immobilization and rest.

The patient's return to activity (whether occupational or sporting) should be monitored. A gradual return is preferable to starting and stopping because the patient has been reinjured. For the recreational tennis player, return to play may be limited to 0.5–1.0 hour of tennis once weekly for the first month, with gradual increases. Seasonal players should be reminded to begin strengthening in the early spring and to pace their return to the game.

Medial Epicondylitis

Medial epicondylitis, frequently referred to as *golfer's elbow*, is essentially the same lesion as lateral epicondylitis. However, this lesion is attributable to cumulative trauma or overuse of the wrist flexors. As opposed to lateral epicondylitis, which commonly occurs in occupational settings, medial epicondylitis is more common in recreational activities, such as throwing or golfing. The same predisposing factors, historic points, and treatment and rehabilitation should be stressed here.

Little League Elbow

The valgus stress of throwing leads to significant abnormalities that are age-dependent. In prepubescent and pubescent boys, the so-called Little League elbow is not uncommon. Generally, children do not develop overuse injuries or CTDs unless they participate in organized sports. Such participation causes children to practice and play at a frequency they would be unlikely to perform on their own. Little Leaguers tend to throw almost as many pitches in a game as does a professional pitcher. They also frequently play other positions on days when they are not pitching.

In 1965, Adams [45] reported that x-ray changes of elbows in boys aged 9–14 years were directly proportional to the amount of throwing the boys did and to whether they threw curve balls. Little League elbow was originally referred to as *medial epicondyle epiphysitis*. Little League elbow has more recently been used to refer to any of the stress-induced changes of the elbow related to overuse or overthrowing. In addition to the valgus stress on the medial part of the joint, lateral compression can lead to osteochondritis desiccans of the capitellum and radial head. These combinations of compression laterally on the joint and avulsion of the epiphysis have led to strict prohibitions of curve balls in young Little League players and overall limitations in their training.

On examination, the characteristic findings are pain and tenderness with loss of full arm extension. In older pitchers, laxity of the medial collateral ligament and traction spurs frequently are noted. Ulnar neuropathies at the elbow are common, owing to the stresses placed on the ulnar nerve as it passes through the medial epicondyle.

The clinical findings associated with an ulnar neuropathy at the wrist are numbness in the fifth digit and the ulnar side of the fourth digit. The workup for this disorder includes electrodiagnostic testing, which is discussed in detail in Chapter 7. Recurrent ulnar neuropathies, either from throwing or from a cubital tunnel syndrome, frequently require surgical treatment, including transposition of the nerve to a more anterior position and covering of the nerve by muscle. Such therapy is usually curative.

Treatment of Little League elbow is predicated primarily on a period of relative rest. At times, splinting or immobilization may be helpful. Detailed treatment of this specific overuse injury is beyond the scope of this text. However, the clinician must retain a high index of suspicion for this disorder in a young pitcher, as early intervention in the form of relative rest and cessation of the offending activity is the best treatment.

Olecranon Bursitis

An olecranon bursitis can result either from trauma or from overuse. This condition is generally characterized by tenderness and swelling posterior to the olecranon and is usually relieved by avoidance of pressure on the area, ice, and anti-inflammatory agents. Corticosteroid injection into the bursa is usually beneficial. Infection must be ruled out, especially if the area appears warm.

Other Common Overuse Injuries of the Elbow

Whereas medial and lateral epicondylitis are the most common overuse injuries seen in the elbow region, many other less common overuse injuries occur in this region. Nirschl [41] refers to a posterior tennis elbow or tendinosis, which is a degenerative lesion of the insertion of the triceps tendon.

Shoulder Disorders

It is generally accepted that CTDs of the lower extremities are primarily sport and activity related, whereas CTDs of the upper extremities are primarily occupation related. There are, of course, numerous exceptions for most body regions, but the rule generally is valid. Most of the lower-extremity musculotendinous and ligamentous injuries we see are related to sports activities or walking or running. In the upper extremities, we much more often see overuse injuries of the wrist and forearm, elbow, and upper trapezius muscle due to abnormal sitting postures. Although there are numerous sports-related injuries to the wrist and especially to the epicondylar regions of the elbow, in volume they are probably far outnumbered by occupational injuries.

A glaring exception to this rule is shoulder injury. For our discussion, we consider the shoulder to include the glenohumeral joint, the scapulothoracic articulations, the acromioclavicular and sternoclavicular joints, and the tendons that approximate the subacromial region. Cumulative sports injuries play a much more prominent role than occupational injuries in the etiology of shoulder problems, owing primarily to the unique anatomy of the shoulder and the fact that the greatest stresses fall on the structures in the subacromial space with overhead movements. Furthermore, in sports, these stresses are compounded with forceful movements, especially forceful eccentric movements.

Anatomy of the Shoulder

Calliet [46] describes seven joints that make up the shoulder: glenohumeral, suprahumeral, acromioclavicular, scapulocostal, sternoclavicular, sternocostal, and costovertebral. According to Reid [21], the shoulder girdle is traditionally considered to comprise the following joints: sternoclavicular, acromioclavicular, and glenohumeral and the scapulothoracic articulation. Reid [21] proposed that the pathologic unit, in addition to the bony articulations just mentioned, also includes the biceps tendon, the coracoacromial arch, and the thoracic outlet and first costosternal and costovertebral joints.

The sternoclavicular joint is the articulation of the proximal end of the clavicle with the sternum and, as such, is the only bony contact of the upper limb with the axial skeleton. At its distal end, the clavicle articulates with the acromion at the acromioclavicular joint. The coracoacromial ligament travels from the inferior part of the acromioclavicular joint to the coracoid process and is usually confluent with the inferior capsule of that joint.

These structures, especially the acromioclavicular joint, are frequently injured in trauma. These structures are also important in CTDs of the shoulder. The rotator cuff and subacromial bursa are frequently squeezed between the humeral head and the undersurface of the acromion and coracoacromial ligament.

The glenohumeral joint is the ball-and-socket part of the shoulder. However, because of the large amount of movement permitted in this region, the shoulder joint is much less of a true ball and socket than is the hip joint. In addition to rotation of the humeral head against a fixed glenoid socket, there is also gliding within the joint without rotation, and rolling (rotation with a shifting axis of rotation).

Generally, if the arm is to abduct a full 180 degrees, approximately 120 degrees of abduction occurs at the glenohumeral joint. The remaining 60 degrees is scapulothoracic motion [47]. Most of the articulating surface of the humeral head is smooth and spherical. The head is mounted on the neck of the humerus, which has both a greater and a lesser tuberosity. The former is located superolaterally, whereas the latter is located anteromedially. Between these tuberosities lies the bicipital groove, in which the biceps tendon travels.

The glenoid labrum is a fibrocartilaginous rim that functionally deepens the glenoid and adds stability to the glenohumeral joint [48]. The glenohumeral joint capsule is a fibrous structure having sufficient laxity to permit the normal wide range of shoulder movement. However, at various positions, different fibers within this capsule are taut and limit further movement, thus enhancing stability.

The scapulothoracic articulation is not a true joint but a complex functioning of bony, muscular, and ligamentous structures working together to permit gliding of the scapula against the thoracic wall while maintaining a very stable platform for the upper extremity. This anatomic makeup permits enormous loads to be placed on the upper extremity, despite the near-complete absence of a bony articulation between that upper extremity and the trunk or axial skeleton. The only bony articulation found there is a small sternoclavicular articulation, separated from the axial skeleton by the costosternal and costovertebral articulations.

The rotator cuff consists of the muscles and associated tendinous insertions of the supraspinatus, infraspinatus, subscapularis, and teres minor muscles. The supraspinatus muscle lies on the dorsal surface of the scapula above the scapular spine. It continues laterally into the shoulder region, where it passes between the humeral head and the acromion and inserts on the greater tuberosity. The infraspinatus and teres minor muscles also insert on the same region, forming the rotator cuff. The action of the infraspinatus and teres minor muscles is primarily one of external rotation, whereas the supraspinatus muscle is primarily an abductor.

Shoulder Pain

Numerous high-powered tests, including magnetic resonance imaging, arthrography, computed tomography with and without contrast, bone scanning, and arthroscopy, are available to the examiner. Although these tests can be important in ruling out or confirming suspected diagnoses, the initial evaluation centers on an adequate history. Such patient factors as age, the type of sport played, and the level of participation are important in making a diagnosis. As discussed earlier in this chapter, a patient's training pattern—including duration of play, frequency of training, and amount of time allotted for rest between training sessions—is always crucial in determining training errors that can be causative factors in CTDs.

According to Job [49], shoulder pain in athletes can generally be divided into three groups: (1) post-traumatic, (2) instability complex, and (3) neurovascular. Post-traumatic problems are usually obvious on the basis of the history. With regard to CTDs, the differential diagnosis falls primarily between instability complexes and neurovascular problems.

The location of the pain, specific activities that initiate it, and its timing relative to the workout (during activity or some time after activity) all help to clarify the diagnosis. The duration of the pain and its persistence at night are highly significant in shoulder injuries. Classically, a rotator cuff tendinitis is painful during overhead activities such as throwing and serving, whereas nocturnal and rest pain are common in a rotator cuff tear [50].

Generally, young athletes (<35 years) who engage in sports requiring overhead activities tend to present with anterior shoulder symptoms secondary to instability and impingement. In older athletes, the likelihood of degenerative changes at the rotator cuff and associated structures increases [49].

Subacromial Pain Syndrome and Impingement Syndrome

Impingement syndrome usually refers to an impingement or compression of the rotator cuff

tendons or the subacromial bursa (as well as the biceps tendon) in the subacromial space between the acromion, acromioclavicular joint, or coracoacromial ligament and the greater tuberosity of the humerus. In the past, the term *impingement syndrome* (impingement of the supraspinatus tendon by the coracoacromial ligament) was used as a wastebasket term to refer to any anterior shoulder pain. A more accurate term for anterior shoulder pain is *subacromial pain syndrome* (SPS). Certainly, impingement syndrome is a significant part of SPS. However, in cases in which the impingement is not secondary to arthritic factors but is secondary to instability, the instability itself should be considered the primary diagnosis.

Impingement leads to rotator cuff tendinitis. Although the rotator cuff is probably the main culprit in SPS, other structures—including the biceps tendon, subscapularis tendon, pectoralis major tendon, triceps tendon [51], and subacromial bursa—are frequently the causes of pain on overhead movement. The complex interactions of the muscles and tendons of the shoulder, including the rotator cuff and scapula stabilizers, are necessary to maintain shoulder stability, especially with forceful overhead movements. Lack of coordination of these complex muscular functions has been implicated in impingement syndrome [52].

Baseball Pitching and Tennis Serving. The common factors in SPS, be it in young athletes or in older professional athletes and recreational players, are overhead activities. Baseball pitching is a common cause of SPS or impingement syndrome. Generally, baseball pitching is limited to younger athletes. For the most part, baseball is not a lifetime sport, and we rarely see people in their thirties, forties, and fifties who continue to play baseball at an intense level. The great majority of people who continue to play generally switch to softball, which uses an underhand pitching style that rarely causes shoulder problems.

Despite the advent of senior baseball leagues, the number of shoulder injuries in older recreational baseball players is dwarfed by the number of tennis injuries seen by clinicians. The tennis serve is implicated in most SPSs. Tennis players can continue playing through all phases of life. Middle-aged and older players are more likely to have osteoarthritic shoulder abnormalities, poor vascularity, and poorer tissue healing than their younger counterparts. All these factors make the shoulder less likely to resist overuse injury.

The tennis serve is probably much less noxious and injurious to the shoulder than is pitching in baseball, as revealed by a study of the number of serves that can be performed by a professional tennis player versus the number of pitches that can be performed by a professional baseball player [20]. A starting pitcher generally pitches 120 balls per game. He will invariably refrain from pitching for 1 day or longer after pitching a full game. A tennis player, on the other hand, frequently hits upward of 100 serves in a match and, conceivably, as many as 150 serves in a hard-fought match. The velocity of the tennis serve is frequently clocked at more than 120 mph, though some serves have been recorded at more than 130 mph [20]. Nonetheless, professional tennis players commonly play at this level several days in a row or with no more than a 1-day break between matches. A professional baseball pitcher could not approach this frequency.

Swimming. Although there are many differences in the mechanics of the pitching and serving movements, a major one appears to be the extremes of external rotation performed in baseball pitching, which are generally not matched in tennis [20]. Other activities, including swimming, commonly cause SPS. Swimming differs from the other two cited overhead activities in that we rarely see the same degree of eccentric strain in swimming that we do in baseball pitching or tennis serving. Throughout swimming, there is a concentric contraction against active resistance—in this case water—and there is much less inertial force with which the shoulder muscles must contend. For this reason, more than an overload tendinitis is commonly implicated in swimming impingement.

Significance of the Supraspinatus Tendon. Neer [53] studied a series of anterior acromioplasties for chronic impingement syndrome in 1972. The area described by Neer [53] as impinging was found by Rathbun and MacNab [54] to be an avascular or watershed zone within the supraspinatus tendon. These investigators demonstrated a similar avascular area in the biceps tendon as it traverses the subacromial space.

Over time, impingement syndrome or other SPSs can lead to partial or complete tears of the rotator cuff. In addition, the pain elicited from an active impingement syndrome causes further incoordination of muscle firing and can lead to additional irritation or tearing of the muscle.

Most authors report that shoulder pain in younger athletes may be more a complication of instability and overload tendinitis than of mechanical impingement. The fundamental structural abnormalities reported are fatigue of the supraspinatus tendon and abnormal muscular activity, leading to overloading of the tendon. Generally, because the greatest stress is during the eccentric contraction or during deceleration of the arm in sports requiring overhead actions, it is believed that most of the damage occurs at this stage of throwing. In most cases, the instabilities are subtle and difficult to detect on a conventional shoulder examination.

Physical Examination. Numerous physical examination tests have been described to assess shoulder pain. For further detail, the interested reader is referred to Magee's *Orthopedic Physical Assessment* [55]. Some of the more widely used tests are the Neer anterior impingement test, the Hawkin's test, Speed's and Yergason's tests (both for bicipital tendinitis), the apprehension sign, the anterior instability test, and relocation tests [22]. With impingement syndrome and other SPSs, one is looking primarily for an area of pain with overhead motion, especially in extremes of rotation combined with elevation that will rotate the greater tuberosity into the acromion and coracoacromial arch regions. Generally, there should be near pain-free passive range of motion below approximately 80 degrees of elevation, with the exception of severe inflammation. Pain in the elevated arm is characteristically aggravated by resistance to abduction. In the extremes of inflammation or rotator cuff tear, a drop-arm test may be positive. A positive drop-arm test is defined as the inability to maintain the arm abducted approximately 90 degrees owing to pain during range of motion.

Treatment. The treatment for the impingement syndrome and SPSs in general can be broadly broken down into two large phases. Phase 1 consists of resolution of the inflammation; phase 2 consists of strengthening of the overall complex to permit the patient to return to the offending activity without inflicting further damage.

Generally, the external rotators of the shoulder are imbalanced as compared with the internal rotators. The supraspinatus combined with the other rotator cuff muscles and, to some degree, the subscapularis maintain the humeral head in a functional part of the glenoid fossa and minimize its anterosuperior translation against the coracoacromial arch and acromion. When these muscles are overloaded or fatigued, the likelihood of impingement is greater, and the imbalances are more likely to produce an overload tendinitis. The type of strengthening exercise—isometric, isokinetic, or isotonic—that is best for such injuries is debated in the literature. Each type has its advantages and disadvantages. However, isokinetic exercise makes it easier to quantify strength and follow improvements in strength. Nonetheless, the optimal means of strengthening is still disputed.

Much attention has been paid to strengthening the external rotators. Because of the muscular actions in athletes, the external rotators generally appear to be underdeveloped in relation to their antagonists. Overall strengthening of both muscle groups is beneficial and avoids having to determine a specific ratio of external rotator to internal rotator strength.

Wolf [51] divides SPS into four stages, each of which is treated differently. Stage 1 is passively reversible tendinitis and bursitis. Stage 2 involves secondary changes that Wolf characterizes as "actively reversible." These changes require more aggressive treatment than stage 1 injuries and, occasionally, some refractory cases require surgical therapy. Stage 3 is characterized by tertiary, surgically correctable structural changes, such as partial or full-thickness rotator cuff tears or anatomic changes to the subacromial space. Stage 4 is end-stage uncorrectable but treatable structural change. Clearly, SPSs are best evaluated and identified at stage 1. At this stage, little more than relative rest (cessation of the offending activity) combined with anti-inflammatory medications is necessary. Frequently, recreational tennis players can be permitted to return to tennis at this stage, with the restriction that they not perform any overhead activities.

In more advanced stages, other therapeutic interventions might be necessary. One intervention that is both diagnostic and therapeutic is a subacromial injection of lidocaine, generally in combination with a corticosteroid. Usually, there is a notable decrease in the patient's perception of pain because of the anesthetic effect of the lidocaine. It should be stressed to the patient that there has been no healing but merely a blocking of the pain. Activities should be limited after the injection. Without pain to limit the activity, the possibility of causing further damage increases. The cortisone component generally starts to take effect after the lidocaine wears off and, in that sense, the injection is primarily therapeutic. Many authors recommend limiting the number of injections in SPSs to no more than three per year [49]. Each additional injection is believed to increase the likelihood of tendon rupture. Clinically, if a patient is not helped by three injections, it is unlikely that additional injections will be beneficial. Often one injection is very helpful, though an additional injection may be necessary.

In certain refractory cases, surgical intervention is an option. However, in the majority of cases that are diagnosed at a relatively early stage, an operation should not be necessary.

Several authors have postulated that dynamic isokinetic testing of internal and external rotators is useful to look for muscular imbalances that would predispose to instability, which could result in traction overload tendinitis [51]. Chandler et al. [56], in a study of the internal and external rotators of the shoulder of college-level tennis players, found the internal rotators to be dominant. They theorized that the ability of the external rotators to handle the force loads created in a repetitive internal rotation movement, such as the tennis serve, might predispose the athlete to shoulder injury. They further recommended exercises to increase the external rotation strength [56]. Currently, these recommendations are considered a mainstay of an SPS rehabilitation program.

Although these muscle imbalances are seen frequently in throwing athletes and it is hypothesized that the imbalances are a factor in the etiology of shoulder injury in such athletes, few well-controlled prospective studies prove these factors to be the precipitating agents. Nonetheless, it is unlikely that any harm will come of actively strengthening the shoulder muscles. Empirically, such treatment makes good sense.

Bicipital Tendinitis

Bicipital tendinitis is frequently associated with supraspinatus tendinitis or SPS. Yergason's and

Speed's signs are helpful in diagnosing this syndrome, although often the only finding on physical examination is tenderness over the bicipital tendon in the bicipital groove. As with SPS, a local cortisone injection is generally helpful. The injection should be around the tendon sheath or in the tendon sheath but not in the substance of the tendon itself.

It has been postulated that shoulder overuse can cause vascular abnormalities. Rohrer et al. [56] describe the case of a 28-year-old major league baseball pitcher who sustained an axillary artery thrombosis. To determine whether the condition was sports related, baseball pitchers were studied. In examining asymptomatic limbs of the pitchers, the authors found a greater than 20–mm Hg blood pressure drop to the pitching arm in a throwing position in 56% of the pitchers studied. In 13% of the extremities, a loss of detectable blood pressure occurred. The investigators documented compression of the axillary artery by the humeral head in 83% of the extremities. They postulated that repeated pressure and compression of the axillary artery led to the thrombosis. Although axillary artery thrombosis due to pitching is relatively rare, examiners should be aware of it.

Cumulative Trauma Disorders in Children

As mentioned elsewhere, CTDs or overuse injuries in children are traditionally rare, as children have better recuperative powers than do adults and naturally alter activities to cross-train without any conscious effort. However, when overuse injuries do occur, they tend to affect children in such organized athletic activities as Little League baseball or gymnastics, tennis, or any other activity in which the child is forced or strongly encouraged to commit hours to one specific discipline. Albert and Drvaric [58] reported a case of Little League shoulder that showed widening of the physeal plate accompanied by metaphyseal fragmentation due to repetitive pitching motion. In the case report, the patient was restricted from athletic activities and was re-examined after 8 weeks, at which time the shoulder was found to be normal. More often than not, however, the offending factor is the parent or coach, who pushes the physical (and psychological) limits of the child beyond what is medically (or socially) appropriate.

References

1. Skully TJ, Besterman G. Stress fracture: a preventable training injury. Mil Med 1982;147:285.
2. Gill RMF, Hopkins GO. Stress fracture in parachute regiment recruits. J R Army Med Corps 1988;134:91.
3. Giladi M, Milgrom C, Simkin A. Stress fractures: identifiable risk factors. Am J Sports Med 1991;19:647.
4. Sahi T. Stress fractures. Rev Int Serv Sante Armees Terre Mer l'Air 1984;57:311.
5. Miller GJ, Purkey WW Jr. The geometric properties of paired human tibiae. J Biomech 1980;13:1.
6. Protzman TR, Griffis CG. Stress fractures in men and women undergoing military training. J Bone Joint Surg Am 1977;59:825.
7. Lagergen C, Lindholm A. Vascular distribution in Achilles tendon—an angiographic and microangiographic study. Acta Chir Scand 1958;116:491.
8. Edwards P, Myerson MS. Exertional compartment syndrome of the leg: steps for expedient return to activity. Phys Sports Med 1996;24:4.
9. Rorabeck CH. Exertional tibialis posterior compartment syndrome. Clin Orthop 1986;208:61.
10. Rorabeck CH, Bourne RB, Fowler PJ, et al. The role of tissue pressure measurement in diagnosing chronic anterior compartment syndrome. Am J Sports Med 1988;16:143.
11. Rorabeck CH, Fowler PJ, Nott L. The results of fasciotomy in the management of chronic exertional compartment syndrome. Am J Sports Med 1988;16:224.
12. Fronek J, Mubarak SJ, Hargens AR, et al. Management of chronic exertional anterior compartment syndrome of the lower extremity. Clin Orthop 1987;220:217.
13. Pedowitz RA, Toutounghi FM. Chronic exertional compartment syndrome of the forearm flexor muscles. J Hand Surg [Am] 1988;13:694.
14. Nirschl RP. Patterns of Failed Healing in Tendon Injury. In WB Leadbetter, JA Buckwalter, SL Gordon (eds), Sports Induced Inflammation: Clinical and Basic Science Concepts. Park Ridge, IL: American Academy of Orthopedic Surgery, 1989.
15. Martens M, Wouters P, Burssens A, Muller JC. Patellar tendinitis: pathology and results of treatment. Acta Orthop Scand 1982;53:445.
16. King JB, Perry DJ, Mourad K, Kumar SJ. Lesions of the patellar ligament. J Bone Joint Surg Br 1990;72:46.
17. Blazina MB, Kerlan RK, Jobe FW, et al. Jumper's knee. Orthop Clin North Am 1973;4:665.
18. Roels J, Martens M, Muller JC, Burssens A. Patellar tendinitis (jumper's knee). Am J Sports Med 1978;6:362.
19. Nichols CE. Patellar tendon injuries. Clin Sports Med 1992;11:807.

20. Kulund DN. The Injured Athlete (2nd ed). Philadelphia: Lippincott, 1988.
21. Reid DC. Sports Injury Assessment and Rehabilitation. Edinburgh: Churchill Livingstone, 1992;199.
22. Magee DJ. Orthopedic Physical Assessment. Philadelphia: Saunders, 1987;380.
23. Milgrom C, Finestone A, Eldad A, Shlamkovitch N. Patellofemoral pain caused by overactivity. A prospective study of risk factors in infantry recruits. J Bone Joint Surg 1991;73:1041.
24. Kujala UM, Kvist M, Österman K, et al. Factors predisposing army conscripts to knee exertion injuries in a physical training program. Clin Orthop 1986;210:203.
25. Weissman BN, Sledge CB. Orthopedic Radiology. Philadelphia: Saunders, 1986;508.
26. Conklin JE, White WL. Stenosing tenosynovitis and its possible relation to the carpal tunnel syndrome. Surg Clin North Am 1960;40:531.
27. Wood MB, Dobyns JH. Sports related extra-articular wrist syndromes. Clin Orthop 1986;202:93.
28. Froimson AI. Tenosynovitis and Tennis Elbow. In DP Green (ed), Operation Hand Surgery. New York: Churchill Livingstone, 1988;2118.
29. Kiefhaber TJ, Stern PJ. Upper extremity tendinitis and overuse syndromes in the athlete. Clin Sports Med 1992;11:39.
30. Pyne JIB, Adams BD. Hand tendon injuries in athletics. Clin Sports Med 1992;11:833.
31. Hosterman AL, Moskow L, Lowe DW. Soft tissue injuries of the hand and wrist in racquet sports. Clin Sports Med 1988;7:329.
32. Grundberg AB, Regan DS. Pathologic anatomy of the forearm, intersection syndrome. J Hand Surg 1985;10:299.
33. Dums F. Uber Trommlerlahmungen. Dtsh Militarztliche Z 1986;25:144.
34. Lipscomb PR. Tenosynovitis of the hand and wrist: carpal tunnel syndrome, de Quervain's disease, trigger digit. Clin Orthop 1959;13:165.
35. Koh TJ, Grabiner MD, Weiker GG. Technique and ground reaction forces in the back handspring. Am J Sports Med 1992;20:61.
36. Weiker GG. Hand and wrist problems in the gymnast. Clin Sports Med 1992;11:189.
37. Yocum LA. The diagnosis in non-operative treatment of elbow problems in the athlete. Clin Sports Med 1989;8:439.
38. Beals RR. The normal carrying angle of the elbow. Clin Orthop 1976;119:194.
39. Morris H. The rider's sprain. Lancet 1882;2:133.
40. Nirschl RP, Pettrone FA. Tennis elbow: the surgical treatment of lateral epicondylitis. J Bone Joint Surg Am 1979;61:832.
41. Nirschl RP. Elbow tendinosis/tennis elbow. Clin Sports Med 1992;11:851.
42. Nirschl RP. Soft tissue injuries about the elbow. Clin Sports Med 1986;5:637.
43. Goldberg EJ, Abraham E, Siegel I. The surgical treatment of lateral humeral epicondylitis by common extensor release. Clin Orthop 1988;233:208.
44. Conrad RW, Hopper WR. Tennis elbow: its course, nature, history, conservative and surgical management. J Bone Joint Surg Am 1973;53:117.
45. Adams JE. Injury to the throwing arm. A study of traumatic changes in the elbow joints of boy baseball players. Calif Med 1965;102:127.
46. Calliet R. Shoulder Pain (3rd ed). Philadelphia: Davis, 1991.
47. Freedman L, Monroe RR. Abduction of the arm in the scapular plane, scapular and glenohumeral movements: a roentgenographic study. J Bone Joint Surg Am 1968;48:1403.
48. Reid DC. Assessment and Treatment of the Injured Athlete [teaching manual]. Edmonton: University of Alberta, 1989.
49. Job FW, Bradley JP. The diagnosis and nonoperative treatment of shoulder injuries in athletics. Clin Sports Med 1989;8:420.
50. Shields CL, Glousman RE. Open Management of Rotator Cuff Tears. In W Grana, JA Lombardo, BJ Sharkey, JA Stone (eds), Advances in Sports Medicine and Fitness, vol 2. Chicago: Year Book Medical, 1989;223.
51. Wolf WB. Shoulder tendinoses. Clin Sports Med 1992;11:871
52. Perry J. Biomechanics of the Shoulder. In CR Enroe (ed), The Shoulder. New York: Churchill Livingstone, 1988.
53. Neer CS. Anterior acromioplasty for the chronic impingement in the shoulder. J Bone Joint Surg Am 1972;54:41.
54. Rathbun JB, MacNab I. Microvascular pattern of the rotator cuff. J Bone Joint Surg Br 1970;52:541.
55. Magee DJ. Orthopedic Physical Assessment (2nd ed). Philadelphia: Saunders, 1992.
56. Chandler TJ, Kibler B, Stracener EC, et al. Shoulder strength, power and endurance in college tennis players. Am J Sports Med 1992;24:455.
57. Rohrer MJ, Cardullo PA. Axillary artery compression and thrombosis in throwing athletes. J Vasc Surg 1990;11:761.
58. Albert MJ, Drvaric DM. Little League shoulder: case report. J Orthop 1990;13:779.

Chapter 9

Cumulative Trauma Disorders in Musicians and Dancers

Arminius Cassvan

Historical Perspectives

There is an extensive body of literature on repetitive strain injuries or cumulative trauma disorders (CTDs) in musicians and dancers. Historical reviews relating to CTDs in musicians are more plentiful than those relating to dancers [1–3] and date back to Bernardino Ramazzini (1633–1714). One year before his death, Ramazzini [4] published his most notable book, *De Morbis Artificans* (*Diseases of Workers),* in which he mentions ailments of singers but also of "flautists" and "those who play the pipes." The infirmities incurred by these musicians were attributed by Ramazzini [4] to overuse: The singers developed hoarseness, severe colds, and hernias, whereas the two types of instrumentalists he discussed displayed puffed-out cheeks and were prone to "ruptures of the vessels of the chest."

Writer's Cramp and Related Disorders in Piano Players

George Vivian Poore [5], in his fifth and last contribution to the study of so-called writer's cramp and related disorders, published in 1887, addressed "certain conditions of the hand and arm which interfere with the performance of professional acts, especially piano-playing." Poore described a group of patients who were experiencing difficulty in playing the piano, "a condition which has in many instances been apparently brought about by the over-exercise of their professional functions as pianists." He explained that "the machinery involved in the delicate manipulation necessary for a pianist is, indeed, so complicated that the wonder is break-down does not oftener occur" [5]. Poore's study included 21 patients, far fewer than his study of patients with writing failure; Poore deduced that writing was much more in demand than piano playing.

At the time that Poore was conducting his studies, the so-called Stuttgart method defined how a pianist should hold the hands during piano playing (Figure 9-1). This method required extension of the wrist in the most rigid manner at all times and extension of the near phalanges of the fingers except when the respective finger or fingers would hit a key. A large number of piano players experienced symptoms related to such muscles as the extensor digitorum communis, extensor indicis proprius, or extensor digiti minimi. Poore [5] described nine cases of "piano failure": In almost all, the patient experienced nerve tenderness and associated conditions including muscular disability that could be present in activities other than piano playing, "more or less tremor," pain or early fatigue during muscular exertion, and "a sense of discomfort in the limb (not exactly pain), which is worse at night and makes it difficult to put the limb in a comfortable position in bed and often keeps the patient awake." On the basis of these and other cases, Poore [5] concluded that "in no two cases was the cause of break-down precisely the same," and so he did not see any justification for a unifying term such as *pianist's cramp.*

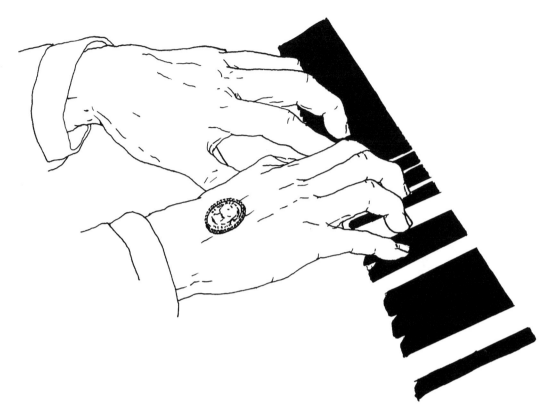

Figure 9-1. Stuttgart method of piano playing.

Poore [5] made an interesting distinction between the disorders of piano players and those of the writers in that the muscles prone to what he called *breakdown in piano playing* are larger and more numerous and "in more common requisition for general purposes than are the muscles (most commonly the interossei) whose breakdown causes writer's cramp." The result is that, while writer's cramp generally affects only the act of writing, the piano-playing failure generally involves other activities, too. This could serve to refute Lucire [6,7], the most prominent proponent of the psychogenic-psychosocial hypothesis, who concluded that writer's cramp and related conditions cannot be recognized as organic conditions because they affect a given group of muscles during a particular activity but often not during another activity. In writing, a very restricted number of muscles are affected, whereas in piano playing, more numerous muscles are involved and so other activities are also perturbed by a disturbance of these muscles.

Poore [5] considered further the diagnosis and prognosis in these piano playing–induced morbid entities. He believed that the prognosis was good with only nerve tenderness and local muscle weakness and recommended rest. To this measure he added a prescription of arsenic (sic) and of counterirritants by means of "blisters" and such other remedies as were popular in Poore's day. Massage was to be used with caution to avoid a frequently overzealous approach by professionals, which certainly was to be avoided in the presence of nerve tenderness. Because the ring finger is recognized as the physiologically weakest one, if its capacity to rise and then hit a key were reduced for anatomic reasons, a surgical procedure was advocated—namely, a sort of tenotomy in which the bands connecting the extensor tendon of the ring finger with the extensor tendons on either side of it were cut. Like other means of management used at the time (i.e., late 1800s), this surgical intervention evidently was abandoned owing to unwanted effects, which exceeded the advantages.

Cumulative Trauma Disorders: A Nineteenth-Century Disease

In the late 1800s, CTDs were recognized in the United Kingdom, the United States, and continental Europe. Not until the twentieth century was Australia added to the list of affected countries. In 1892, referring to CTDs and repetitive strain or overuse syndromes, Riggs [8] expressed the opinion that all "these occupational disorders may safely be called a 19th century disease."

Terminology

In the nineteenth-century, the entities currently considered CTDs were known as *occupational cramp* and *occupational neurosis*. The former term applied well to musicians' cramp, particularly violinists' or pianists' cramp. Despite Poore's opposition to this term as an acceptable diagnosis, the appellation gained general acceptance. The term *occupational neurosis* apparently was not connected at the time to psychiatric disorders but rather meant a neurologic condition occurring as a consequence of "a deranged action in the centres concerned in the act of writing" [9]. Other terms used in the late nineteenth century for the same disorder included *professional impotence* [10], *craft palsy, occupational overstrain,* and *fatigue disease.*

The celebrated clinician Osler [11] defined the condition as "the continuous and excessive use of the muscles in performing a certain movement . . . followed by an irregular, involuntary spasm or cramp, which may completely check the performance of the action." Probably the first adequate clinical description of a CTD in musicians was made by Duchenne [10], who described an affected concert pianist. The initial recorder of "telegrapher's cramp," Onimus [12], acknowledged that the disorder was already known in musicians. A similar condition was then recognized in dancers [13–17]. In 1886, Lewis [18] stated (and Fry [1] reiterated) that "writers, telegraph operators and musicians are those which by far are the most frequently affected, the others being almost curiosities." The overuse syndrome, though recorded in musicians in general, was particularly noted in pianists and violinists and involved either the fingering or bowing arm (Figure 9-2). A somewhat large number of authors considered the left hand to be the more severely affected [13,14,18,19].

Overuse Syndromes in Musicians

Fry [1] was preoccupied with the views on these entities, particularly the "overuse syndrome in musicians." He reviewed no fewer than 21 books and 54 articles on the topic, published between 1830 and 1911. There were, according to the author, two prevalent theories to explain all the conditions included in this rather vast occupation-related topic. The *central theory* (see Chapter 2) regarded the lesion as occurring in the central nervous system, whereas the *peripheral theory* implied a primary muscle disorder. The psychogenic origin was not given much consideration, "though emotional factors were believed to aggravate the condition" [1].

Prevalence. Fry [1] elucidated an important point that helped to explain the prevalence of the overuse syndrome in musicians in the nineteenth century. At that time, advances in musical instrument manufacture (e.g., the concert piano and the clarinet) were significant. From a medical practice viewpoint, CTDs were among the standard conditions for which a patient would consult a physician in the last part of the nineteenth century. The patient population was composed mainly of writers (i.e., people who had to write by hand in order to make a living, such as scriveners) and musicians.

Symptoms. A musician's inability to play the instrument in question was determined by the presence of pain, weakness, and deficient control. Spasm was present only occasionally, according to Poore [20], who recommended that terms such as *paresis* or *palsy* be avoided when referring to musicians [21]. However, Aitken [22], who published in the same period, described the condition as a "local palsy or paralysis." Reynolds [23] claimed that abnormal sensations might occur in the affected limb and usually preceded the cramp; this author described these sensations as "vague in character" and as a "feeling of weight, tightness, numbness, or coldness."

Pianists seem to be more severely affected than other players, and rather dramatic cases are presented in the literature. For instance, Graham [18] described the symptoms of a professional piano player who practiced an excessive number of hours before a recital and, as a result, developed swelling, weakness, and aching of the hands. Particularly dif-

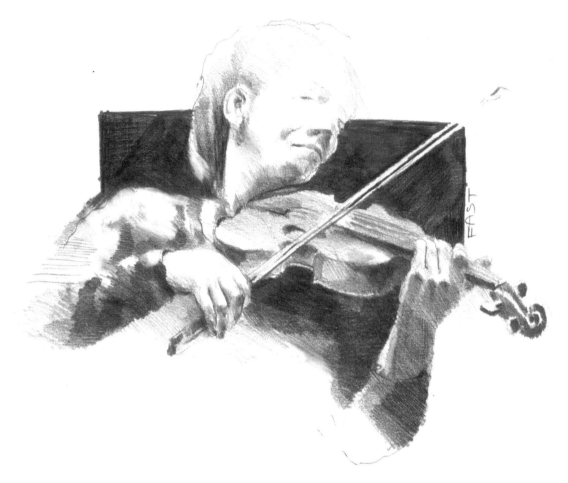

Figure 9-2. Violinists are affected by cumulative trauma disorders mainly in the bowing arm.

ficult pieces, or passages within such pieces, were especially conducive to the development of various symptoms, which would appear suddenly when the offending passages were played or attempted [18].

According to Oppenheim [24], who played a significant role in our understanding of CTDs, the "flute player cramp" affects a few fingers or the entire hand, the left hand being more often affected than the right, as is true for pianists. Bianchi [25] described loss of control of the left ring finger in flute players, which resulted in an alteration of intonation.

The spread of symptoms to other muscles, more proximal than those activating the fingers, and to additional activities was mentioned by a few authors, of whom Poore [20] was the first. Poore [20] noted that at times only the act of playing the instrument seemed to be affected, whereas at other times, corresponding to more severe cases, "some other act or acts is affected." Spread to more proximal muscles was noted by Gowers [9] and Vance [26]. Despite their limited knowledge of human anatomy and physiology, relative to what we know today, authors described the spreading of symptoms to the contralateral extremity [5,9,20,27]. Another clinical manifestation was tenderness in the affected areas, which Poore [5] noted in the extensor muscles of the wrist, the fingers, and the forearm. Like today's experts on fibromyalgia, he noted tender areas in particular muscles, such as the levator scapulae, as well as direct tenderness of the nerves themselves [5]. Erb [28] used electrotherapy and rest to treat the tender areas.

Poore [29] blamed muscle failure as the primary condition, because "the nervous system was bypassed when the muscle was stimulated directly by electricity." Although Poore did not undertake to do so, the study of biopsy specimens obtained from the muscle to which Poore paid the most attention, the first dorsal interosseous muscle, would be the next step in the process of understanding CTDs in musicians [5]. Poore [5] postulated that fatty and fibroid changes were also associated with painful, tender, or stiff muscles, and he rather arbitrarily labeled these patients as suffering from *muscular rheumatism* or *myalgia*.

Treatment and Prognosis. The treatment and prognosis of CTDs in musicians has evolved from rest, which is advocated by nearly all contributors in this field, through "splinting the limb" [30]. Drug therapy [31], exercise therapy [22], surgery [27,32], and emphasis on posture [33] were also mentioned. Many of these therapeutic options have failed. Fry and Rowley [34] conclude that "total avoidance of pain-inducing activities" is the only truly effective treatment.

It is also vital that musicians receive appropriate training from their teachers. Faulkner and Sharpey-Schafer [35] exposed the often erroneous views of even fine teachers on important matters such as lip position and *embouchure*, a term meaning both the mouthpiece of a wind instrument and the way the mouth, lips, and tongue are used in playing. Use of the diaphragm by flute players is another controversial issue: Although some authors advocate tensing the diaphragm during playing, allegedly to assure breath support, electromyographic studies demonstrate that good breath support actually results in a relaxed diaphragm [36].

Cumulative Trauma Disorders in Musicians in the Twentieth Century

Occupational diseases in musicians were rarely reflected in the literature before the twentieth century. Albert [37] reported recurrent swelling of the parotid glands in trumpet players, and Stone [38] associated emphysema with the playing of instruments. Aside from numerous case reports and letters, writings dedicated to occupation-related diseases in musicians have rarely been collected even in this century. Two that did appear—*Diseases of the Musical Profession* [39] and *Occupation and*

Health, a publication of the International Labor Office [40]—were criticized for different reasons, primarily because musicians were considered generally healthy. This viewpoint is reflected in the title of a paper published in 1955 [41]: "Musicians are a healthy lot."

At the turn of the century, Turner [42] identified the distal muscles involved when the fingers-only Stuttgart method was used by professional piano players: the extensor digitorum communis, dorsal interossei, extensor indicis, and extensor digiti minimi. The interosseous muscles reportedly are the only ones also used in writing, whereas the larger muscles named by Turner are specifically used by musicians, particularly piano players. Turner [42] mentioned also the problem of tongue overuse in wind instrument players, referring specifically to "cornet players' cramp."

In a review of the literature on occupational diseases of instrumental musicians, Harman [3] noted that in the second half of the twentieth century the United States became more than a blue-collar, manufacturing society: In 1967, it was estimated that 64 of 100 workers were employed in "service" occupations [43]. A *Handbook of Medical Specialties* published in 1976 indicates that the appellation *industrial medicine* was broadened by that time to *occupational medicine* and included additional categories of workers, such as professional instrumental musicians [44]. Special emphasis was placed by some authors of the same time on wind instrumentalists, as their effort in playing their instruments appeared to be greater than that of other musicians. Bouhuys [45], for example, considered the playing of wind instruments to be "one of the most strenuous respiratory activities." The author based this description on the exceedingly high air pressure that exists within the respiratory tract while a wind instrument is being played.

Acceptance by the Medical Community

Not until April 8, 1983, when the *Journal of the American Medical Association* published an article entitled "Hand Difficulties Among Musicians," did the medical community at large begin to take stock of the serious consequences that can ensue from the professional playing of instruments [46]. The first musicians' clinic, conducted at Massachusetts General Hospital in Boston, reflected the medical community's genuine concern for the major occurrence of CTDs in musicians [47]. If one considers, for example, that the number of separate motor actions per second that might be necessary to play piano at a level of recognized virtuosity is as high as 600 [48], one begins to understand that pianists might be more vulnerable than other professionals to the development of CTDs. Hochberg, in his study of 100 instrumentalists, reported that more than one-third lost control of their playing and a significant number (47) had to abandon their careers.

In Fry's experience [34], the common condition reported in all cases that preceded the publication of Hochberg and colleagues' article [46] was generally labeled *tenosynovitis*, which later became known as *musculoligamentous overuse*, and then *overuse syndromes, repetitive strain injuries*, and *cumulative trauma disorders*. According to the same author, CTDs in musicians were not publicly recognized earlier primarily because, although some physicians were aware of their existence, the medical community at large had not yet accepted CTD as a viable diagnosis, and doctors feared losing their jobs and reputations as a result of advocating such acceptance [34]. As CTDs in some musicians progressed to severe disability, performances would be canceled, although the musicians would not admit the true reason for such cancellations, fearing that they would be perceived as unreliable [34].

The 1983 report by Hochberg et al. [46] released doctors and musicians from some of these fears: It became easier to discuss diseases related to playing musical instruments professionally, conditions that previously were mentioned rarely. Subsequent publication of a number of articles brought to the attention of physicians and the public other related conditions, such as those affecting the face, palate, throat, and respiratory muscles of musicians who play wind instruments.

Classification of Occupational Hazards for Musicians

Harman's Classification

Harman [3], in an attempt to classify the various occupational hazards facing musicians, divided the hazards into six basic categories: dermatitides, nerve compression syndromes, occupational cramps, intraoral pressure problems, cardiac abnormalities, and miscellaneous conditions. In a review of CTDs in musicians, the nerve compression syndromes are primarily of interest. It is easy to understand that repetitive pressure by instruments against different parts of the body might compress nerves and thus produce sensations such as paresthesias, pins and needles, or numbness. Affected areas of the body can include lips, shoulders, hands, arms, or legs. Aside from suffering unpleasant sensations, the affected musicians experience difficulties in moving the affected part. These nerve compression syndromes were named according to the involved instrument or playing (e.g., *viol paresthesia* [49], *paralyzed embouchure* [50,51]).

Another condition affecting musicians and closely related to the nerve compression syndromes are so-called occupational cramps, which are somewhat reminiscent of true writer's cramp (discussed in Chapter 2). However, instead of nerves, muscles seem to be the target in this condition. Hunter [52] refers to occupational cramps as *psychoneuroses* and explains that they occur when the "necessary coordination of movement breaks down." The player of the respective instrument experiences "spasm, tremor, pain, weakness and loss of control." Occupational cramps in musicians have been described in guitarists [53], pianists, violinists, flutists, cellists, harpists, organists, and drummers [39,40,52].

CTDs in wind instrumentalists in particular might affect the cardiovascular system, which is a part of the neuromusculoskeletal apparatus that is not usually affected by CTDs. The basic physiologic features of playing a wind instrument could predispose the musician to cardiac abnormalities. Reported effects of playing wind instruments include "wandering pacemaker activity" [54] and premature ventricular contractions [55].

Of course, accidental morbid conditions can also occur as a result of playing a musical instrument, but these are much more peripheral to our interest in studying CTDs.

Lederman's and Calabrese's Classification

In 1986, Lederman and Calabrese [56] published a comprehensive review of overuse syndromes in instrumentalists. On the basis of the predominant pathophysiologic manifestations, the authors divided the conditions into five categories, according to the part of the body involved: bones, joints, and bursae; the musculotendinous unit; muscle (primary muscular pain or cramp); nerves (nerve entrapment); and miscellaneous conditions (the group known generically as *occupational palsies*).

Bones, Joints, and Bursae. The most serious overuse injury of bone results from repetitive impact loading, which leads to microfractures or stress fractures. Such injuries are noted mostly in the lower limbs of runners and ballet dancers but not, as a rule, in musicians or instrumentalists. A radiographic study of hand osteoarthropathy among 20 piano players disclosed the presence of degenerative changes of the right hand more than of the left hand, particularly in the ring and little fingers, which are generally the most stressed digits in professional piano playing [57].

Musculotendinous Unit. Ligamentous laxity and pain were reported in musicians as a result of repetitive efforts. Wind instrumentalists seem more affected than other musicians (e.g., strain of the collateral ligament of the thumb in a clarinetist [46] and swelling and tenderness of the radial collateral ligament in horn players [58]). Muscle and tendon syndromes appear to be common in musicians [46,59]. In Finland between 1975 and 1979, Kivi [60] described musicians affected by these morbid entities mainly at the wrist, hand, or proximal forearm levels. Not unlike industrial workers, musicians are affected mainly in extensor rather than flexor muscles [61].

Muscles. The third category of overuse syndromes, according to Lederman and Calabrese [56], refers to muscular pain. Conditions comprised by this category are complex and difficult to define [62]. Such different terms as *myofascial pain, tension myalgia, fibromyalgia,* and *fibrositis*, used to describe muscular conditions, further complicate the issue [63–65]. Fibromyalgia or fibrositic syndrome is rarely seen in musicians, who are less prone than other workers to diffuse muscular pain, multifocal trigger-point sites, and sleep disturbances. Instead, instrumentalists are prone to a more localized form of muscle pain, a referred type of pain syndrome involving acute; subacute; or, at times, chronic cervical, upper-neck, or low-back

derangement that occurs as a result of long hours of practice. Carrying heavy instruments and working in uncomfortable quarters are contributing factors. Muscle cramps are frequently the common denominator in these cases [66], and they appear to be universally distributed and not locally confined.

Nerves. The inclusion of nerve entrapment syndromes as CTDs appears logical today but was questionable as recently as 1986 [56]: "One may argue with the decision to include entrapment neuropathies among the overuse syndromes. However, symptoms of nerve compression may mimic or overlap those of musculoskeletal origin (e.g., radial tunnel syndrome), nerve entrapment may be associated with or precipitated by musculotendinous injury (e.g., carpal tunnel syndrome [CTS]), and repetitive movement against resistance may at times lead directly to compression of nerve at specific locations." It is well known that entrapments occur at sites where the nerve can be easily trapped while passing between relatively rigid structures such as bones, tendons, ligaments, or even muscles. A nerve can also be compressed externally when it passes close to the body's surface.

Besides pain, which is a fairly nonspecific complaint, symptoms such as numbness, tingling, and pins and needles in the distribution of the respective nerve are important indicators of possible impending damage. Sensory loss generally does not occur, and weakness is a late phenomenon. Tapping or pressing the site of the involved nerve usually produces an electric shock type of sensation along the nerve's course.

Clinical maneuvers such as Tinel's, Phalen's, or a specific nerve compression test are helpful in establishing the diagnosis. These tests can be misleading, however, as they depend on a patient's subjective response, which can be influenced by a variety of factors. A truly objective, quantitative examination includes electrophysiologic studies and nerve conduction testing, which are indispensable in the evaluation of nerve entrapment syndromes. These studies establish the diagnosis and pinpoint the exact location of the entrapped nerve.

Fry's Classification of Muscle Failure

Fry distinguishes two types of muscle failure due to overuse [34]. The first type, musculoligamentous failure, comprises conditions that result from excessive or unusual efforts, in which tissues are forced beyond their biological limits, most often during periods of prolonged hours of practice (e.g., in preparation for a special performance) and shortened rests, if any. A major contributing factor is the musician's desire to master particularly difficult passages, which frequently require that the fingers be brought into strenuous positions. Experience shows that this type of muscle failure responds better to rest than to surgery, corticosteroid injections, or psychiatric evaluations [48].

The second type of muscle failure secondary to CTD, much less common than the musculoligamentous one, is known as *focal dystonia* or *cramp* [67,68]. Such failure consists of painless incoordination that generally affects the hands. In addition to loss of control, involuntary movements of the fingers are typical, primarily the ulnar fingers, which can go into complete flexion. Another pathognomonic feature is substitute movements, whereby an intended motion results in an unintended one. The agonist muscles might as well contract synchronously with the antagonists. The distortion of motion appears erratic, but careful consideration reveals a kind of rogue program, mostly predictable but drastically different from the expected sequence.

Cocontraction of agonist and antagonist muscles of the extremity engaged in most CTD-prone repetitions in musicians, particularly in the performance of difficult passages, creates tension and pain and, consequently, major technique impairment. The loss of ability to play was reported in violinists engaged in a major competition [69]. In another report, no fewer than six different types of "loss of facility in playing" were recognized [70]. Fry reported on an impressive number of orchestra players (485) with "loss of technique" [71]. In a national survey reported by Fishbein et al. [72], 23% of instrumentalists complained of diminished motor control and an even larger group (38%) felt weakness of the left hand. Finally, another extensive contribution by Lockwood [73] emphasized the "loss of fine motor control" and, expectedly, "poor motor control," which caused the musicians difficulty in playing their respective instruments. In another study by the same author, this time in secondary school–aged musicians,

loss of control or dexterity was attributed to "painful overuse" [74]. Some loss of technique with painful overuse in musicians has been reported elsewhere [75].

Neuropathy in Performing Artists

Lederman reported on neuropathy in performing artists [76] and noted that particularly the playing of musical instruments had recently been recognized as a potential risk factor for mononeuropathies [77]. A substantial percentage of neuropathic conditions seen in medical practice are indeed presented by instrumentalists [77,78]. Of these, CTS was the most common entrapment neuropathy in players of musical instruments [77].

Koppell and Thompson describe a patient in whom an occupational cramp or focal dystonia interfered with piano playing [79]. A violinist ("fiddler"), the victim of another, more proximal, median nerve entrapment—namely the pronator syndrome—was one of seven patients with this rather rare condition [80].

Occupational cubital tunnel syndrome, an ulnar neuropathy, was considered to be the result of repetitive stress or cumulative trauma in instrumental musicians generally and, more specifically, the outcome of traumatic events combined with prolonged elbow flexion in string players [81]. Charness et al. reported on 13 instrumentalists with cubital tunnel syndrome, including four with bilateral involvement [81]. According to these authors, the symptoms might precede electrodiagnostic abnormalities in all of these cases. Distal compression of the ulnar nerve was also reported in two flutists [82].

Although it is the most resistant to compression, the radial nerve, too, has been involved in compression neuropathies. Radial tunnel syndrome, known also as *posterior interosseous syndrome* and resulting from the entrapment of the radial nerve in the forearm, was seen in a piano player [83] and a flute player [84] and was treated successfully in the latter by surgical means. Digital neuropathies, caused by the cumulative pressure of an instrument against the instrumentalist's fingers, were described in a violist [85] and a flutist [86]. Both cases involved the index finger pressed against the respective instrument.

Thoracic Outlet Syndrome

Despite the controversies surrounding its very existence, the thoracic outlet syndrome (TOS) has been reported more often than expected in instrumentalists. At the same Cleveland Clinic Foundation where Wilbourn [87] contested the presence of this syndrome except in very rare cases, Lederman [88] diagnosed the TOS in 17 symptomatic instrumentalists. Other authors also describe musicians afflicted by this condition [46,89], though Lederman [88] did not grant credibility to any of these studies. More credible, according to this same critic [88], is the study by Roos [90], which reported on 11 string players who underwent successful surgical therapy for TOS that invariably affected the left arm. In addition, a flutist with left-arm involvement was described by Lascelles et al. [91]. A unique case of a drummer affected by a "posterior cutaneous neuropathy of the right arm" attributable to the cumulative effect of percussive action was described by Makin and Brown in 1985 [92].

An Extensive Study of Neuropathy in Musicians

An extensive study of 141 instrumentalists, among whom a definitive diagnosis was established in all cases, was published by Lederman in 1987 [93]. The predominant diagnostic category was peripheral nervous system disorders, which accounted for 30% of the cases.

Of major interest is the fact that all but two patients suffered from conditions affecting the upper limbs. Violinists and violists had mostly left-arm involvement, whereas piano players were affected in the right hand and arm. The wind instrumentalists did not show any clear predilection in terms of lateralization. The most common diagnoses were, in order of frequency, the controversial TOS, median neuropathies, ulnar nerve entrapments, cervical radiculopathy, digital mononeuropathies, and radial mononeuropathy.

Electrophysiologic studies were performed in the six patients with cervical radiculopathy, 10 of 18 with TOS, nine of 12 with median nerve entrapments, eight of nine with ulnar neuropathies, three of four with digital neuropathies, and in the one case of radial neuropathy. In addition to routine studies, in six patients somatosensory evoked potentials were also performed and were normal in every case, despite the use of various arm positions; routine diagnostic studies were noncontributory also. In the patients with CTS (nine of 12 patients with median neuropathy), nerve conduction studies confirmed the clinical diagnosis in eight. Of electrodiagnostic studies in eight patients with suspected ulnar entrapment neuropathies, four revealed normal conduction velocities.

It must be noted that not all the diagnoses were established firmly as, in conditions such as CTS or ulnar nerve entrapment, the electrodiagnostic abnormalities were the only findings on which a diagnosis was being made. For instance, the author reported positive electromyographic results in all six patients with suspected cervical radiculopathy but, even in the face of negative or normal electromyographic results, the diagnosis can be confirmed by magnetic resonance imaging or computed tomography scanning.

All 141 of these cases were managed conservatively, at least initially. Two TOS patients were treated surgically and reported to do well, whereas another 12 similarly afflicted patients recovered with only conservative management. Treatment failures were recorded in three patients, and only one was lost to follow-up. Of the nine patients with CTS, one had already undergone surgery and another five underwent surgery later, all with good results. Three musicians chose to wear splints or change their playing technique, which met with generally good results.

There are instrumentalists who, despite well-documented entrapment neuropathies, continue to play their instruments full-time. Such was the case with a harp player suffering from the relatively rare pronator teres syndrome, a piano player with a traumatic median neuropathy, a violinist with an anterior interosseous entrapment neuropathy and focal dystonia, and another violinist with distal ulnar entrapment neuropathy. In contrast, surgery was necessary in other instrumentalists—for example, in one patient with ulnar mononeuropathy and one with cervical radiculopathy, both of whom had reportedly excellent results with this treatment modality [76]. Taking into account all 43 patients studied who had peripheral nerve disorders [76], recovery was good to excellent in 33 (77%), only equivocal in five, and poor or unimproved in the other five.

Lederman [76] concluded that when both the clinical picture and electrodiagnostic abnormalities are taken into account, performing artists appear to be more affected by their symptoms than are other corresponding groups. This can be explained by the unusually high demands placed on the neuromuscular apparatus of concert musicians especially. Because the slightest impairment could ruin or hamper a performance, early detection in these individuals is paramount. However, despite the obvious logic of the preceding statement, there are authors (among them Harman [3]) who present the view that musicians who play an instrument do not suffer major health problems related to that activity or, if they do suffer such health problems, are afflicted only rarely.

Overuse Syndromes in Children

A Melbourne-generated study in secondary school children introduced gender as a possible factor in overuse syndromes in musicians [75]. The article reported that the instrumentalists' technique was affected adversely by overuse in almost one-third of the girls and one-fifth of the boys but, when current pain exclusively was considered, there was a male prevalence (five of seven [71%], as compared to 11 of 26 girls [42%] who cited the same complaint). On the basis of the study by Fry et al. [75], we can conclude that even if school-aged girls are more vulnerable to pain from playing instruments, once boys become afflicted with similar pain, they generally become more impaired. Therefore, in evaluating CTDs in musicians who play instruments, one must consider genetic factors also.

Of course, some individuals experiencing pain can play for much longer periods of time than can others. Rest, generally consisting of a few months of abstinence from playing the instrument, is regarded as the only effective management measure in cases of focal dystonia, although according to Newmark and Hochberg [94], physical therapy can also be valuable in such cases. Further research is urged to define more exactly the early signs of CTDs due to excessive instrument playing.

Cumulative Trauma Disorders in Dancers

Ballet dancers with CTDs are far from rare. To manage such disorders successfully, one must have an intimate knowledge of dancing in general and ballet in particular, an awareness of all the anatomic details, and knowledge of a number of morbid conditions that affect dancers. In a review of the literature addressing CTDs in ballet dancers, Khan et al. [95] found that turnout is the "single most fundamental physical attribute in classical ballet," and "forcing turnout" is a frequent contributor to overuse injuries in ballet dancers. The foot and ankle are the parts of the body injured most often (Figure 9-3). Injuries at these levels include those at the first metatarsophalangeal joint, second metatarsal stress fractures, flexor hallucis longus tendinitis, and anterior and posterior ankle impingement syndromes. The shin might be involved in dancers, and shin pain in these cases is frequently secondary to chronic compartment syndrome or stress fractures of the posteromedial or anterior aspect of the tibia. Pain at the knee level can be generated by a patellofemoral syndrome, patellar tendon insertional conditions, or a combination of these two. Hip and back areas also are not spared in dancers.

A team approach to the management of dancers' injuries is often mandatory if rapid recovery is to be achieved. An accurate diagnosis is vital, and the correction of certain details of a dancer's technique might be necessary. Manual therapy to different joints and soft tissues might be necessary in association with exercises for strengthening and fitness. Nutritional instruction should be incorporated in the management program. In this author's experience, most ballet-related overuse injuries respond reasonably well to conservative measures. When surgical procedures cannot be avoided, a rehabilitation program should follow.

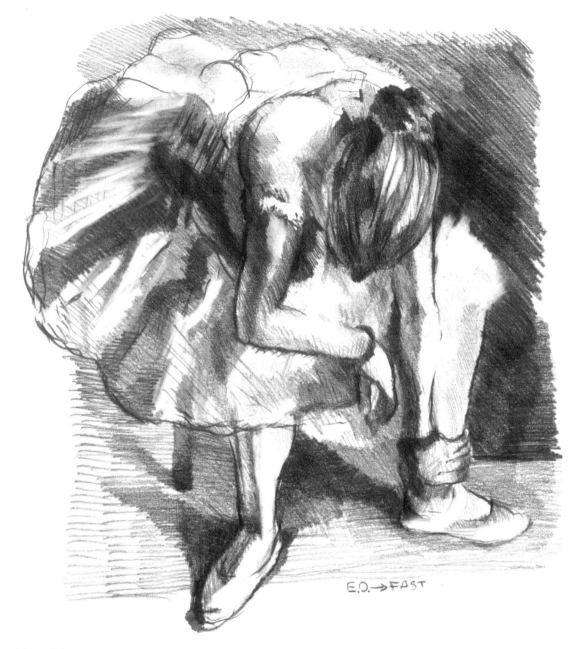

Figure 9-3. Ankle injuries are common in dancers.

References

1. Fry HJH. Overuse syndrome in musicians—100 years ago. Med J Aust 1986;145:620.
2. Fry HJH. The effect of overuse on the musician's technique. Int J Arts Med 1991;1(1):46.
3. Harman SE. Occupational diseases of instrumental musicians. Literature review. Md State Med J 1982;31(6):39.
4. Ramazzini B. Diseases of Workers (WC Wright, trans). New York: Hafner, 1964. (Original work published in 1700 and 1713.)
5. Poore GV. Clinical lecture on certain conditions of the hand and arm which interfere with performance of professional acts, especially piano playing. BMJ 1887;1:441.
6. Lucire Y. Neurosis in the workplace. Med J Aust 1886;145:323.

7. Lucire Y. Social iatrogenesis of the Australian disease "RSI." Community Health Studies 1988;12:146.

8. Riggs CE. Nervous Disorders and Paralyses from Excessive Use of the Parts Affected: Vertigo, Tremor, and Lead-Poisoning. In HA Hare (ed), A System of Practical Therapeutics, vol 3. Philadelphia: Lea & Febiger, 1892;419.

9. Gowers WR. A Manual of Diseases of the Nervous System, vol 2. London: Churchill, 1888;656.

10. Duchenne GB. De L'électrisation Localisée et de son Application á la Pathologie et á la Thérapeutique (2nd ed). Paris: Baillière, 1861;928.

11. Osler W. The Principles and Practice of Medicine (4th ed). New York: Appleton, 1902;1107.

12. Onimus E. Cramps des employés au Telegraphe. Comptes Rendus Seances Memoires Soc Biol [series 6] 1875;2(27):120.

13. Wilkes S. Lectures on Diseases of the Nervous System. London: Churchill, 1878;455.

14. Gould GM, Pyle WL (eds). A Cyclopedia of Practical Medicine and Surgery. Philadelphia: Blakiston's, 1901.

15. Wolff J. The treatment of writer's cramp and allied muscular affections [communicated by D Ferrier]. BMJ 1890;2:165.

16. Poore GV. Clinical memoranda—dancers' cramp. BMJ 1875;2:640.

17. Dancers'cramp [editorial]. BMJ 1875;2:615.

18. Lewis MJ. The Neural Disorders of Writers and Artisans. In W Pepper (ed), A System of Practical Medicine, vol 5. London: Sampson, Low, Marston, Searle & Rivington, 1886;504.

19. Wood H. Occupation Neuroses. In W Pepper (ed), A Textbook of the Theory and Practice of Medicine, vol 1. Philadelphia: Saunders, 1896;651.

20. Poore GV. Craft Palsies. In TC Albutt (ed), A System of Medicine, vol 3. London: Macmillan, 1899;3.

21. Poore GV. Writer's Cramp. In R Quain (ed), A Dictionary of Medicine, part 2. London: Longmans Green, 1885;1792.

22. Aitken W. The Science and Practice of Medicine, vol 2 (6th ed). London: Griffin, 1872;279.

23. Reynolds JR (ed). A System of Medicine, vol 2. London: Macmillan, 1878;243.

24. Oppenheim H. Textbook of Nervous Diseases for Physicians and Students (5th ed) [A Bruce, trans]. Edinburgh: Schulze, 1911;548. (Original work published in 1894.)

25. Bianchi L. A contribution on the treatment of the professional dyscinesiae. BMJ 1878;1:87.

26. Vance R. Writers' cramp, or scriveners' palsy. Boston Med Surg J 1873;88:251.

27. Jelliffe SE. Migraine Neuralgia, Professional Spasms, Occupation Neurosis, Tetany. In W Osler (ed), Modern Medicine: Its Theory and Practice, vol 7. Philadelphia: Lea & Febiger, 1910;786.

28. Erb W. Electro-Therapeutics. In A De Watteville, J Cagney (trans), Von Ziemssen' Handbook of General Therapeutics, vol 6. London: Smith, Elder, 1887;608.

29. Poore GV. An analysis of seventy-five cases of "writers' cramp" and impaired writing power. Med Chirurg Trans 1878;43:111.

30. Fraser D. Proceedings of the Meeting of the Pathological and Clinical Society. Glasgow Med J 1879;11:75.

31. De Watteville A. The cure of writers' cramp. BMJ 1885;1:323.

32. Haward W. Note on pianist's cramp. BMJ 1887;1:672.

33. Colman WS. An unusual case of writers' cramp. Lancet 1896;1:415.

34. Fry HJH, Rowley G. Instrumental musicians showing technique impairment with painful overuse. Md Med J 1992;41:899.

35. Faulkner M, Sharpey-Schafer EP. Circulatory effects of trumpet playing. BMJ 1959;1:685.

36. The way to high D [letter]. Lancet 1973;797:242.

37. Albert E. Sur une cause de rechutes dans les oreillons et une complication possible de ces rechutes. Rev Med 1895;15.

38. Stone WH. On wind-pressure in the human lungs during performance of wind instruments. Phil Mag 1874;48(series 4):113.

39. Singer K. Diseases of the Musical Profession: A Systematic Presentation Their Causes, Symptoms and Methods of Treatment [W Lakend, trans]. New York: Greenberg, 1932.

40. International Labor Office. Occupation and Health. Encyclopedia of Hygiene, Pathology and Social Welfare. Geneva: International Labor Office, 1934.

41. Schweisheimer W. Musicians are a healthy lot. Music J 1955;13:9.

42. Turner WA. Occupational Neuroses. In GA Gibson (ed), Text-Book of Medicine, vol 2. Edinburgh: Young J Petland, 1901;828.

43. Felton JS. 200 years of occupational medicine in the US. J Occup Med 1976;18:809.

44. Wechsler H. Handbook of Medical Specialties. New York: Human Science, 1976.

45. Bouhuys A. Lung volumes and breathing patterns in wind-instrument players. J Appl Physiol 1964;19:967.

46. Hochberg FH, Leffert RD, Heller MD, et al. Hand difficulties among musicians. JAMA 1983;249:1869.

47. The music clinic [editorial]. Lancet 1985;1:1309.

48. Fry HJH. Overuse syndrome in musicians: prevention and management. Lancet 1986;2:728.

49. Schwartz E, Hodson A. A viol paresthesia. Lancet 1980;2:156.

50. Morgan T. Musician warns men of paralyzed embouchure. Downbeat 1950;17:6.

51. Morgan T. Paralyzed embouchure: it can happen to anyone. Downbeat 1950;17:13, 19.

52. Hunter D. The Diseases of Occupations (6th ed). London: Hodder & Stoughton, 1978.

53. Brattberg A, Fagius J. Guitarist's cramp—analogous to writer's cramp. Lakartidningen 1978;75:403.

54. Nizet PM, Borgia JF, Horvath SM. Wandering atrial pacemaker: prevalence in French hornists. J Electrocardiol 1976;9:5.

55. Borgia JF, Horvath SM, Dunn FR, et al. Some physiological observations on French horn musicians. J Occup Med 1975;17:696.

56. Lederman RJ, Calabrese LH. Overuse syndromes in instrumentalists. Med Probl Perform Art 1986;1:7.

57. Bard CC, Sylvestre JJ, Dussault RG. Hand osteoarthropathy in pianists. J Can Assoc Radiol 1984;35:154.

58. Shulman IA, Milberg P. English horn player's thumb. J Hand Surg 1982;7:424.

59. Cauldron PH, Calabrese LH, Lederman RJ, et al. A survey of musculoskeletal problems encountered in high-level musicians. Arthritis Rheum 1985;78(suppl 4):597.

60. Kivi P. Rheumatic disorders of the upper limbs associated with repetitive occupational tasks in Finland in 1975–1979. Scand J Rheumatol 1984;13:101.

61. Wilson RN, Wilson S. Tenosynovitis in industry. Practitioner 1957;178:612.

62. Mills KR, Edwards RHT. Investigative strategies for muscle pain. J Neurol Sci 1983;58:73.

63. Smythe HA. Nonarticular Rheumatism and Psychogenic Musculoskeletal Syndromes. In DJ McCarty (ed), Arthritis and Allied Conditions: A Textbook of Rheumatology (11th ed). Philadelphia: Lea & Febiger, 1985;1083.

64. Simons DG. Muscle pain syndromes, part 2. Am J Phys Med 1976;55:15.

65. Wilke WS, Mackenzie AH. Proposed pathogenesis of fibrositis. Cleve Clin Q 1985;52:147.

66. Layzer RB, Rowland LP. Cramps. N Engl J Med 1971;285:31.

67. Cohen LG, Hallett M. Hand cramps: clinical features and electromyographic patterns in a focal dystonia. Neurology 1988;8:1005.

68. Fry HJH, Hallett M. Focal dystonia (occupational cramp) masquerading as nerve entrapment or hysteria. Plast Reconstr Surg 1988;82:908.

69. Hiner SL, Brandt KD, Katz BP, et al. Performance related medical problems amongst premier violinists. Med Probl Perform Art 1987;2(2):67.

70. Couldron PH, Calabrese LH, Clough JD, et al. A survey of musculoskeletal problems encountered in high-level musicians. Med Probl Perform Art 1986;1(4):136.

71. Fry HJH. The incidence of overuse syndrome in the symphony orchestra. Med Probl Perform Art 1986;1:51.

72. Fishbein M, Middlestadt SE, Ottati V, et al. Medical problems amongst ICSOM musicians: overview of a national survey. Med Probl Perform Art 1988;3(1):1.

73. Lockwood AH. Medical problems of musicians. N Engl J Med 1989;320:221.

74. Lockwood AH. Medical problems in secondary school–aged musicians. Med Probl Perform Art 1988;3(4):129.

75. Fry HJH, Ross P, Rutherford M. Music-related overuse in secondary schools. Med Probl Perform Art 1988;3(4):129.

76. Lederman RJ. Neuromuscular problems. Muscle Nerve 1994;17:569.

77. Lederman RJ. Nerve entrapment syndromes in instrumental musicians. Med Probl Perform Art 1986;1:45.

78. Knishkowy B, Lederman RJ. Instrumental musicians with upper extremity disorders: a follow-up study. Med Probl Perform Art 1986;1:85.

79. Koppell HP, Thompson WAL. Pronator syndrome: a confirmed case and its diagnosis. N Engl J Med 1958;259:713.

80. Morris HH, Peters BH. Pronator syndrome: clinical and electrophysiological features in seven cases. J Neurol Neurosurg Psychiatry 1976;39:461.

81. Charness ME, Barbaro NM, Olney RK, Parry GJ. Occupational cubital tunnel syndrome in instrumental musicians. Neurology 1987;37(suppl 1):115.

82. Wainapel SF, Cole JL. The not-so-magic flute: two cases of distal ulnar nerve entrapment. Med Probl Perform Art 1986;3:63.

83. Woltman HW, Learmonth JR. Progressive paralysis of the nervus interosseous dorsalis. Brain 1934;57:25.

84. Charness ME, Parry GJ, Markison RE, et al. Entrapment neuropathies in musicians. Neurology 1985;35(suppl 1):74.

85. Spaans F. Occupational Nerve Lesions. In PJ Vinken, GW Bruyn (eds), Handbook of Clinical Neurology, vol 7. New York: American Elsevier, 1970;326.

86. Cynamon KG. Flutist's neuropathy. N Engl J Med 1981;305:961.

87. Wilbourn AJ, Porter M. Thoracic outlet syndrome. Spine 1988;2:597.

88. Lederman RJ. Thoracic outlet syndrome: review of the controversies and a report of 17 instrumental musicians. Med Probl Perform Art 1987;2:87.

89. Newmark J, Hochberg FH. Isolated painless manual incoordination in 57 musicians. J Neurol Neurosurg Psychiatry 1987;50:291.

90. Roos DB. Thoracic outlet syndrome: symptoms, diagnosis, anatomy and surgical treatment. Med Probl Perform Art 1986;1:90.

91. Lascelles RG, Mohr PD, Neary D, Bloor K. The thoracic outlet syndrome. Brain 1977;100:601.

92. Makin GJV, Brown WF. Entrapment of the posterior cutaneous nerve of the arm. Neurology 1985;35:1677.

93. Lederman RJ. Peripheral nerve disorders in instrumental musicians. Ann Neurol 1987;2:125.

94. Newmark J, Hochberg FH. "Doctor it hurts when I play." Painful disorders amongst instrumental musicians. Med Probl Perform Art 1987;2(3):93.

95. Khan K, Brown J, Way S, et al. Overuse injuries in classical ballet. Sports Med 1995;19:341.

Appendix 9.1
Update to Chapter 9

The reference list provided for this chapter covers materials published through 1995. There is a relative paucity of published information concerning cumulative trauma disorders (CTDs) in dancers before 1996. I felt therefore compelled to update the chapter with more recent materials, to include more information concerning disorders affecting dancers, in addition to a more recent article concerning CTDs in musicians. A separate reference list accompanies this update.

New Reports on Cumulative Trauma in Dancers

In a paper published in 1996 in the *Journal of Bone and Joint Surgery*, the authors discussed the differential diagnosis and operative treatment of pain in the ankle of dancers [1]. Thirty-seven dancers (comprising 41 procedures) treated surgically for stenosing tenosynovitis of the flexor hallucis longus tendon or posterior impingement syndrome were followed for an average of 7 years. Twenty-six of the operations were for tendinitis and posterior impingement, nine for only tendinitis, and six for impingement alone. Thirty ankles had a good or excellent outcome, six had a fair result, and, in four ankles, the outcome was poor. The results were good or excellent in 28 of the 34 ankles of professional dancers, as opposed to the good or excellent result in only two of six ankles in amateur dancers.

The "dancer's fracture" (i.e., of the distal shaft of the fifth metatarsal) is analyzed in an article published in the *American Journal of Sports Medicine* [2]. Thirty-five dancers with this type of fracture are studied. The common pattern is a spiral, oblique fracture starting distal and lateral to the fifth metatarsal and running proximally-medially. The majority of the patients (24) were treated with an elastic wrap. Open reduction and internal fixation were used in two cases, closed reduction and percutaneous fixation in another two, and short leg weightbearing casts in the remaining seven. The average time to pain-free ambulation was 6.1 weeks, to return to barre exercises 11.6 weeks, and to performance 19 weeks, without limitation or pain reported.

Proprioception in classical ballet dancers suffering from ankle sprain was discussed in another paper published in 1996 [3] and authored by a group of doctors from the Karolinska Institute in Stockholm. Fifty-three professional dancers from the Royal Swedish Ballet and 23 controls were included in this study that recorded the dancers' postural sway using a stabilimeter with a specially designed, portable, computer-assisted foot plate. The results appear gender dependent: Male dancers demonstrated a smaller total area of sway. Both male and female dancers had a smaller mean sway on the left foot than on the right, and there was no mean difference in sway between the left and right feet in the control group. The dancers' postural stability was impaired for several weeks following the ankle sprains, with gradual improvement during rehabilitation, which continued for several weeks after professional dancing resumed.

Another article on ballet dancers published in September 1996 [4] deals with the same isolated stenosing tenosynovitis treated surgically with release of the flexor hallucis longus tendon, as discussed above. Thirteen female dancers underwent the procedure after failing to respond to nonoperative management. Their symptoms had been present for a mean of 6 months. All patients returned to professional dancing within a mean of 5 months, 11 reaching a level of full participation in dancing without restriction.

According to a study published in the *American Journal of Public Health* [5], "no less than 55.5% of Broadway performers are prone to injuries." The mean value was 1.08 injuries per performer in this series of 313 subjects appearing in 23 Broadway companies. Lower-extremity injuries were, as expected, the most common. Sixty-two percent of performers believed that their injuries were preventable. The article identifies factors that significantly increase the risk of injury for dancers and actors and emphasizes the need to heighten application of measures aimed at reducing the incidence of injuries to professional performers, theatrical students, and nonprofessionals.

New Reports on Cumulative Trauma in Musicians

A review article on "Musculoskeletal and neuromuscular conditions of instrumental musicians" with 108 references, covering the previous 10 years, was also published in 1996 [6]. According to the authors, "although nearly all of these conditions are the same ones seen in the general work force, it is clear that their occurrence patterns in the professional musician are unique, as is their impact on the life and livelihood of the patient." The article also acknowledges that the lack of research done in a true blind, random case-controlled fashion does not allow a real critical review. Many statements in the literature are based only on clinical experience.

References

1. Hamilton WG, Geppert MJ, Thompson FM. Pain in the posterior aspect of the ankle in dancers. Differential diagnosis and operative treatment. J Bone Joint Surg Am 1996;78:1491.
2. O'Malley MJ, Hamilton WG, Munyak J. Fractures of the shaft of the fifth metatarsal. "Dancer's fracture." Am J Sports Med 1996;24:240.
3. Leanderson J, Eriksson E, Nilsson C, Wykman A. Proprioception in classical ballet dancers. A prospective study of the influence of an ankle sprain on proprioception in the ankle joint. Am J Sports Med 1996;24:370.
4. Kolettis GJ, Micheli LJ, Klein JD. Release of the flexor hallucis longus tendon in ballet dancers. J Bone Joint Surg Am 1996;78:1386.
5. Evans RW, Evans RI, Carvajal S, Perry S. A survey of injuries among Broadway performers. Am J Public Health 1996;86:77.
6. Bejjani FJ, Kaye GM, Benham M. Musculoskeletal and neuromuscular conditions of instrumental musicians. Arch Phys Med Rehabil 1995;77:406.

Chapter 10

Low-Back Pain Due to Cumulative Trauma Disorders

Jay Mitchell Weiss

Cumulative trauma disorders (CTDs) have been cited as causes of industrial low-back pain and injury. Various studies have proposed risk factors for back injury, including heavy physical labor [1–3], smoking, and vibration [4]. Others consider psychosocial factors to be among the most significant predisposing factors for low-back pain and injury.

There has been a tremendous increase in the number of reported cases of industrial low-back pain since the early 1970s, so much so that it has been referred to as an epidemic. Frymoyer and Cats-Baril [5] note that in the 1960s, there was very little information about or interest in the epidemiologic features or cost of low-back pain. These authors estimated the direct costs of low-back pain in the United States in 1990 (including medical costs but not costs related to lost work time) to be more than $24 billion. This number continues to escalate. Investigators are asking, "Is the work significantly more stressful now than it was 30 or 40 years ago?" If the answer to this question is no, the next logical question is, "Are the workers of today significantly less prepared or less capable of performing the work than were workers of 30 or 40 years ago?"

Certainly, no simple answers to these questions currently exist. Nonetheless, it appears highly unlikely that a significant percentage of the current increased incidence of back disability is attributable to either of these two factors. Although there may be small populations in which back pain is caused purely by mechanical overload or muscular insuffi-ciency, surely these causes cannot explain the epidemic of reports of low-back pain.

For years, industrial managers had a vested interest in predicting which workers were most susceptible to back injury. In the first half of this century, numerous screening programs were used. Initially, predictions of workers at risk for low-back *injury* were based on lumbar spine x-rays. Unfortunately, these studies had very little predictive value in determining who would develop low-back *pain*. According to Rowe [6], "Routine spinal roentgenograms of industrial workers are not cost or risk benefit effective." Other authors, including Gibson [7], have reached the same conclusion. Consequently, numerous other factors have been investigated.

One of the best-designed and most definitive studies of risk factors for low-back pain and injury was a prospective study by Bigos et al. [8] of 3,020 aircraft employees at Boeing Aircraft in Seattle. These investigators followed most employees over a 3-year period. Risk factors examined include demographics (age, gender, race, marital status, smoking history, medical history of back injuries or back surgery), work history (including job satisfaction), psychosocial factors (with the Minnesota Multiphasic Personality Inventory [MMPI]), physical characteristics, straight-leg raising ability, and physical capacities. The factor most predictive of future injury was found to be job satisfaction and the hysteria component of the MMPI. It was reported that subjects scoring highest on the hysteria scale of the MMPI were two times more likely to report a back injury than were subjects with low scores on this scale.

Waddell [9] considered the question, "Is low-back pain a Western phenomenon?" He found that back pain was not considered a significant health problem in the country of Oman, but when a back clinic was opened in that country, it became widely used. Waddell [9] concluded that although back pain is likely to be ubiquitous, people in certain cultures consider it a normal facet of life and are unaware that it can be treated; hence, they do not seek treatment.

We can infer from these epidemiologic and research data that the *reporting* of back pain and injury is at epidemic proportions, but this does not necessarily correlate with a true epidemic of back disability. Myriad psychosocial and economic factors exist that might make the reporting of back injury advantageous to the worker. This situation will probably be magnified when an employee has a perceived grievance against the employer or when layoffs are being anticipated. Hence, although mechanical factors must be considered, and some empiric data stress the importance of a worker's strength and flexibility, the evaluation of back pain cannot be considered a purely medical problem. In the industrial setting, it must also be considered a social and economic problem.

Prevalence of Back Pain

Epidemiologic studies report that nearly all adults will experience back pain at some point in their lives [10,11]. Other studies cite the presence of back pain in up to 25% of individuals between the ages of 30 and 50 years at the time these persons were surveyed [12]. Clearly, then, if all workers who experienced some degree of low-back pain were to report it, the numbers would be even higher than they currently are. The incidence of industrial low-back pain is estimated at 2–5% of workers in the United States annually [5]. However, to examine back pain using only the conventional disease model of illness would be inadequate. It is conceivable that some back injuries reported as work-related injuries are non-industrial injuries or normally occurring complaints of back pain that are being attributed to an industrial origin.

Evaluation of Back Pain and Injury

The vast majority of examinations for back pain do not reach a definitive diagnosis. Also, most back pain is of short duration and is self-limited. As such, avoiding prolongation of the disability is an important goal of medical intervention.

Clinical Examination

A good clinical history should address such factors as frequency of lifting, the types of loads that are lifted, and the perception of the weight lifted (as opposed to the actual weight that is being lifted). As is true for most medical disorders, a good history yields the most important information. The ergonomic environment must be assessed, including the workstation, personal protective gear, tools, and materials used. Neurologic dysfunction must be ruled out. Radiographs should be obtained if trauma is involved.

Radiographic Studies

Generally, in cases of low-back pain due to CTDs, the yield of radiographic evaluation is low. According to Borenstein and Wiesel [13], medical evaluation, including laboratory and radiographic tests, of patients with low-back pain should be initiated only if the patient has significant symptoms and signs of an underlying medical illness on initial presentation. These investigators recommend that those individuals without evidence of a medical etiology or cauda equina syndrome initially be treated conservatively. If after 6 weeks the pain remains unresponsive, they recommend that the physician consider obtaining plain-film radiographs.

Differential Diagnosis

A detailed discussion of all the differential diagnoses of back pain is beyond the scope of this book. For additional information on this topic, the interested reader is referred to references 14–16.

Preventing Back Pain

Industry managers seek to prevent back disability and absenteeism. However, it is unlikely, given the epidemiologic factors noted earlier, that any one intervention can prevent all back pain in the workplace. A realistic goal is to decrease the incidence of back injury. It can be argued that the concept of injury is a misnomer and that the pain may be a muscular response to overload, implying that an injury may convince the worker that the level of anatomic damage is greater than it actually is. To some degree, this misconception may be counterproductive to a worker's rapid return to activities (both vocational and avocational).

Because no single course of intervention appears to decrease morbidity and mortality significantly in low-back injuries, most interventions have both their proponents and their opponents. Some authors report that increasing the employees' awareness of hazards at work might, paradoxically, increase rather than decrease the number and cost of back injuries [17].

Back Schools

Back schools are among the interventions that have been tried. Such schools began in Sweden and Canada and, on the basis of early promising reports [18], this concept spread rapidly. Unfortunately, no consistent criteria were applied to defining a back school. Although most schools concentrated on back anatomy and physiology and independent exercise programs, curricula varied widely. Anecdotal evidence of high cure rates abounded, but very few quality studies demonstrated a significant benefit of back school [19]. Hall [20] has argued for back schools, stating that "the alternative to education is ignorance." Hall maintains that, while far from perfect, back schools might be helpful. In contrast, Hadler [20] believes that back schools "institutionalize the medicalization of regional low-back pain." He maintains that this approach invites more disability and less coping with low-back pain,

which is an essentially ubiquitous phenomenon at some point in most people's lives [20].

Ergonomics

The science of ergonomics was discussed in some depth in Chapter 6. Jacobs and Bettencourt [21] remind us that good principles of ergonomics are noted most when they are absent: Good design is rarely noticed.

Because humans come in varying sizes and shapes, adjustability of the workstation is extremely important. Experts on ergonomics can evaluate a work site and identify causes of recurrent injury. However, prevention of work-related injury is far more desirable. Most work stations can be modified to minimize the amount of required lifting from floor level and keep workers from exerting force far from the body. The mechanical forces are much lower when working within a few inches of the trunk than when working a foot from the body. Similarly, lifting from or lowering to the floor places greater strain on the low-back muscles, bones, and ligaments and can be minimized through efficient workstation design.

Back Strengthening

There is debate in the literature as to whether increased strength is a protective factor in low-back pain or back injury [22]. Also debated in the literature is which of the many methods of testing back strength is optimal. In the author's opinion, back flexibility and job-specific back strength are more important parameters than are isolated strength measurements. Pre-employment screening, although its value is dependent on the prospective employee's degree of effort, can help assess whether minimum standards of strength and flexibility are met, provided that the screening is based on an appropriate job description.

Low-Back Pain Due to Overuse Injuries

Complaints of low-back pain can issue from a multitude of medical causes. What is becoming ever more clear is that numerous psychosocial issues can also play a significant role in the development of low-back pain. Regarding the reporting of back pain and return-to-work productivity, psychosocial factors may play as important a role as do biological factors.

Medical Workup and Treatment

It appears that assessments in the form of medical workup and treatment might actually be counterproductive. Such interventions can reinforce a sense of illness, which might keep a patient from returning to work. Similarly, some of the provisions of the workers' compensation system might be counterproductive. Certainly, the workers' compensation system is a necessity, and employers should be required to provide for medical care as well as to financially compensate individuals who are injured while performing tasks for their employers. However, in many cases of nonspecific low-back pain, the medical workup is negative, and the treatment continues primarily because of complaints of symptoms.

Studies that showed an improvement in return-to-work rates of patients treated with functional restoration programs were flawed from a design point of view, according to Teasell and Harth [23], who noted selection bias. Control groups included either treatment failures or patients who were refused entry into the program, or other factors such as incomplete follow-up were present. For these reasons, Teasell and Harth [23] believed that there were no well-controlled, prospective, randomized clinical trials that proved functional restoration programs to be efficacious.

It can be argued that the role of medical care in the treatment of occupation-related low-back pain, especially nonspecific low-back pain, is to rule out a significant neurologic or skeletal problem. The workup should be sufficient to rule out spinal fracture, neurologic compromise, or other processes affecting the spine that should be aggressively treated. Such other processes affecting the spine could include cancer (either primary or secondary) or infection. It is beyond the scope of this text to discuss the workup for the various etiologies. Nonetheless, it is commonly accepted that low-back pain due to overuse and without evidence of neurologic compromise does not necessitate radiography, magnetic

resonance imaging studies, or laboratory tests [24]. Most cases of musculoskeletal and nonspecific low-back pain will resolve spontaneously within several weeks. At this early stage, it is likely that any minor abnormalities found on conventional radiographs would not contribute significantly to the determination of treatment and might be counterproductive by reinforcing the patient's perception that he or she does, in fact, have a structural problem [24].

Most therapies for nonspecific low-back pain have been found to be either minimally effective or ineffective, depending on where and when they are used. Specific treatment options that have been shown to be effective for nonspecific low-back pain include bed rest for more than 7 days, trigger-point injections, stretching, traction, and surgery [24]. In certain cases, especially in the face of acute low-back pain, treatment such as trigger-point injection might be appropriate. There may be other specific situations in which these treatment options are effective. The problem with studying these interventions, as noted previously, is that it is difficult to assess a purely medical or mechanical intervention without addressing associated problems. Studies of these interventions also look at a symptom (low-back pain) and, although the workup may have been negative, there may be several different underlying disorders. Although far from conclusive, there is evidence that exercise is valuable for treating low-back pain. Mayer et al. [25] reported improved function and a decreased incidence of unemployment in low-back pain patients after they completed a functional restoration program. This value might be attributable to psychological factors that make the patient feel his or her back is strong enough to accomplish the assigned tasks.

Influence of the Workers' Compensation System

The workers' compensation system may actually encourage low-back disability. Recently, Hadler et al. [26] matched a group of patients with back injuries that were reportedly work related to a similar group of low-back pain patients without work-related injuries. These investigators found that those covered by workers' compensation had taken off a greater amount of work time than a matched group that was not eligible for such compensation. Therefore, interventions that are based solely on medical aspects and that completely ignore psychosocial factors are destined to fail. This explains the paucity of data that convincingly show the value of various interventions in treating compensable low-back pain.

Modifying Predisposing Factors

Each industry must assess any repetitive task that may predispose a worker to back injury. Although worker fitness is always desirable, the data as to whether relative fitness will, in fact, prevent injury are conflicting. What appears much more likely, on the basis of the findings presented in this chapter, is that employer policy and handling of workers' complaints is as much a factor in determining injury existence and duration of disability as are medical factors. Light-duty options and accommodation of injured or disabled workers by redesigning and modifying job sites should be applied wherever possible.

An employee's perception that the employer is concerned with his or her health and enjoyment of the job is paramount to a successful return to work. When these factors are present and appropriate medical interventions are used, the likelihood of a successful outcome improves greatly.

Long-Term Disability

The Task Force on Pain in the Workplace, commissioned by the International Association for the Study for Pain, recommends that nonspecific low-back pain be considered a problem of activity intolerance rather than a modern medical condition [24]. The task force makes this recommendation on the basis of the fact that no specific medical pathologic process is found, according to the illness model. Reliance on the illness model ensures that most interventions that do not assess psychological and social factors will fail. The task force recommends that any long-term management program address the following seven objectives [24]:

- Preserve and optimize worker health
- Preserve, as far as is practicable, the health and economic viability of the family unit
- Enable long-disabled patients to return to work, if possible
- Minimize unnecessary health care services

- Minimize the need for workers to seek medical recertification as disabled employees
- Redirect health care services where indicated by rediagnosis
- Reduce litigation

The task force also recommended changes in the workers' compensation system that would limit the period of disability for nonspecific low-back pain to 6 weeks [24]. The authors believe that medical workup and appropriate short-term treatment are necessary. However, without diagnostic evidence that indicates that the problem is something other than nonspecific low-back pain, further justification of disability would be inappropriate. The task force further recommended that after 6 weeks, the worker should be considered unemployed as opposed to disabled [24]. This obviously would require radical revision of the U.S. workers' compensation system. Providers who work extensively with the workers' compensation system are aware that currently it encourages disability. Although such revision of the system might be in the best interests of most patients, numerous powerful and influential groups have a vested stake in maintaining the current system, making any change exceedingly difficult to effect.

Conclusion

As has been shown here, the treatment of most nonspecific low-back pains and injuries under a purely medical model, without assessment of the psychosocial factors, will be incomplete. Because of the workers' compensation system, we frequently deal with the reported incidence of low-back pain as opposed to the actual incidence. Numerous factors such as job satisfaction and other nonmedical issues modify both the incidence of reported back pain and the time taken off from work because of complaints of back pain. It is reasonable to also assume that these same factors, if appropriately addressed, will help to effect an improved treatment response.

Traditionally, medical treatment has been performed in a vacuum, without regard for the nonmedical factors, which explains, at least in part, why our treatments have often been less than effective. This also explains why there are no strict, established treatment protocols and why there is a great deal of anecdotal evidence for the efficacy of all treatments but very little scientific evidence for the efficacy of any.

The recommendations by the Task Force on Pain in the Workplace might be viewed by some as extreme [24]. However, the task force certainly is on the right track when it considers the possibility that the structure of the workers' compensation system itself might be a significant factor in low-back pain. As practitioners, we are obligated to try to help our patients. Interventions that merely reinforce the concept of disability might be counterproductive and not serve the best interests of the patient. It is in the employer's best interest to keep workers satisfied, as a worker who is satisfied with his or her job is far less likely to report low-back pain or to call in sick or take disability leave due to back pain and is more likely to return to work sooner than a worker who is dissatisfied.

References

1. Lloyd MH, Gauld S, Soutar CA. Epidemiologic study of back pain in miners and office workers. Spine 1986;11:136.
2. Riihimaki H, Tola S, Videman T, Hanninen K. Low back pain and occupation. A cross-sectional questionnaire study of men in machine operating, dynamic physical work, and sedentary work. Spine 1989;14:204.
3. Svensson HO, Andersson GBJ. Low back pain in 40 to 47 year old men: work history and work environment factors. Spine 1983;8:272.
4. Battie MC, Bigos SJ. Industrial back pain complaints. A broader perspective. Orthop Clin North Am 1991;22:273.
5. Frymoyer JW, Cats-Baril WL. An overview of the incidences and costs of low back pain. Orthop Clin North Am 1991;22:263.
6. Rowe ML. Are routine spine films on workers in industry cost or risk benefit effective? J Occup Med 1982;24:41.
7. Gibson ES. The value of preplacement screening radiography of the low back. Occup Med 1988;3:91.
8. Bigos SJ, Battie MC, Spengler DM, et al. A prospective study of work perceptions and psychosocial factors affecting the report of back injury. Spine 1991;16:1.
9. Waddell G. A new clinical model for the treatment of low back pain. Spine 1987;12:632.
10. Spengler DM, Bigos SJ, Martin NA, et al. Back injuries in industry: a retrospective study: I. Overview and cost analysis. Spine 1986;11:241.
11. Von Korff M, Dworkin S. An epidemiologic comparison of pain complaints. Pain 1989;32:173.
12. Andersson BJ. Epidemiological aspects of low back pain in injury. Spine 1981;6:53.
13. Borenstein DG, Wiesel SW. Low Back Pain: Medical Diagnosis and Comprehensive Management. Philadelphia: Saunders, 1989;120.
14. Wiesel SW, Weinstein JN, Herkowitz H, et al. (eds). The Lumbar Spine (2nd ed). Philadelphia: Saunders, 1996.
15. Macnab I, McCulloch J. Backache (2nd ed). Baltimore: Williams & Wilkins, 1990.
16. Frymoyer JW, Ducker TB, Hadler NM, et al. (eds). The Adult Spine: Principles and Practice (2nd ed). Philadelphia: Lippincott–Raven, 1997.
17. Robertson L, Keeve J. Worker injuries: the effects of workers' compensation and OSHA inspections. J Health Polit Policy Law 1983;8:581.
18. Berquist-Ullman M, Larsson U. Acute low back pain in industry. A controlled prospective study with special reference to therapy and confounding factors. Acta Orthop Scand 1977;170:117.
19. Cohn JE, Goal V, Frank JW, et al. Group education interventions for people with low back pain: an overview of the literature. Spine 1994;19:1214.
20. Hall H, Hadler NM. Controversy: low back school, education or exercise? Spine 1995;20:1097.
21. Jacobs K, Bettencourt C. Ergonomics for Therapists. Boston: Butterworth–Heinemann, 1995;4.
22. Battie MC, Bigos SJ, Fisher LD, et al. Isometric lifting strength as a predictor of industrial back pain. Spine 1989;14:851.
23. Teasell RW, Harth M. Functional restoration. Returning patients with chronic low back pain to work—revolution or fad? Spine 1996;21:844.
24. Fordyce WE, Task Force on Pain in the Workplace. Back Pain in the Workplace. Seattle: International Association for the Study of Pain Press, 1995.
25. Mayer T, Gatchel R, Mayer H, et al. Objective assessment of spine function following industrial accident: a prospective study with comparison group and one-year follow-up. Spine 1985;10:482.
26. Hadler NM, Carey TS, Garrett J. The influence of indemnification by workers' compensation insurance on recovery from acute backache. Spine 1995;20:2710.

Chapter 11
Reflex Sympathetic Dystrophy Syndrome

Jack L. Rook

The human body normally recovers from injury in a manner that is thoroughly predictable and consistent with the type and severity of trauma. This statement holds true for the vast majority of cumulative trauma disorder (CTD) patients who receive appropriate treatment for their condition. Occasionally, instead of improving, a patient's condition worsens; the patient develops a degree of pain and disability that is disproportionate to the original injury and persists long after the injury has healed [1,2]. This may be attributable to development of the reflex sympathetic dystrophy syndrome (RSDS), a constellation of signs and symptoms first described in 1864 by Weir Mitchell, a Civil War surgeon [3]. Mitchell used the terms *causalgia* (Greek for "burning pain") and *erythromelalgia* (redness and pain) to describe this new syndrome seen in soldiers who had major nerve injuries due to gunshot wounds. Mitchell described the pain and behavior observed in patients suffering from causalgia as follows:

> Its intensity varies from the most trivial burning to a state of torture which can hardly be credited but which reacts on the whole economy until the general health is seriously affected. ... Exposure to the air is avoided by the patient with the care which seems absurd and most of the bad cases keep the hand constantly wet. ... As the pain increases, the general sympathy becomes more marked. The temper changes and grows irritable, the face becomes anxious and has a look of weariness and suffering. The sleep is restless and the constitutional condition reacting on the wounded limb exasperates the hyperesthetic state so that the rattling of a newspaper, a breath of air, another's step cross the ward, the vibrations caused by a military band or the shock of the feet in walking, give rise to intense pain. At last the patient grows hysterical, if we may use the only term which covers the fact. He walks carefully, is tremulous, nervous and has all kinds of expedients for lessening his pain [4].

Since Mitchell's time, numerous names have been applied to RSDS (Table 11-1), suggesting a general lack of understanding about the disease entity and its pathophysiology [3–18]. Most recently, the umbrella term *complex regional pain syndrome* (CRPS) has been adopted [10]. Two types of CRPS have been recognized: Type I corresponds to RSDS and occurs without a definable nerve lesion, whereas type II, formerly called *causalgia*, refers to cases in which a definable nerve lesion is present. These revised categories have been included in the second edition of the International Association for the Study of Pain *Classification of Chronic Pain Syndromes* [19].

Terminology

As mentioned previously, the original terms *erythromelalgia* and *causalgia* were coined by Mitchell in the 1860s [3,4]. At the turn of the twentieth century, Sudeck [11] described bony changes seen with this disorder and, in 1937, DeTakats [12] described reflex dystrophy of the extremities. In the 1940s, causalgia was further subdivided into minor and major types and, in 1947, Evans [16] first used the term *reflex sympathetic dystrophy syndrome*. Even

Table 11-1. Alternative Terms for the Reflex Sympathetic Dystrophy Syndrome

Year	Term	Describer
1864	Erythromelalgia	Mitchell [3,4]
1867	Causalgia	Mitchell [3,4]
1900	Sudeck's atrophy of bone	Sudeck [11]
1929	Peripheral acute trophoneurosis	Zur Verth [5,6]
1931	Traumatic angiospasm	Morton and Scott [5]
1933	Post-traumatic osteoporosis	Fontaine and Herrmann [5]
1934	Traumatic vasospasm	Lehman [18]
1937	Reflex dystrophy of the extremities	DeTakats [12]
1940	Minor causalgia	Homans [13]
1947	Reflex neurovascular dystrophy	Steinbrocker [15]
1947	Reflex sympathetic dystrophy syndrome	Evans [16]
1967	Reflex algodystrophy	Serre [17]
1973	Mimo-causalgia	Patman [14]
1973	Algoneurodystrophy	Glick [7]
1986	Sympathetically maintained pain	Roberts [9]
1995	Complex regional pain syndrome	Stanton-Hicks et al. [10]

since that time, additional terms for this entity have evolved, including *reflex algodystrophy*, *mimo-causalgia*, and *sympathetically maintained pain* [5–7,9,11–15,20].

Causalgia refers to RSDS that occurs after nerve injury, minor causalgia being caused by minor injury to a sensory nerve and major causalgia being caused by injury to a major mixed nerve (e.g., median nerve, brachial plexus). The pain of minor causalgia tends to be less severe and fairly localized, whereas major causalgia may be localized initially but spreads rapidly [2,21].

Shoulder-hand syndrome refers to RSDS that begins in the shoulder and spreads distally, causing swelling and burning pain in the hand. The shoulder-hand syndrome is most frequently associated with hemiparetic stroke syndromes, but it has also been described after shoulder injury and in association with referred shoulder pain due to cervical radiculopathy [2].

The term *Sudeck's atrophy of bone* refers to osteoporotic bony changes that may occur in association with RSDS. Algoneurodystrophy is RSDS that occurs after minor trauma, whereas *reflex dystrophy* and *reflex neurovascular dystrophy* are earlier terms for RSDS. Current common terminology includes *reflex sympathetic dystrophy*, *reflex sym-pathetic dystrophy syndrome* (RSDS), *sympathetically maintained pain* (SMP), and *complex regional pain syndrome*. In this chapter, we use *RSDS* to refer to this entity. Later in this chapter, SMP is discussed briefly as a variant of RSDS.

Epidemiologic Features

Trauma, the most common cause of RSDS, can be accidental or iatrogenic. The injury can be major, minor, or even trivial. In the CTD patient, the traumatic precipitator may be an entrapped nerve (e.g., carpal tunnel syndrome) rather than injury to bone, muscle, or ligament [1,2]. Iatrogenic trauma is usually surgical. RSDS has developed after first-rib resection for treatment of thoracic outlet syndrome [22] and after carpal tunnel surgery, procedures that may be associated with underlying nerve damage. Other potential iatrogenic problems include tight-fitting casts [23] applied after fractures and long-term casting of nonfracture diagnoses (e.g., epicondylitis, severe strain, ulnar neuritis), in which cases the loss of proprioceptive afferent input (which can down-regulate the sympathetic nervous system) could precipitate the development of RSDS (Table 11-2).

Three Stages of the Reflex Sympathetic Dystrophy Syndrome

The symptoms of RSDS might begin gradually, days or weeks after injury, or they may manifest within a few hours. The patient suffers greatly and protects the affected area. This disorder progresses in stages.

The first, *acute* stage, can last up to 3 months. It is characterized by signs and symptoms of sympathetic underactivity. RSDS is normally considered to be a process characterized by excessive activity of the sympathetic nervous system (SNS), with vasoconstriction and decreased blood flow. However, in the acute stage, blood flow actually increases, and there is redness, warmth, and soft swelling of the extremity. Increased blood flow to hair follicles and nail beds leads to increased hair and nail growth. Patients find that pain worsens with heat application and that generalized stiffness can occur owing to soft swelling. Lastly, osteoporosis may commence after approximately 3 weeks, possibly owing to a combination of intraosseous hyperemia and disuse of the extremity [1,2,21,24–34].

The second stage, the *dystrophic* stage, usually occurs between the third and ninth months. In this stage, pain progressively worsens, and the patient begins to develop characteristic psychological and behavioral changes. The swelling spreads and becomes firm and fixed over time (brawny edema). In the dystrophic stage, we begin to see sympathetic overactivity, with decreased blood flow (cyanotic, pale, cool skin), increased sweating (hyperhidrosis), and decreased hair growth. Cold will worsen pain in this stage. The osteoporosis that began in stage 1 becomes marked and diffuse. Owing to a localized lack of nutrition, nails become brittle, skin begins to atrophy, fibrosis of joints commences, and patients develop increasing stiffness in their affected extremity [1,2,12,21,24,25,27,31,32,34,35].

The third stage, the *atrophic* stage, usually occurs after 9 months. The patient's pain reaches a plateau, swelling decreases, and skin appears pale, cool, and dry. The skin begins to atrophy, tightening around the fingers, and patients may develop "pencil-pointing" of the fingertips (extreme tapering of the digits). Osteoporosis, contractures, and muscle wasting now involve most of the extremity. In general, patients with stage 3 RSDS are left with a nonfunctional, contracted extremity [2,12,13,21,24,25,27,32,35,36].

Table 11-2. Common Causes of the Reflex Sympathetic Dystrophy Syndrome in the Cumulative Trauma Disorder Patient

Soft-tissue injury
Fasciitis
Tendinitis
Bursitis
Operative procedures
Brachial plexopathy
Scalenus anticus syndrome
Cervical radiculopathy
Cervical cord injury
Immobilization with cast or splint

Signs and Symptoms

Pain

Pain is the most prominent symptom, distinguished by its intensity. It seems disproportionate to the injury, constant and burning, and tends to spread in a nonanatomic distribution—proximally through the extremity, to the contralateral extremity, or even throughout the body [37–39]. These findings—disproportionate pain that spreads in a nonanatomic distribution—suggest the presence of two positive Waddell signs, but the use of Waddell signs to guide management of affected individuals could prove very harmful as necessary care might be delayed.

The pain is increased by motion of the involved extremity and by anything that increases sympathetic tone (excessive exercise; being startled; and emotional states such as anxiety, fear, or even pleasure) [2,37,40]. Heat or cold will aggravate the pain, depending on the stage of the disorder: Heat aggravates the involved extremity in the first stage and cold in the later stages. *Allodynia* refers to pain that worsens with non-noxious stimuli (e.g., gentle pressure, clothing, or a breeze). Because of this phenomenon, the RSDS patient tends to hold the involved extremity close to the body in a protective fashion [41].

Other Clinical Signs and Symptoms

Edema, localized at first, may spread proximally through the extremity. Early in the process, the edema is soft but, over time, it becomes firm and fixed (i.e., brawny edema) as the proteinaceous edema fluid organizes, resulting in fibrosis and contractures.

Vasomotor instability results in color and temperature changes throughout the extremity. Redness and warmth are characteristic early in the process. Over time, the extremity may appear blotchy, cyanotic, pale, and cool.

Sudomotor changes (abnormalities of sweating) include hyperhidrosis (stage 2) and excessive dryness of the extremity (stages 1 and 3).

Osteoporosis may begin by the third week after onset of the disorder. Initially, it is spotty and periarticular but, over time, it can become homogeneous and diffuse.

Trophic changes occur owing to lack of nutrition to the extremity. The skin becomes shiny, thin, and tight, causing a loss of skin creases. There is atrophy of subcutaneous fat, muscle wasting and, occasionally, pencil-pointing of the fingertips. Over time, fibrosis and contractures will develop if mobility of the extremity is not maintained through physical therapy and independent exercise [2,21].

Some RSDS patients experience involuntary movements such as jerking, twisting, writhing motions, or muscle spasm. The presence of such activity suggests centralization of disease within the central nervous system [39,42].

Psychological and Behavioral Characteristics

A number of psychological and behavioral characteristics might become evident in RSDS patients over time, leading some researchers to describe these patients as having a "causalgic personality," characterized by withdrawn, fearful, and suspicious behavior, a low pain threshold, and preoccupation with protection of the painful extremity [1]. Such patients present as chronic complainers who are depressed and emotionally unstable [2,24,43]. Eighty percent of patients in one series scored high on the hysteria, hypochondriasis, and depression scales of the Minnesota Multiphasic Personality Inventory, a report that has incited debate as to whether RSDS occurs because patients have a predisposing diathesis [44].

Although injuries are very common, only a very small fraction of injured patients go on to develop RSDS. Of patients with nerve injuries, only approximately 2–5% develop causalgia [21], and of patients

with all kinds of trauma, the incidence of RSDs has been estimated at between 5% and 15% [44]. It has been suggested that those individuals who do develop the disease have a predisposing diathesis that might be a physiologic alteration rather than an underlying psychological predisposition (personality diathesis) [1,2]. The *physiologic diathesis* refers to an underlying autonomic imbalance (history of cold hands or feet, pre-existing Raynaud's phenomenon, excessive sweating, fainting, migraine headaches, or blushing) before the onset of RSDS [2].

Personality diathesis refers to a psychological predisposition to development of RSDS. The theoretic model for this suggests that the premorbid presence of depression, anxiety, and life stress may result in sympathetic hyperarousal, which can contribute to the development or maintenance of RSDS. The RSDS personality diathesis is a controversial issue, as many researchers believe that the personality changes are secondary to the chronic, unrelenting pain [40]. However, the disparity between the often minor trauma believed to have initiated RSDS and the extreme pain experienced by the patient can cause health professionals to conclude that the RSDS patient is malingering, neurotic, or emotionally unstable. Certainly, further investigation is needed in this area [45–50].

Diagnosis

Diagnosis is based on clinical criteria, x-rays, techniques that measure skin temperature, bone scans, blood tests, electrodiagnostic studies, and response to sympathetic interruption. A thorough history and physical examination might reveal the characteristic signs and symptoms consistent with a diagnosis of RSDS (Table 11-3). Patients typically complain of pain that is out of proportion to what would be expected, given the degree of injury. Physical examination may demonstrate swelling, stiffness, vasomotor and sudomotor changes and, in late-stage disease, trophic changes, which make the diagnosis more obvious.

Radiographic Studies

X-rays of both involved and uninvolved extremities should be obtained. These may demonstrate periarticular osteoporosis within a few weeks of injury. The radiologic hallmark of RSDS of the limb is unilateral osteoporosis (Sudeck's atrophy). However, osteoporosis can be absent in as many as 33% of cases, particularly during the early course of the disease process. The radiologic appearance of RSDS osteoporosis has been characterized as spotty or patchy. Osteoporosis is manifested by the thinning of the cortices, loss of fine trabeculae, and tunneling of the cortex due to widening of intracortical haversian canals [2,24,38,43,44,51,52]. Although RSDS can exist in the absence of osteoporosis, the diagnosis of RSDS cannot be made on the basis of radiographic appearance or the presence of osteoporosis alone.

Thermography

Thermography, an infrared imaging technique that can measure very subtle temperature differences between involved and uninvolved regions, might provide objective documentation of autonomic dysfunction. Serial thermograms can be used to help determine the effectiveness of treatment over time [24]. Thermography is most useful in identifying early cases of RSDS and, for this purpose, is actually better than triple-phase bone scanning, the sensitivity of which is in the range of 50–75%. Infrared stress studies significantly improve the sensitivity and the specificity of standard thermographic procedures by challenging the integrity of the autonomic nervous system.

The cold-water stress test is performed as follows:

- A baseline quantitative thermal emission of the symptomatic extremity is obtained.
- After baseline imaging, the contralateral or asymptomatic extremity is immersed for 5 minutes in a cold-water bath filled with 10–15°C water.
- At the end of the 5-minute session, a quantitative thermal image of the symptomatic extremity is obtained.
- The quantitative pretest- and post-test-image changes in temperature are calculated. Post-test cooling of the nonimmersed extremity is the expected result. Paroxysmal warming is strongly suggestive of vasomotor instability.

The warm-water stress test is performed in a similar fashion but with opposite results expected. Phys-

Table 11-3. Characteristic Signs and Symptoms of the Reflex Sympathetic Dystrophy Syndrome

Signs
Allodynia
Edema
Vasomotor changes
   Increased sweating (stage 2)
   Decreased sweating (stages 1, 3)
Osteoporosis
Trophic changes
   Shiny, thin skin
   Loss of skin creases
   Atrophy of subcutaneous fat
   Muscle wasting
   Pencil-pointing of digits
Contractures
Increased hair and nail growth (stage 1)
Decreased hair and nail growth (stages 2, 3)
Nail fragility
Involuntary movements
Muscle spasm

Symptoms
Pain
   Out of proportion to injury
   Burning
   Unrelenting
   Spreads in nonanatomic distribution
   Worsens with anxiety or stress
   Worsens with heat (stage 1)
   Worsens with cold (stages 2, 3)
Skin hypersensitivity
Psychological manifestations
   Depression
   Anxiety
Sleep disturbance

iologic thermovascular challenges may demonstrate decreased autonomic function in suspected cases of sympathetically mediated pain. An asymmetric thermovascular rate of change in involved extremities has been deemed clinically useful in the study of RSDS [53–60].

Triple-Phase Bone Scans

Triple-phase bone scans also will demonstrate blood flow abnormalities, providing further supporting objective documentation of the diagnosis, though such scans may be negative in up to 40% of patients in whom RSDS is clinically diagnosed [8,61]. Triple-phase scintigraphy employing radiopharmaceutical technetium coupled with a phosphate complex has been used to help facilitate the diagnosis of RSDS. However, many different conditions can produce osteoporosis, and a triple-phase bone scan does not distinguish between the causes of bone demineralization. In general, then, triple-phase bone scanning may be considered a highly sensitive but not very specific tool. Though it will help to support the diagnosis, clinical acumen and correlation ultimately are required to diagnose RSDS.

Clinical information can be derived from each of the three phases of the triple-phase bone scan after injection of the radiopharmaceutical agents. First is the angiogram phase, as the compound remains intravascular for 1–2 minutes immediately following the injection. Serial images are recorded rapidly. Over the next 5–10 minutes, the radiopharmaceutical compound diffuses into the extracellular fluid spaces of the body. This period reflects the soft-tissue distribution of the compound and is referred to as the *blood pool phase* (phase 2). After 2 or 3 hours, the tracer is maximally bound to bone and will increase in areas where there is stimulus of bone turnover. It is during this time (phase 3) that images of the skeleton or bone are obtained.

In early (stage 1) RSDS, uptake of the tracer during phase 1 is increased. However, in disease stages 2 and 3, uptake during phase 1 can actually be decreased. Likewise, in phase 2, which reflects the soft-tissue vascularity, an increased diffuse uptake may be appreciated during the early course of RSDS. During phase 3, one will see diffuse bony uptake in the involved limb, reflecting bone turnover secondary to osteoporosis [43,44,62–70].

Blood Tests

Blood tests that should be obtained include a complete blood cell count, erythrocyte sedimentation rate, muscle enzyme studies, and rheumatoid factor. In RSDS, these are usually normal, but they do help to differentiate RSDS from other disorders that might present with a similar clinical picture [43,44,68].

Electrodiagnostic Studies

Electrodiagnostic studies, including electromyography and nerve conduction velocities, generally are not very helpful. Occasionally, severe nerve entrapment or radiculopathy may be causing the RSDS and, in such cases, electromyography and nerve conduction velocities would assist in identifying the underlying lesion [1].

Sympathetic Blockade

Many authorities consider the diagnosis of RSDS to be confirmed *only* if the patient improves after sympathetic blockade (i.e., stellate ganglion block, Bier block, phentolamine test) [2,8,21,71]. Such improvement would imply an abnormality of the SNS, thus helping to confirm the diagnosis of RSDS or a sympathetically maintained pain state. It is recommended that three diagnostic stellate ganglion blocks or Bier blocks be done. At least 50% relief should be experienced for the duration of the local anesthetic. Placebo effects should be checked by injection of sodium chloride solution or by using local anesthetics possessing different durations of action (i.e., procaine, lidocaine, bupivacaine). However, it should be noted that with RSDS, it is not unusual for the relief to last longer than the duration of the local anesthetic. After the administration of a diagnostic block (or blocks), the patient should not be physically stressed or sent to physical therapy if one wishes to assess accurately the results of the procedure.

Recently, the phentolamine test was introduced as a diagnostic tool for RSDS. Phentolamine is an alpha-adrenoceptor antagonist (alpha$_1$, alpha$_2$). Up to 30 mg phentolamine and 100 ml saline are infused intravenously over approximately 20 minutes, or 5–15 mg are infused over 5–10 minutes. Pain is measured using a visual analog scale. If pain is reduced, the SNS is likely to be involved in the generation of pain [72–74].

Pathophysiologic Features

RSDS is characterized by dysfunction of the autonomic nervous system. Pupillary changes, heart rate, blood pressure, gastrointestinal peristalsis, and bowel and bladder function all represent involuntary reactions controlled by the autonomic nervous system, which has two divisions, sympathetic and parasympathetic.

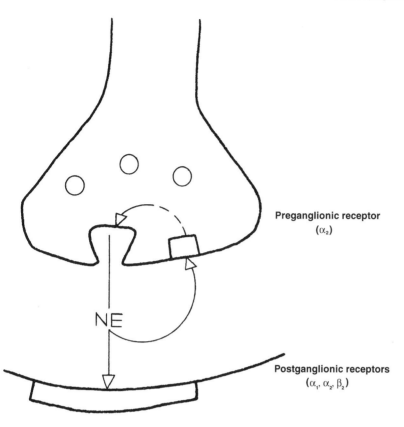

Figure 11-1. Preganglionic and postganglionic receptors at the ending of a noradrenergic neuron. The preganglionic receptor is alpha$_2$; the postganglionic receptors can be alpha$_1$, alpha$_2$, or beta$_2$. (NE = norepinephrine.)

Preganglionic receptor
(α_2)

NE

Postganglionic receptors
(α_1, α_2, β_2)

The parasympathetic division is concerned with conservation of energy. For example, with activity of the parasympathetic nervous system (PNS), there will be a decrease in heart rate and blood pressure, bronchiolar and pupillary constriction, and stimulation of the gastrointestinal tract so that reabsorption of nutrients can occur during this resting phase.

The energy stored during activity of the PNS can be used on activation of the SNS, which is concerned with energy expenditure. With increased sympathetic activity, there is an elevation of heart rate and blood pressure, bronchiolar dilatation (to provide muscles with greater oxygenation), and pupillary dilatation (to enhance peripheral vision). Most importantly, there is a redistribution of blood flow *away* from the skin and gastrointestinal tract and toward muscles.

During stress, sympathetic activity increases, preparing the organism for the so-called fight-or-flight response. In contrast, injury to an arm, leg, hand, or foot may evoke a sympathetic reflex with vasoconstriction in only the injured extremity. This type of sympathetic reflex results in minimized blood loss and swelling. However, the sympathetic reflex will need to diminish over time so that healing can commence [1,2].

The sympathetic neurotransmitter norepinephrine (NE) causes vasoconstriction of blood vessels and the secretion of sweat from sweat glands. The SNS originates from the intermediolateral gray area of the spinal cord. Myelinated nerve fibers from cell bodies in this region travel out to the sympathetic ganglion, where there is a synaptic connection with an unmyelinated sympathetic nerve that travels outward toward the periphery. The target tissues for adrenergic peripheral neurons have two types of catecholamine receptors—alpha and beta. The alpha receptor mediates vasoconstriction and the beta receptor mediates vasodilatation. There are two subtypes of alpha (alpha$_1$ and alpha$_2$) and beta (beta$_1$ and beta$_2$) receptors. The postganglionic receptors are of the beta$_2$ type (Figure 11-1).

Target tissues of particular interest in the RSDS patient include arterioles, systemic veins, and skin (pilomotor muscles and sweat glands). Alpha-receptor stimulation leads to vasoconstriction of arterioles and veins, whereas beta$_2$-receptor stimulation causes dilatation. Alpha-receptor stimulation of pilomotor muscles and sweat glands causes piloerection and sweat secretion, respectively [75].

RSDS results from an abnormality of sympathetic activity. Over the years, many different pathophysiologic theories have been proposed to explain the various clinical signs and symptoms seen in the typical RSDS patient. An optimal pathophysiologic model would be able to explain autonomic changes, allodynia, spread of the disease, and psychological manifestations. The following theories explain many of these manifestations.

Activation of the Nociceptive Afferent System

One model suggests that peripheral trauma causes activation of nociceptive afferent (C and A delta) fibers. The nociceptive impulses enter the dorsal horn, where there is activation of second-order pain transmission cells in layers I (nociceptor-specific pain transmission cells [NSPTCs]) and V (wide, dynamic-range neurons [WDRNs]). Increased dorsal horn activity is relayed to the nearby intermediolateral gray region, the origin of the SNS. Increased sympathetic efferent activity causes sensitization of peripheral sensory receptors. The sensitized peripheral nociceptors and mechanoreceptors bombard the dorsal horn, and nociceptive input causes sensitization of NSPTCs and WDRNs. The sensitized WDRN, which responds to a wide range of stimuli, produces the phenomenon of allodynia (Figure 11-2) [9,76–78].

Injury to the Sympathetic Efferent System

A more recent hypothesis implies that the initial injury is to the sympathetic efferents and not to the nociceptive afferent system. Such an injury results in decreased sympathetic outflow and the classic description of stage 1 RSDS (hot, red, dry limb with increased nail growth). This hyposympathetic phase causes subsequent upregulation of receptors in the peripheral tissues that could then result in a pathologic response to circulating catecholamines or to NE released from both surviving and reinnervated sympathetic efferents. This hypersensitivity phase would produce the clinical picture of stage 2 RSDS, representing not increased efferent sympathetic activity but rather an exaggerated response to normal levels of circulating catecholamines or residual sympathetic outflow. The intense nociception could be explained by either the upregulation of existing, normally quiescent adrenergic receptors or the development of new pathologic receptors on the nociceptive afferents. This ongoing intense nociceptive barrage might cause altered central processing, with sensitization of the second-order pain transmission cells, including the WDRN, and resultant allodynia [79].

Activation of Ascending Pain Pathways

Impulses spread cephalad via axons from sensitized second-order pain transmission cells traveling in the spinothalamic tract (STT) [80]. The STT is believed to exhibit somatotopic organization, fibers from the WDRN being medially located and fibers from the nociceptor-specific cells occupying a more lateral position as they ascend toward the brain. Two distinct pathways have been identified anatomically once the STT enters the brain: the medial paleospinothalamic tract (PSTT), extending to the frontal lobes and limbic system, and the lateral neospinothalamic tract (NSTT), traveling to the somatosensory cortex. It is believed that the medial system modulated by the WDRN is more active in RSDS, the result of which is poorly localized, diffuse, noxious pain with emotional features. The STT, PSTT, and NSTT characterize the ascending system [78,80,81].

The pain of RSDS is diffuse, burning, intolerable, and unpleasant. Other findings that remain fairly consistent from case to case include strong emotional reactions, a sense of emotional alarm, chronic anxiety, chronic insomnia, depression, and other chronic pain behaviors. However, increased activity in the PSTT pathway might account for such behaviors on a physiologic, rather than on a purely psychological, basis.

The PSTT, a more primitive pathway than the NSTT, is the principal pathway for nociceptive messages in lower vertebrates, fish, and amphibians. Activation of this system in humans results in a sense of alarm, thereby increasing activity of

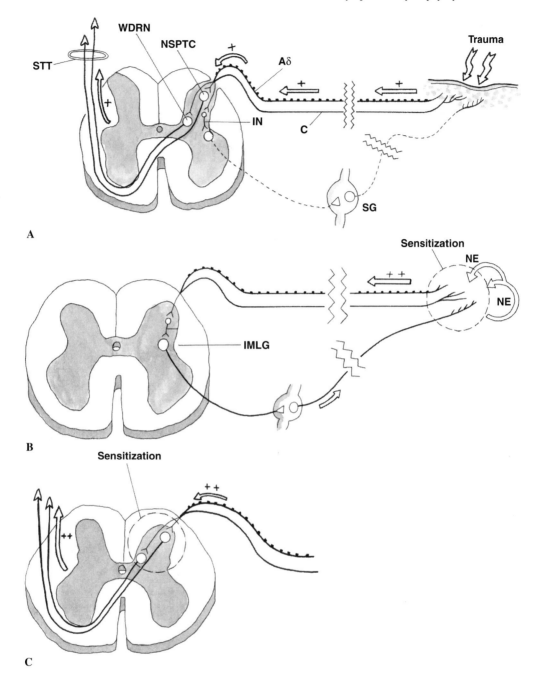

Figure 11-2. Pathophysiologic model for the development of reflex sympathetic dystrophy syndrome. A. Peripheral trauma causes activation of nociceptive afferent (C and A delta) fibers. The nociceptive impulses enter the dorsal horn, where there is activation of second-order pain transmission cells in layers I (NSPTC) and V (WDRN). B. Increased dorsal horn activity is relayed to the nearby IMLG, the origin of the sympathetic nervous system. Increased sympathetic efferent activity causes sensitization of peripheral sensory receptors. C. The sensitized peripheral nociceptors and mechanoreceptors bombard the dorsal horn with nociceptive input, causing sensitization of second-order pain transmission cells. The sensitized WDRN produces the phenomenon of allodynia. (Aδ, C = A delta and C nociceptive fibers; WDRN = wide dynamic-range neuron; NSPTC = nociceptor-specific pain transmission cell; STT = spinothalamic tract; IN = interneuron; IMLG = intermediolateral gray area; SG = sympathetic ganglion; NE = norepinephrine; + = nociceptive transmission; ++ = sensitized nociceptive transmission.)

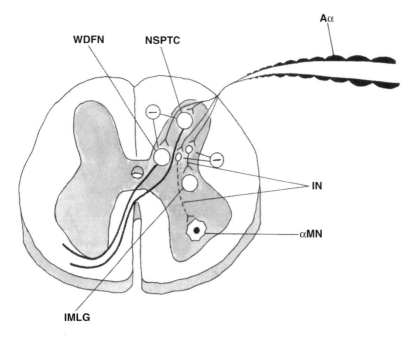

Figure 11-3. Down-regulation by large A-alpha proprioceptive fibers. Increased movement in an extremity relays proprioceptive information to the spinal cord, which down-regulates second-order pain transmission cells, intermediolateral gray cells (sympathetic nervous system), and alpha motor neurons. (Aα = A-alpha myelinated nociceptive fiber; NSPTC = nociceptor-specific pain transmission cell; WDRN = wide dynamic-range neuron; IN = interneuron; αMN = alpha motor neuron; – = inhibitory impulse; IMLG = intermediolateral gray area.)

the SNS and mediating fight-or-flight response behaviors [78].

Activation of Anterior Horn Cells

Nociceptive impulses stimulate the SNS (see Figure 11-2B). Likewise, pain impulses via C and A delta fibers, through interneurons, have a stimulating effect on anterior horn cells, possibly resulting in reactive muscle spasm (Livingston's vicious cycle). Muscle spasm is a painful process, and pain fibers originating in the muscle further propagate nociceptive impulses back to the spinal cord, thereby perpetuating the cycle of muscle spasm [76,77] (see Figure 4-3).

A-Alpha Proprioceptive Fiber Pain Modulation

There is, however, a counterbalancing effect from A-alpha proprioceptive fibers. Increased movement in an extremity relays proprioceptive information into the spinal cord, which down-regulates second-order pain transmission cells, interomediolateral cells (SNS), and alpha motor neurons (Figure 11-3). Therefore, increased proprioceptive input in an RSDS patient can decrease pain, sympathetic outflow, and muscle spasm [78]. Unfortu-

nately, patients with RSDS tend to avoid use of the involved extremity. With decreased proprioceptive input, the pain impulses become uninhibited, and there is no modulation of the SNS. For this reason, among others, physical therapy (to keep the extremity moving) is of great importance in managing RSDS.

Sympathetically Maintained Pain

The term *sympathetically maintained pain* (SMP) refers to the effect of NE on nerve terminals in the periphery. The three major physiologic changes in SMP include (1) increased activity of the SNS, which causes (2) sensitization of peripheral nociceptors and mechanoreceptors and (3) subsequent sensitization of the WDRN.

Increased activity of the SNS results in the release of NE in the periphery. It is believed that NE may increase the baseline tonic firing rate of the A-mechanoreceptors and nociceptors in the periphery to the point at which they begin firing spontaneously, even in the absence of noxious or nonnoxious stimuli. The sensitized WDRN now perceives this increased firing rate as representing a painful stimulus. At this point, the patient is experiencing pain even in the absence of any cutaneous stimulation: This is SMP [9].

Table 11-4. Summary of Currently Available Treatment Modalities for Managing the Reflex Sympathetic Dystrophy Syndrome

Sympatholytic medications
    Alpha blockers
    Beta blockers
Calcium channel blockers
Sympathetic blockade
    Stellate ganglion block
    Bier block
Physical therapy modalities
    Massage
    Splinting
    Range-of-motion exercises
    Functional activities
    Stress loading
    Contrast baths
Cold packs
Hot packs
Thermoelastic gloves
Transcutaneous electrical nerve stimulation
Acupuncture
Psychotherapy
    Treatment of depression
    Relaxation training
    Biofeedback
    Hypnosis
Nonsympatholytic medications
    Nonsteroidal anti-inflammatory drugs
    Corticosteroids
    Tricyclic antidepressants
    Baclofen
    Mexiletine
    Capsaicin cream
Sympathectomy
Opioid analgesics
Opioid pump implantation
Spinal cord stimulation

Treatment

Most RSDS patients require treatment to relieve pain and prevent disability. Untreated, the pain mechanisms may become centralized or irreversibly implanted within the central nervous system. The sooner treatment is begun, the better the prognosis. Of course, implicit in this is the fact that the patient's physician must be capable of making a quick and appropriate diagnosis.

Basic treatment principles include elimination of precipitating factors, relief of pain, and establish-

Table 11-5. Common Beta Blockers

Generic Name	Trade Names
Labetalol	Normodyne, Trandate[a,b]
Nadolol	Corgard[a]
Pindolol	Visken[a]
Propranolol	Inderal[a]
Timolol	Blocadren[a]

[a]Nonselective beta$_1$- and beta$_2$-adrenergic antagonist.
[b]Labetalol also is a potent alpha$_1$-adrenergic antagonist.
Note: Beta$_2$ receptors mediate vasodilatation and, in stage 1 disease, a beta blocker is the drug of choice.

ment of an active physical therapy program [1]. The hallmark of treatment is to shut down the SNS. Sympathetic interruption can be accomplished either in the periphery through sympatholytic medications, Bier blocks, or centrally via sympathetic ganglion blockade or invasive surgical procedures such as sympathectomy. The goal of such treatment is to desensitize the peripheral sensory receptors and WDRNs.

Some patients will suffer indefinitely from unrelenting neurogenic pain that has become unresponsive to traditional sympatholytic techniques and conservative interventions. Occasionally, such patients may be candidates for pain management via oral opioids (see Chapter 12), opioid pump implantation (see Chapter 13), or spinal cord stimulation (see Chapter 14) (Table 11-4).

Sympatholytic Medications

Peripheral interruption of the SNS is accomplished via blockade of sympathetic receptors. The sympathetic neurotransmitter NE binds to alpha$_1$ and alpha$_2$ receptors on blood vessels, producing vasoconstriction. However, stage 1 RSDS is characterized by vasodilatation, soft edema, and erythema, either due to underactivity of the SNS or overactivity with selective noradrenergic stimulation of beta$_2$ receptors. Whereas alpha receptors mediate constriction of blood vessels, beta$_2$ receptors mediate vasodilation. Hence, in stage 1 disease, a beta blocker is the drug of choice [24,27,71,82] (Table 11-5).

In contrast, disease stages 2 and 3 are characterized by decreased blood flow due to excessive noradrenergic stimulation of alpha receptors. In late-stage

Table 11-6. Alpha Blockers

Generic Name	Trade Name	Mode of Action
Doxazosin mesylate	Cardura	Selective alpha$_1$-receptor blocker
Phenoxybenzamine HCl	Dibenzyline	Alpha$_1$-, alpha$_2$-receptor blocker
Guanethidine monosulfate	Esimil, Ismelin	Interferes with release of the sympathetic neurotransmitter norepinephrine
Prazosin HCl	Minipress	Alpha$_1$-, alpha$_2$-receptor blocker
Clonidine HCl	Catapres	Central nervous system alpha$_2$ agonist that decreases sympathetic outflow

Note: In late-stage disease, alpha-blocking agents may improve blood flow and minimize trophic changes.

disease, alpha-blocking agents might improve blood flow and minimize trophic changes [2,6,24,75,83] (Table 11-6). Calcium channel blockers such as verapamil or nifedipine also might prove useful in increasing blood flow and decreasing the pain associated with ischemia in late-stage disease [84].

Bier Blocks

Bier blocks are performed using medications that work either by interfering with NE storage (reserpine, guanethidine) or by preventing NE release from sympathetic nerve endings (guanethidine, bretylium) [75].

In the Bier blocking procedure, a tourniquet is placed proximally on the involved extremity, and a distal intravenous line is used to exsanguinate the extremity, after which the respective medication (guanethidine, reserpine, or bretylium, with anesthetics or steroids) is infused. After 15–20 minutes, the tourniquet is released. By that time, most of the medication has been absorbed by the tissues, and very little enters the general circulation to exert systemic effects. Patients may experience significant pain relief that can last from 1 to several days or even months at a time. During the period of pain relief, physical therapy should be instituted [24,34,71,85–97].

Sympathetic Ganglion Blockade

General Considerations

If a Bier block fails, or in severe long-standing cases of RSDS, a ganglion block is frequently successful [98–106]. A *ganglion* is a group of nerve cells located outside the central nervous system. The sympathetic ganglia are paired chains of nervous tissue lying on either side of the spinal cord, extending from the neck to the pelvis (Figure 11-4) [1,2].

With each sympathetic ganglion block, the SNS shuts down for the duration of the anesthetic agent's effective period, there is inhibition of NE release in the periphery, and sensitized mechanoreceptors and nociceptors are able to desensitize. In turn, fewer impulses are transmitted to the WDRNs, allowing them to rest and desensitize. In the *ideal* situation, aggressive shutdown of the SNS for a prolonged period (perhaps through a series of sympathetic blocks) will enable the central pathophysiologic abnormalities to return to their baseline (i.e., normal) level.

Basic Principles of Stellate Ganglion Blockade

Infiltration of the appropriate ganglion with local anesthetic interrupts transmission of sympathetic impulses to the painful area. For upper-extremity RSDS, it is necessary to infiltrate the stellate ganglion. The stellate ganglion is the relay station for sympathetic nerves traveling to the head, neck, and upper extremity. If effected early in the course of disease, a single block may produce lasting relief. However, usually five to seven and perhaps even more blocks are necessary [1,2,21,71].

Stellate ganglion blockade is usually performed by anesthesiologists specially trained in invasive pain management techniques. It is necessary to retract the carotid sheath so that the needle can be cleanly inserted down to the stellate ganglion, which overlies a cervical transverse process. There are a number of critical structures adjacent to the stellate ganglion, including the common carotid artery, internal jugular vein, vagus nerve (housed within the carotid sheath), and recurrent laryngeal nerve (which controls the larynx and vocal cords) (Figure 11-5).

The carotid sheath must be retracted before needle insertion (Figure 11-6). The anesthetic can then be injected, most likely without the threat of hemorrhage or vascular collapse [107]. After successful stellate ganglion block, a painful, cold, pale extremity will become pink and warm, and there will be a marked decrease in pain [2,21,24]. The patient also will develop a Horner's syndrome, characterized by ptosis (drooping of the eyelid), miosis (constriction of the pupil), anhidrosis (lack of sweating on the blocked side of the face and arm), eye redness, and nasal congestion [2,24].

It might take several sympathetic blocks to relieve a patient's symptoms for a prolonged period. The absence of pain relief with a block might indicate that the diagnosis is in error or that the RSDS has become centralized [2,39].

Complications of Stellate Ganglion Blockade

There are a host of possible complications of stellate ganglion blockade, including injection of anesthetic directly into an artery (carotid or vertebral), causing seizure activity; infiltration of the recurrent laryngeal nerve, resulting in transient hoarseness and increased risk for aspiration; perforation of the lung apex, causing pneumothorax that could necessitate hospitalization for chest tube placement; and bradycardia. If the anesthetic trickles into the spinal canal, a high spinal cord block can occur, which might necessitate rapid intubation and short-term hospitalization until the anesthetic wears off. Other possible complications are hypotension and allergic or toxic reaction to the anesthetic [1,24].

Protocol for Stellate Ganglion Blockade

Early in the treatment program, blocks should be done frequently and before the rehabilitative treatments (daily, every other day, or two times per day, depending on the patient's response). During the first six to 12 blocks, the patient should be making notable progress in his or her rehabilitation program and achieving an increasingly longer duration of relief between blocks. If appropriate outcomes are

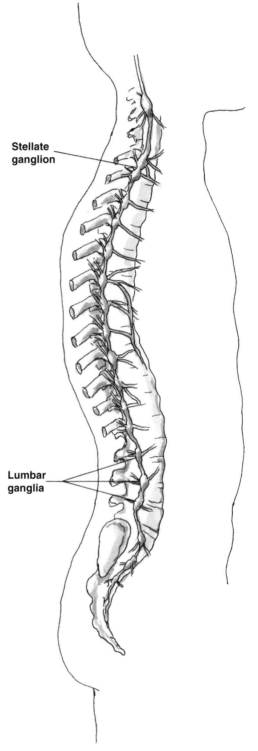

Figure 11-4. The sympathetic ganglia are paired chains of nervous tissue lying on either side of the spinal cord, extending from the neck to the pelvis.

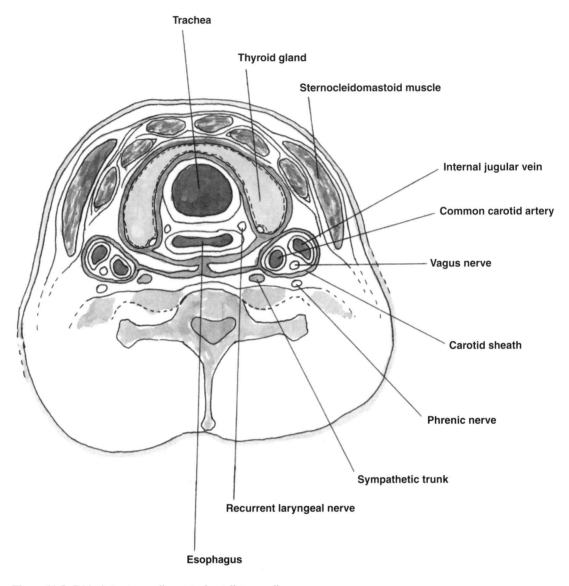

Figure 11-5. Critical structures adjacent to the stellate ganglion.

not achieved within this treatment period, changes should be made in the treatment regimen. Often, continued blocks are needed, but the duration between the blocks should increase if they are being used as maintenance therapy.

Maintenance blocks are considered appropriate if they provide relief or decrease pain for 6–12 weeks at a time. An effective maintenance therapeutic regimen should involve only four to eight blocks during the course of a year. Maintenance blocks are usually combined with and enhanced by appropriate neuropharmacologic medications and other care (e.g., self-directed home exercise program, transcutaneous electrical nerve stimulation [TENS], relaxation techniques). It is anticipated that the frequency of maintenance blocks may need to be increased in cold winter months and decreased in the warmer summer months.

For best results, sympathetic interruption needs to be done as early as possible in the course of RSDS. Nonetheless, long-standing disease does not preclude attempts at sympathetic interruption; yet if irreversible fibrosis already has occurred, the patient will experience some permanent disability.

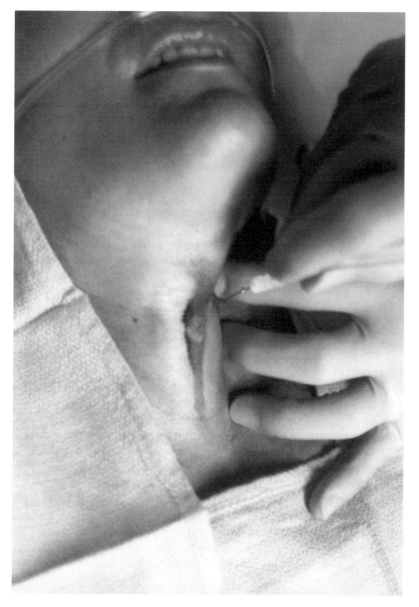

Figure 11-6. The stellate ganglion block. The carotid sheath must be retracted prior to needle insertion.

Sympathectomy

If sympathetic ganglion blocks produce good but only temporary relief, surgical or chemical sympathectomy may be indicated, although this is controversial [2,14,24,71,99,108–118]. Much of the research on the effectiveness of sympathectomy is based on short-term postoperative data [118]. Long-term experience suggests only temporary relief with this neuroablative procedure [32,78]. Destruction of part of the SNS should be considered only rarely and

very carefully, as long-term success with this treatment is poor [28,119]. Destructive treatment is very rarely contemplated if intermittent therapeutic and maintenance blocks are effective.

Chemical or surgical sympathectomy can be considered if a patient demonstrates single-extremity RSDS and distal pain only. This procedure should *not* be done if the proximal part of the extremity is involved. In addition, destructive sympathectomy should be considered only if the local anesthetic consistently gives excellent (75–100%) but temporary relief each time a technically good block is performed.

Physical Therapy

Physical therapy is an essential part of the RSDS treatment protocol and needs to be instituted early. However, in severe cases, physical therapy should be done under sympathetic interruption (via medications or blocking procedures). The concept of "no pain, no gain" does not hold for patients in whom RSDS has been diagnosed. The disease will worsen and spread faster if excessive exercise is performed without appropriate sympathetic interruption.

The basic principles of physical therapy for RSDS patients include gentle, repetitive, active motion and massage and weight-bearing activities. Passive motion is not recommended. Between exercising, splinting occasionally is needed to prevent contractures.

Exercise will improve mobility, prevent contractures, and reduce pain. Once some degree of active range of motion has been restored, functional activities can be introduced, practicing simple tasks initially and progressing gradually to more complex activities [1,2,68,109,120–122].

Stress-loading exercise [123,124], paraffin baths, and contrast baths may be helpful tools in the RSDS therapy protocol, both in supervised treatment and as part of an independent self-treatment regimen. Stress loading consists of active traction (carrying activities) and compression exercises (scrubbing) that provide stressful stimuli to the extremity without joint motion.

Contrast baths are done by alternating immersion of extremities in media (generally water) at contrasting (hot and cold) temperatures. Such baths may be useful in decreasing edema, improving peripheral circulation, and decreasing joint pain and stiffness.

Other Treatment Modalities

Other adjunctive treatments that might help the RSDS patient include cold, heat, thermoelastic gloves, TENS, acupuncture, psychotherapy, nonsympatholytic medications, opioid analgesics, spinal cord stimulation, and opioid pump implantation.

Cold packs are useful in stage 1 disease, whereas warm moist packs are more helpful in stages 2 and 3, when there is an overall decrease in blood flow. Hot packs decrease muscle spasm and improve blood flow [125,126].

Thermoelastic gloves provide compression, warmth, and protection [1,2]. TENS or even acupuncture appears to help some individuals with RSDS [2,21,24,71,127–134].

Psychotherapy is an extremely important modality for RSDS patients. Depression, anxiety, financial concerns, and fears about the future are common problems encountered in this population. RSDS patients frequently need aggressive treatment of depression through therapy and medications. Biofeedback and hypnosis are occasionally helpful in promoting relaxation, decreasing muscle spasm, and improving circulation through reduction of sympathetic tone [125,135,136]. Relaxation training is important, as a chronically anxious state with high levels of circulating NE from the adrenal glands (which respond in this manner to chronic anxiety) certainly will worsen the pain of RSDS.

Nonsympatholytic medications that might provide analgesic relief for these individuals include nonsteroidal anti-inflammatory drugs, corticosteroids, tricyclic antidepressants, anticonvulsants, baclofen, mexiletine, capsaicin cream, and opioid analgesics.

The primary usefulness of nonsteroidal anti-inflammatory drugs is to deal with the myofascial discomfort associated with physical and occupational treatment, which typically can cause myofascial pain secondary to prior disuse syndromes [24,43]. Gastrointestinal side effects should be monitored.

The use of corticosteroids has been advocated in the literature particularly if there are any contraindications to sympathetic blocks or if the latter are not helpful. Various protocols have been recommended (e.g., 30 mg/day for 12 weeks or 100–200 mg/day for 2–3 weeks) [7,21,24,71,137–142].

Tricyclic antidepressants (amitriptyline, imipramine, and nortriptyline) are frequently helpful in promoting better-quality sleep, in decreasing neurogenic pain, and in treating depression [143–149]. Anticonvulsants (e.g., phenytoin, carbamazepine, gabapentin, valproic acid) are often helpful in decreasing neurogenic pain, including the pain of RSDS [21,150,151]. Anticonvulsants are suggested to deal with the patient's complaints of lancinating, shooting, spontaneous, electrical-like pain. In some patients, the typical burning associated with RSDS may also be favorably affected. Biannual serum studies for anticonvulsant level, liver function, and blood counts should be used to monitor patients maintained on anticonvulsant therapy.

Baclofen (40–80 mg/day in divided doses) is useful for sympathetically related abnormalities of tone, especially dyskinesia or dystonia [42]. Mexiletine (oral lidocaine) is increasingly being used for various types of neurogenic pain, including the pain of RSDS [152–154]. Capsaicin cream depletes nerve terminals of substance P, feels quite warm, and may be soothing for patients with later-stage disease.

The use of oral opioid analgesics, opioid pump implantation, and spinal cord stimulation should be considered if traditional modalities have failed to relieve pain and improve function and quality of life for the suffering RSDS patient. Because of the controversial (opioid analgesics) and costly (opioid pump implantation, spinal cord stimulation) nature of these modalities, separate chapters are devoted to discussion of each (see Chapters 12–14).

Finally, patients should be instructed to stop smoking, as nicotine, a potent vasoconstrictor, often worsens the symptoms of RSDS [25,43].

Conclusion

RSDS is a neuropathic condition that must be identified and treated early in the course of disease. The disorder, which is difficult both to diagnose and to treat, can prove frustrating for the physician and for third-party payers (owing to the staggering health care costs associated with diagnosis and treatment). Ultimately, however, it is the patient and his or her family who must deal with a number of unfortunate realities including extreme lifelong pain, prolonged family disruption, disability and unemployment, misdiagnosis by and disbelief of inexperienced physicians, improper treatment, multiple operations, unsuccessful surgery, diminished quality of life, and increased health care costs.

References

1. Mausner PA. Reflex sympathetic dystrophy. Trial Talk 1987;36:92.

2. Lankford LL. Reflex Sympathetic Dystrophy. In CM Evarts (ed), Surgery of the Musculoskeletal System. New York: Churchill Livingstone, 1983;145.

3. Mitchell SW, Morehouse GR, Keen WW. Gunshot Wounds and Other Injuries of Nerves. New York: Lippincott, 1864.

4. Mitchell SW. Injuries of Nerves and Their Consequences. New York: Lippincott, 1872.

5. Shelton RM, Lewis CW. Reflex sympathetic dystrophy: a review. J Am Acad Dermatol 1990;22:513.

6. Escobar PL. Reflex sympathetic dystrophy. Orthop Rev 1986;15:646.

7. Glick EN. Reflex dystrophy (algoneurodystrophy): results of treatment by corticosteroids. Rheumatol Rehabil 1973;12:84.

8. Schwartzman RJ, McLellan TL. Reflex sympathetic dystrophy—a review. Arch Neurol 1987;44:555.

9. Roberts WJ. A hypothesis on the physiological basis for causalgia and related pains. Pain 1986;24:297.

10. Stanton-Hicks M, Janig W, Hassenbusch S, et al. Reflex sympathetic dystrophy: changing concepts and taxonomy. Pain 1995;63:127.

11. Sudeck P. Dietrophische extremitantensgroung durch periphere (infetoise and traumatische) Reize Dtsch Z Chir 1931;234:596.

12. DeTakats G. Reflex dystrophy of the extremities. Arch Surg 1937;34:939.

13. Homans J. Minor causalgia: a hyperesthetic neurovascular syndrome. N Engl J Med 1940;222:870.

14. Patman RD, Thompson JE, Persson AV. Management of posttraumatic pain syndromes: a report of 113 cases. Ann Surg 1973;177:780.

15. Steinbrocker O. The shoulder-hand syndrome. Am J Med 1947;3:402.

16. Evans JA. Reflex sympathetic dystrophy. Surg Clin North Am 1946;26:780.

17. Serre H, Simon L, Claustie J. Sympathetic dystrophy of the foot. Rev Rheum 1967;34:722.

18. Lehman EP. Traumatic vasospasm: a study of four cases of vasospasm in the upper extremity. Arch Surg 1934;29:92.

19. International Association for the Study of Pain (IASP). Classification of Chronic Pain: Descriptions of Chronic Pain Syndromes and Definitions of Pain Terms (2nd ed). Seattle: IASP Press, 1994.

20. Steinbrocker O, Argyros TG. The shoulder-hand syndrome: present status as a diagnostic and therapeutic entity. Med Clin North Am 1958;42:1533.

21. Warfield CA. The sympathetic dystrophies. Hosp Pract 1984;19(5):52C.

22. Horowitz SH. Brachial plexus injuries with causalgia resulting from transaxillary rib resection. Arch Surg 1985;20:1189.

23. Goldner JD. Causes and prevention of reflex sympathetic dystrophy. J Hand Surg 1980;5:295.

24. Rowlingson JC. The sympathetic dystrophies. Int Anesthesiol Clin 1983;21(4):117.

25. Lankford LL, Thompson JE. Reflex Sympathetic Dystrophy: Upper and Lower Extremity: Diagnosis and Management. In The American Academy of Orthopaedic Surgeons Instructional Course Lectures, vol 26. St. Louis: Mosby, 1977;63.
26. Kleinert HE, Cole NM, Wayne L, et al. Post-traumatic sympathetic dystrophy. Orthop Clin North Am 1973;4:917.
27. Hodges DL, McGuire TJ. Burning and pain after injury. Is it causalgia or reflex sympathetic dystrophy? Postgrad Med 1988;83:185.
28. Richards RL. Causalgia. Arch Neurol 1967;16:339.
29. Mayfield FH. Causalgia. Springfield, IL: Thomas, 1951;3.
30. DeTakats G. Causalgic states in peace and war. JAMA 1945;128:669.
31. Sylvest J, Jensen EM, Siggaard-Andersen J, et al. Reflex dystrophy. Scand J Rehabil Med 1977;9:25.
32. Bonica JJ. Causalgia and other reflex sympathetic dystrophies. Postgrad Med 1973;53:143.
33. Richards RL. Vasomotor and nutritional disturbances after injuries to peripheral nerves. Med Res Council Spec Rep Ser 1954;282:25.
34. Jaeger SH, Singer DI, Whitenack SH. Nerve injury complications. Management of neurogenic pain syndromes. Hand Clin 1986;2:217.
35. DeTakats G. Nature of painful vasodilatation in causalgic states. Arch Neurol Psychiatry 1943;50:318.
36. Doupe J, Cullen CH, Chance GQ. Post-traumatic pain and the causalgic syndrome. J Neurol Neurosurg Psychiatry 1944;7:33.
37. Seddon H. Surgical Disorders of the Peripheral Nerves. New York: Churchill Livingstone, 1972;139.
38. Turek SL. Orthopaedics: Principles and Their Application. Philadelphia: Lippincott, 1984;796.
39. Schott GD. Mechanisms of causalgia and related clinical conditions: the role of the central and of the sympathetic nervous systems. Brain 1986;109:717.
40. Mayfield FH, Devine JW. Causalgia. Surg Gynecol Obstet 1945;80:631.
41. Meyer RA, Campbell JN, Raja S. Peripheral neural mechanisms of cutaneous hyperalgesia. Adv Pain Res Ther 1985;9:53.
42. Schwartzman RJ, Kerrigan J. The movement disorder of reflex sympathetic dystrophy. Neurology 1990;40:57.
43. Tietjen R. Reflex sympathetic dystrophy of the knee. Clin Orthop 1986;209:234.
44. Markoff M, Farole A. Reflex sympathetic dystrophy syndrome: case report with a review of the literature. Oral Surg Oral Med Oral Pathol 1986;61:23.
45. Weiss WU. Psychophysiologic aspects of reflex sympathetic dystrophy syndrome. Am J Pain Manage 1994;4:67.
46. Lynch ME. Psychologic aspects of reflex sympathetic dystrophy: a review of the adult and paediatric literature. Pain 1992;49:337.
47. Van Houdenhove B, Vasquez G, Onghena P, et al. Etiopathogenesis of reflex sympathetic dystrophy: a review and biopsychosocial hypothesis. Clin J Pain 1992;8:300.
48. Bruehl S, Carlson CR. Predisposing psychological factors in the development of reflex sympathetic dystrophy—a review of the empirical evidence. Clin J Pain 1992;8:287.
49. Egle UT, Hoffman SO. Psychosomatic Aspects of Reflex Sympathetic Dystrophy. In M Stanton-Hicks, W Janig, RA Boas (eds), Reflex Sympathetic Dystrophy. Boston: Kluwer Academic, 1990.
50. Van Houdenhove B. Neuroalgodystrophy: a psychiatrist's view. Clin Rheumatol 1986;5:399.
51. Bickerstaff DR, Charlesworth D, Kanis JA. Changes in cortical and trabecular bone in algodystrophy. Br J Rheumatol 1993;32:46.
52. Kozin F, Genant HK, Bekerman C, et al. The reflex sympathetic dystrophy syndrome: 2. Roentgenographic and scintigraphic evidence of bilaterality and of periarticular accentuation. Am J Med 1976;60:332.
53. Hobbins WB. Differential Diagnosis of Painful Conditions and Thermography. In WCV Parris (ed), Contemporary Issues in Chronic Pain Management. Boston: Kluwer Academic, 1991;251.
54. Hobbins WB. Pain Management in Thermography. In PP Raj (ed), Practical Management of Pain (2nd ed). St. Louis: Mosby–Year Book, 1992;181.
55. Green J. A preliminary note: dynamic thermography may offer a key to the early recognition of reflex sympathetic dystrophy. J Acad Neuromusc Thermogr 1989;8:104.
56. Green J. The pathophysiology of reflex sympathetic dystrophy as demonstrated by dynamic thermography. J Acad Neuromusc Thermogr 1989;8:121.
57. Green J. Tutorial 12: thermography medical infrared imaging. Pain Dig 1993;3:268.
58. Uematsu S, Jankel WR. Skin temperature response of the foot to cold stress of the hand: a test to evaluate somatosympathetic response. Thermology 1988;3:41.
59. Feldman F. Thermography of the hand and wrist: practical applications. Hand Clin 1991;7:99.
60. Karstetter KW, Sherman RA. Use of thermography for initial detection of early reflex sympathetic dystrophy. J Am Podiatr Med Assoc 1991;81:198.
61. Kozin F, Soin JS, Ryan LM, et al. Bone scintigraphy in the reflex sympathetic dystrophy syndrome. Radiology 1981;138:437.
62. Weiss L, Alfano A, Bardfeld P, et al. Prognostic value of triple phase bone scanning for reflex sympathetic dystrophy in hemiplegia. Arch Phys Med Rehabil 1993;74:716.
63. Davidoff G, Werner R, Cremer S, et al. Predictive value of the three-phase technetium bone scan in diagnosis of reflex sympathetic dystrophy syndrome. Arch Phys Med Rehabil 1989;70:135.
64. Intenzo C, Kim S, Millin J, et al. Scintigraphic patterns of the reflex sympathetic dystrophy syndrome of the lower extremities. Clin Nucl Med 1989;14:657.

65. Constantinesco A, Brunot B, Demangeat J, et al. Three-phase bone scanning as an aid to early diagnosis in reflex sympathetic dystrophy of the hand: a study of 89 cases. Ann Chir Main Memb Super 1986;5:93.

66. Greyson N, Tepperman P. Three-phase bone studies in hemiplegia with reflex sympathetic dystrophy and the effect of disuse. J Nucl Med 1984;25:423.

67. Demangeat J, Constantinesco A, Brunot B, et al. Three-phase bone scanning in reflex sympathetic dystrophy of the hand. J Nucl Med 1988;29:26.

68. Berstein BH, Singsen BH, Kent JT, et al. Reflex neurovascular dystrophy in childhood. J Pediatr 1978;93:211.

69. Laxer RM, Malleson PN, Morrison RT. Technetium 99m–methylene diphosphonate bone scans in children with reflex neurovascular dystrophy. J Pediatr 1985;106:437.

70. Holder LE, Mackinnon SE. Reflex sympathetic dystrophy in the hands: clinical and scintigraphic criteria. Radiology 1984;152:517.

71. Schutzer SF, Gossling HR. The treatment of reflex sympathetic dystrophy syndrome. J Bone Joint Surg Am 1984;66:625.

72. Arner S. Intravenous phentolamine test: diagnostic and prognostic use in reflex sympathetic dystrophy. Pain 1991;46:17.

73. Raja SN, Treede RD, Davis KD, et al. Systemic alpha-adrenergic blockade with phentolamine: a diagnostic test for sympathetically maintained pain. Anesthesiology 1991;74:691.

74. Campbell JN, Meyer RA, Raja SN. Is nociceptor activation by alpha-1 adrenoreceptors the culprit in sympathetically maintained pain? Am Pain Soc J 1992;1:3.

75. deGroot J. The Autonomic Nervous System. In J de Groot (ed), Correlative Neuroanatomy. East Norwalk, CT: Appleton & Lange, 1991;193.

76. Fields HL. Painful Dysfunction of the Nervous System. In HL Fields (ed), Pain. New York: McGraw-Hill, 1987;133.

77. Livingston WK. Pain Mechanisms. New York: Macmillan, 1943.

78. Hooshmand H. Chronic Pain: Reflex Sympathetic Dystrophy Prevention and Management. Boca Raton, FL: CRC Press, 1993.

79. Harden RN, Duc TA, Williams TR, et al. Norepinephrine and epinephrine levels in affected versus unaffected limbs in sympathetically maintained pain. Clin J Pain 1994;10:324.

80. Fields HL. Pain Pathways in the Central Nervous System. In HL Fields (ed), Pain. New York: McGraw-Hill, 1987;41.

81. Melzack R, Casey KL. Sensory, Motivational, and Central Control Determinants of Pain. A New Conceptual Model. In D Kenshalo (ed), The Skin Senses. Springfield, IL: Thomas, 1968;423.

82. Visitsunthorn U, Prete P. Reflex sympathetic dystrophy of the lower extremity: a complication of herpes zoster

with dramatic response to propranolol. West J Med 1981;135:62.

83. Ghostine SY, Comair YG, Turner DM, et al. Phenoxybenzamine in the treatment of causalgia: report of 40 cases. J Neurosurg 1984;60:1263.

84. Prough DS, McLeskey CH, Poehling GG, et al. Efficiency of oral nifedipine in the treatment of reflex sympathetic dystrophy. Anesthesiology 1985;62:796.

85. Pak TJ, Martin GM, Magness JL, et al. Reflex sympathetic dystrophy. Minn Med 1970;53:507.

86. Tabira T, Shibasaki H, Kuroiwa Y. Reflex sympathetic dystrophy (causalgia). Treatment with guanethidine. Arch Neurol 1983;40:430.

87. Hannington-Kiff JG. Intravenous regional sympathetic block with guanethidine. Lancet 1974;1:1019.

88. Hannington-Kiff JG. Relief of Sudeck's atrophy by regional intravenous guanethidine. Lancet 1977;1:1132.

89. Hannington-Kiff JG. Relief of causalgia in limbs by regional intravenous guanethidine. BMJ 1979;2:367.

90. Hannington-Kiff JG. Hyperadrenergic-affected limb causalgia: relief by IV pharmacologic norepinephrine blockade. Am Heart J 1982;103:152.

91. Glynn CJ, Basedow RW, Walsh JA. Pain relief following postganglionic sympathetic blockade with IV guanethidine. Br J Anaesth 1981;53:1297.

92. Loh L, Nathan PW, Schott GD, et al. Effects of guanethidine infusion in certain painful states. J Neurol Neurosurg Psychiatry 1980;43:446.

93. Bonnelli S, Conoscente F, Movilia PG, et al. Regional intravenous guanethidine vs. stellate ganglion block in reflex sympathetic dystrophies. A randomized trial. Pain 1983;16:297.

94. Holland AJC, Davies KH, Wallace DH. Sympathetic blockade of isolated limbs by intravenous guanethidine. Can Anaesth Soc J 1977;24:597.

95. Chuinard RG, Dabezies FJ, Gould JS, et al. Intravenous reserpine for treatment of reflex sympathetic dystrophy. South Med J 1981;74:1481.

96. Benzon HT, Chomka CM, Brunner EA. Treatment of reflex sympathetic dystrophy with regional intravenous reserpine. Anesth Analg 1980;59:500.

97. Poplawski ZJ, Wiley AM, Murray JF. Post-traumatic dystrophy of the extremities. J Bone Joint Surg Am 1983;65:642.

98. DeTakats G. The nature of painful vasodilatation in causalgic states. Arch Neurol 1943;50:318.

99. Wettrell G, Hallbook T, Hultquist C. Reflex sympathetic dystrophy in two young females. Acta Paediatr Scand 1979;68:923.

100. Carron H, McCue F. Reflex sympathetic dystrophy in a 10-year-old. South Med J 1972;65:631.

101. Guntheroth WG, Chakmakjian S, Brena SC, et al. Post-traumatic sympathetic dystrophy: dissociation of pain and vasomotor changes. Am J Dis Children 1971;121:511.

102. Loh L, Nathan PW. Painful peripheral states and sympathetic blocks. J Neurol Neurosurg Psychiatry 1978;41:661.

103. Loh L, Nathan PW, Schott GD. Pain due to lesions of central nervous system removed by sympathetic block. BMJ 1981;2:1026.

104. Steinbrocker O. The shoulder-hand syndrome. Present perspective. Arch Phys Med Rehabil 1968;49:388.

105. Steinbrocker O, Neustadt D, Lapin L. Shoulder-hand syndrome. Sympathetic block compared with corticotropin and cortisone therapy. JAMA 1946;153:788.

106. Subbarao J, Stillwell GK. Reflex sympathetic dystrophy syndrome of the upper extremity: analysis of total outcome of management of 125 cases. Arch Phys Med Rehabil 1981;62:549.

107. Ferrante FM. Techniques for blockade of the sympathetic nervous system. Curr Rev Clin Anesth 1991;12:1.

108. Wirth FP, Rutherford RB. A civilian experience with causalgia. Arch Surg 1970;100:633.

109. Shumacker HB, Abramson DI. Posttraumatic vasomotor disorders: with particular reference to late manifestations and treatment. Surg Gynecol Obstet 1949;88:417.

110. Holden WD. Sympathetic dystrophy. Arch Surg 1948;57:373.

111. Echlin F, Owens FM, Wells WL. Observations on 'major' and 'minor' causalgia. Arch Neurol 1945;62:183.

112. Szeinfeld M, Palleres VS. Considerations in the treatment of causalgia. Anesthesiology 1983;58:294.

113. Rasmussen TB, Freedman H. Treatment of causalgia: an analysis of 100 cases. J Neurosurg 1946;3:165.

114. Spurling RG. Causalgia of the upper extremity: treatment by dorsal sympathetic ganglionectomy. Arch Neurol 1930;23:784.

115. Barnes R. The role of sympathectomy in the treatment of causalgia. J Bone Joint Surg Br 1953;35:172.

116. Evans JA. Sympathectomy for reflex sympathetic dystrophy: report of 29 cases. JAMA 1946;132:620.

117. Hardy WG, Posch JL, Webster JE, et al. The problem of major and minor causalgia. Am J Surg 1958;95:545.

118. Olcott C, Eltherington LG, Wilcosky BR, et al. Reflex sympathetic dystrophy—the surgeon's role in management. J Vasc Surg 1991;14:488.

119. Bingham JA. Some problems of causalgic pain. A clinical and experimental study. BMJ 1948;2:334.

120. Ruggeri SB, Athreya BH, Doughty R, et al. Reflex sympathetic dystrophy in children. Clin Orthop 1982;163:225.

121. Goodman CR. Treatment of shoulder-hand syndrome. N Y State J Med 1971;71:559.

122. Johnson EW, Pannozzo AN. Management of shoulder-hand syndrome. JAMA 1966;195:152.

123. Watson HK, Carlson LK. Stress loading treatment for reflex sympathetic dystrophy. Complications Orthop 1990;2:19.

124. Watson HK, Carlson L. Treatment of reflex sympathetic dystrophy of the hand with an active "stress loading" program. J Hand Surg [Am] 1987;12:779.

125. Blanchard EB. The use of temperature biofeedback in the treatment of chronic pain due to causalgia. Biofeedback Self Regul 1979;4:183.

126. Fermaglich DR. Reflex sympathetic dystrophy in children. Pediatrics 1977;60:881.

127. Richlin DM, Carron H, Rowlingson JC, et al. Reflex sympathetic dystrophy: successful treatment by transcutaneous nerve stimulation. J Pediatr 1978;95:84.

128. Owens S, Atkinson ER, Lees DE. Thermographic evidence of reduced sympathetic tone with transcutaneous nerve stimulation. Anesthesiology 1979;50:62.

129. Ebersold MJ, Laws ER, Albers JW. Measurements of autonomic function before, during, and after transcutaneous stimulation in patients with chronic pain and control subjects. Mayo Clin Proc 1977;52:228.

130. Meyer GA, Fields HL. Causalgia treated by selective large fibre stimulation of peripheral nerve. Brain 1972;95:163.

131. Chan CS, Chow SP. Electroacupuncture in the treatment of post-traumatic sympathetic dystrophy (Sudeck's atrophy). Br J Anaesth 1981;53:899.

132. Leo KC. Use of electrical stimulation at acupuncture points for the treatment of reflex sympathetic dystrophy in a child. Phys Ther 1983;63:957.

133. Fialka V, Resch KL, Ritter-Dietrich D, et al. Acupuncture for reflex sympathetic dystrophy. Arch Intern Med 1993;153:661.

134. Hill SD, Sheng LM, Chandler PJ. Reflex sympathetic dystrophy and electroacupuncture. Tex Med J 1991;87:76.

135. Lauer JW. Hypnosis in the relief of pain. Med Clin North Am 1968;52:217.

136. Gainer MJ. Hypnotherapy for reflex sympathetic dystrophy. Am J Clin Hypn 1992;34:227.

137. Kozin F, McCarty DJ, Sims J, et al. The reflex sympathetic dystrophy syndrome: I. Clinical and histologic studies. Evidence for bilaterality, response to corticosteroids and articular involvement. Am J Med 1976;60:321.

138. Ingram GJ, Scher RK, Lally EV. Reflex sympathetic dystrophy following nail biopsy. J Am Acad Dermatol 1987;16:253.

139. Kozin F, Ryan L, Carerra G, et al. The reflex sympathetic dystrophy syndrome (RSDS): III. Scintigraphic studies, further evidence for the therapeutic efficacy of systemic corticosteroids and proposed diagnostic criteria. Am J Med 1981;70:23.

140. DeTakats G. Sympathetic reflex dystrophy. Med Clin North Am 1965;49:117.

141. Mowat AG. Treatment of the shoulder-hand syndrome with corticosteroids. Ann Rheum Dis 1974;33:120.

142. Christensen K, Jensen EM, Noer I. The reflex sympathetic dystrophy syndrome. Response to treatment with systemic corticosteroids. Acta Chir Scand 1982;148:653.

143. Watson CP, Evans RJ, Reed K, et al. Amitriptyline versus placebo in postherpetic neuralgia. Neurology 1982;32:671.

144. Gomez-Perez FJ, Rull JA, Dies H, Guillermo J. Nortriptyline and fluphenazine in the symptomatic treatment of diabetic neuropathy. A double-blind crossover study. Pain 1985;23:395.

145. Kvinesdal B, Molin J, Froland A, Gram LF. Imipramine treatment of painful diabetic neuropathy. JAMA 1984;251:1727.
146. Turkington RW. Depression masquerading as diabetic neuropathy. JAMA 1980;243:1147.
147. Gringras M. A clinical trial of Tofranil in rheumatic pain in general practice. J Int Med Res 1976;4:41.
148. Scott WAM. The relief of pain with an antidepressant in arthritis. Practitioner 1969;202:802.
149. Kehoe WA. Antidepressants for chronic pain: selection and dosing considerations. Am J Pain Manage 1993;3:161.
150. Chaturvedi SK. Phenytoin in reflex sympathetic dystrophy. Pain 1989;36:379.
151. Mellick GA, Mellicy LB, Mellick LB. Gabapentin in the management of reflex sympathetic dystrophy. J Pain Symptom Manage 1995;10:265.
152. Davis RW. Phantom sensation, phantom pain, and stump pain. Arch Phys Med Rehabil 1993;74:79.
153. Chabal C, Russell LC, Burchiel KJ. The effect of intravenous lidocaine, tocainide, and mexiletine on spontaneously active fibers originating in rat sciatic neuromas. Pain 1989;38:333.
154. Dejgaard A, Petersen P, Kastrup J. Mexiletine for the treatment of chronic painful diabetic neuropathy. Lancet 1988;29:9.

Chapter 12
Opioid Analgesia

Jack L. Rook

A small subset of cumulative trauma disorder or reflex sympathetic dystrophy syndrome patients might benefit physically, functionally, and emotionally from the use of opioid analgesic maintenance therapy for management of chronic unrelenting pain. The use of opioids for treatment of chronic nonmalignant pain (CNMP) is a fairly hot topic both in the literature and at pain seminars. Thus far, no double-blind, randomized, controlled studies have focused on the use of these medications for chronic pain management. Nevertheless, anecdotal reports and case studies in the literature support their use if stringent prescribing guidelines are followed and if patients are seen regularly for assessment of efficacy.

The use of opioids for CNMP is a controversial issue throughout the world. For every physician who believes that narcotic analgesics are indicated for those patients with chronic pain, objective pathologic processes, and failure of conservative and sometimes even surgical interventions, numerous opponents (medical and lay people, government agencies) believe that such management is detrimental to the patient and to society. Indeed, many physicians go to great lengths to avoid the use of opioids. Multiple pharmacologic combinations with poorly tolerated medications, costly pain clinics, multiple surgical procedures, spinal-cord stimulator implantation, and neuroablative procedures (e.g., rhizotomy, sympathectomy, neurectomy) might all be considered preferred treatments as opposed to around-the-clock opioid analgesic maintenance therapy.

The varying opinions regarding the use of opioids have developed for a number of reasons. The topic of pain management is addressed poorly in most medical schools, and knowledge of opioid pharmacology is lacking in the medical community (i.e., among physicians, nurses, and pharmacists). Many opioids have a half-life of only 2–3 hours, yet they are given on an every 4- to 6-hour schedule, leaving most patients (who are suffering acutely or chronically) to endure several hours of uncontrolled pain. Attempts by patients to increase dosage or frequency in such situations is often perceived as abuse or drug-seeking behavior, when in effect it represents the patient's response to waning levels of medication and breakthrough pain. A typical scenario may be one of inappropriately low doses of opioids at intervals that are longer than their duration of action, which results in undertreatment.

Reservations regarding the use of opioids also focus on the risk of opioid toxicity, although typically the development of addiction is overestimated. Also, pain assessment and monitoring techniques from month to month are inadequate. Medications may have to be titrated (upward or downward) on the basis of the patient's response from visit to visit.

Knowledge of salient terminology (e.g., *addiction, tolerance, dependence, pseudoaddiction*) is deficient throughout the medical community and society. Also, physicians who prescribe opioids for CNMP must often deal with the perception in the medical community that they order these medications too liberally. It is the perceived risk of sanctions by governmental and medical agencies that has the greatest effect on prescribing practices [1]. Although no statutory limitations apply to the treatment of pain with opioid drugs [2], many physicians perceive an unacceptable degree of personal risk in the prescription of such medications to patients with CNMP. Perceived sanctions might include investigation by the U.S. Drug Enforcement Agency, a state medical board, or local peer review committees. Also, concern arises over liability if the patient does become iatrogenically addicted. Such perceived risks have a powerful conscious or subconscious effect on the prescribing habits of virtually all physicians.

Physicians choosing to undertake prescription of opioid maintenance therapy for CNMP should follow a series of strict prescribing guidelines and ensure a good understanding of the literature in support of the use of this therapy for this patient population.

Background Studies

Since 1982, eight published clinical studies encompassing 642 patients have focused on opioid use for CNMP (Table 12-1) [1,3–9]. In the first and largest survey yet published, Taub [3] describes 313 treated patients who had chronic intractable pain and were maintained on a variety of opioids (methadone, oxycodone, codeine, meperidine [Demerol]) for up to 6 years. The average daily dose was equivalent to 10–20 mg oral methadone per day. No significant side effects or toxicity were observed. Overall efficacy was considered good, as no patients suffered uncontrolled spontaneous pain while on therapy. Tolerance was not a major problem, and only 13 patients presented management problems (i.e., prescription forgery, heroin abuse, loss or theft of medication, and excessive dose escalation), eight of whom had a history of substance abuse in some capacity.

In 1984, a second report by France et al. [4] described the use of chronic opioid therapy as a component of multidisciplinary pain treatment in 16 patients, most of whom had chronic back pain. Drugs used included methadone, codeine, and oxycodone, the mean equianalgesic dose being 8 mg oral methadone per day. At the time of discharge from the program, all patients had either good (50–74%) or excellent (75–99%) pain relief. Twelve

of the 16 patients returned to work, and none of the patients developed management problems.

In 1986, Urban et al. [5] performed a small survey of five patients with phantom limb pain. This survey is of particular importance because it demonstrates the potential for sustained benefit in patients with refractory neuropathic pain. The five patients were treated with methadone (10–20 mg/day) for a mean period of 22 months. At follow-up, all patients reported greater than 50% pain relief, and all experienced a recurrence of pain on attempted withdrawal of the opioid. No management problems (i.e., toxicity or abuse) arose in this study.

In 1983, Tennant and Uelman [6] described 118 patients who had CNMP and had failed a variety of pain clinic approaches. Following initiation of chronic opioid therapy, 15 were able to return to work, and all reduced medical visits.

A second survey by Tennant et al. [7], conducted in 1988, described 52 patients with chronic pain and treated with opioids (equianalgesic dosage of 10–240 mg oral methadone) for an average of 12 years. Efficacy was reported as good in 88% and partial in 12%. Abuse behaviors developed in nine patients, and the principal side effect experienced was constipation. This survey is significant for its long duration of opioid treatment and its high rate of reported efficacy.

In 1988, Wan Lu et al. [8] described 76 patients, most of whom had low-back pain. These patients were treated principally with methadone (maximum daily dosage, 20 mg orally) for an average of 29 months (range, 6–76 months). Efficacy was reported as greater than 25% pain relief in 87% of patients. In all cases, relief was sustained at the last follow-up, and no dose escalation was required. Abuse behaviors developed in seven patients.

Two surveys of patients given chronic opioid therapy for nonmalignant pain have been reported by Portenoy [1]. The report described a total of 58 patients with varying diagnoses, including chronic back pain (20), chronic pain of unknown etiology (13), and neuropathic pain (12). Of the neuropathic pain population, two had causalgia. Outcome data were available for 39 of the 58 patients, and pain relief for 32 of the 39 was either adequate (16) or partial (16). Only seven patients continued to have sustained periods of severe pain. Fluctuation in pain over time often was mirrored by transitory increases in opioid dosage with eventual

Table 12-1. Published Clinical Studies on Opioid Use for Chronic Nonmalignant Pain

Study	No. of Patients	Diagnosis	Average Duration of Therapy	Drug	Efficacy	Problems (No. of patients)
Taub [4]	313	—	≤6 yrs	Methadone, oxycodone, codeine, meperidine	Good	Management problems; abuse (13)
France et al. [4]	16	Back pain	6.5 yrs (2–14 yrs)	Methadone, codeine, oxycodone	3 Good, 13 very good, 12 returned to work	None
Urban et al. [5]	5	Phantom pain	22 mos (12–26 mos)	Methadone	Good	None
Tennant and Uelman [6]	118	Arthritis/bursitis, post-trauma pain, headache, back/spine disorder, postsurgical pain, miscellaneous	7 mos	Oxycodone, hydromorphone, meperidine, methadone, codeine, morphine	Good	—
Tennant et al. [7]	52	Degenerative arthritis, traumatic injuries	Mean: 12 yrs	—	88% Good, 12% partial	Abuse (9), constipation
Wan Lu et al. [8]	76	Back pain	29 mos (6–76 mos)	Methadone	>25% Pain relief in 87%	Abuse (7)
Portenoy [1]	58	Back pain, neuropathic pain, others	6 mos–20 yrs	Oxycodone, methadone, levorphanol, meperidine, others	Information from 39: 16 (41%) good, 16 (41%) partial, 7 (18%) no benefit	Personality change (2), myoclonus (2), abuse (4)
Zenz [9]	100	Neuropathic back pain, osteoporosis, head-facial ischemic pain, rheumatic pain	≥1 yr (n = 23), ≤1 yr (n = 77)	Buprenorphine, sustained-release morphine, sustained-release dihydrocodeine	51% Good, 28% partial, 21% no benefit	Constipation (46), addiction (0), respiratory depression (0), euphoria (0)

return to baseline, which in all cases was accomplished with guidance from the treating physician. Four patients developed persistent and distressing side effects, and four others developed abuse behaviors.

Zenz et al. [9] surveyed 100 patients with non-malignant pain, 53 of whom had neuropathic pain. Medications used included sustained-release dihydrocodeine, buprenorphine, and sustained-release morphine. Pain reduction was measured via visual analog scales, and the Karnofsky performance status scale was used to assess function. Outcome data included good pain relief (50% or greater) in 51 patients and partial relief (25–50%) in 28 patients. Twenty-one patients had no beneficial effects from opioid therapy. Pain reduction was associated with an increase in performance. The most common side effects were constipation and nausea. There were no cases of addiction to the opioids.

Data from the Zenz et al. study [9] indicated that opioids were effective in treatment of neuropathic pain. More than one-half of the patients with neuropathic pain obtained good pain reduction with lower opioid doses than those used by patients with non-neuropathic pain. Signs of dependence, disability, or increasing depression were absent during opioid treatment. The authors concluded that despite statements in the literature holding that opioids were ineffective for treatment of chronic neuropathic pain [10], their data supported the use of such medications in this population if no therapeutic alternatives existed.

Function of Opioids in Relieving Pain

Such opiate analgesics as morphine are believed to relieve pain by activating the descending pain-modulatory network. (Ascending and descending pain transmission pathways are reviewed in Chapter 3.) The descending pain-modulatory network extends from the cortex and limbic system to the brain stem and, ultimately, to the spinal cord dorsal horn [11–13]. Important work leading to a better understanding of these pathways included research on electrical stimulation–produced analgesia [14–16], discovery of specific opiate receptors within the central nervous system (CNS) [17,18], and discovery of endogenous opioids [19–21].

Stimulation-Produced Analgesia

The concept that there was an independent and specific CNS network that modified pain sensation was first suggested by the observation that electrical stimulation of the midbrain in rats selectively suppressed responses to painful stimuli [22,23]. This phenomenon—stimulation-produced analgesia—was reproduced in humans when neurosurgeons placed electrodes in homologous sites and demonstrated how electrical stimulation produced a striking reduction of severe pain [15,24,25].

The periaqueductal gray area (PAG) and the rostroventral medulla (RVM) are regions in which electrical stimulation is highly effective in producing analgesia [16,26–28]. Both PAG and RVM are believed to be part of the descending pain network.

Opiates produce analgesia by a direct action on the CNS. In animal studies, microinjection of small amounts of narcotics into the brain stem can produce potent analgesia [29,30]. The brain stem regions that produce analgesia when electrically stimulated largely overlap those at which opiate microinjection produces analgesia (PAG, RVM). Similarly, application of opioids to the outer layers of the spinal cord has an additive analgesic effect [31]. Opiate-sensitive systems at both spinal cord and brain stem levels clearly seem to contribute to the narcotic analgesic effect [32].

Opiate Receptors

The analgesia produced by opiate drugs depends on their ability to bind with opiate receptors on neuronal cell membranes. Often, the opioid receptor function is described as a *lock-and-key phenomenon*. Opiates bind to their receptors with varying affinity. The stronger the attachment, the greater the analgesic potency of the drug. For example, codeine (a mild narcotic) binds weakly to opioid receptors, whereas morphine, a drug with greater analgesic potency, has greater affinity for the same receptor [17,18,33,34].

Localization of opiate receptors throughout the body was made possible through the use of radioactively labeled opiates. Dense concentrations of opiate-binding sites have been localized to the amygdala, hypothalamus, midbrain (PAG), medulla (RVM, nucleus raphe magnus), and spinal cord dorsal horn

Table 12-2. Contrasting Features of Endogenous Versus Exogenous Opioids

Effect	Endogenous Opioids	Exogenous Opioids
Pain relief	Yes	Yes
Antidepressant	Yes	No
Strength	100 times stronger	100 times weaker
Dose required	Tiny	Flooding dosage
Effect on hormones	Stimulates sex hormones, thyroid hormones	Blocks secretion of hormones
Appetite	Increased	Reduced
Sexual desire	Increased	Reduced
Duration of effect	Very brief with no significant withdrawal	Prolonged with withdrawal
Sympathetic function	Reduced; warm extremities and normalized blood pressure	Increased during withdrawal; cold extremities and hypertension
Effect on limbic system	Stimulates and normalizes better sleep, better memory	Inhibits insomnia, amnesia, poor judgment

Note: It is believed that chronic administration of exogenous opioids will inhibit markedly the production of endogenous opioids.
Source: Modified from H Hooshmand. Chronic Pain: Reflex Sympathetic Dystrophy Prevention and Management. Boca Raton, FL: CRC Press, 1993.

[17,18,32,33]. All these regions are believed to be part of the descending pain-modulatory network. However, opioids produce a variety of *other* biological actions aside from analgesia, including respiratory depression, pupillary constriction, decreased body temperature, and decreased gastrointestinal tract motility and constipation. These effects result from the presence of opiate receptors in tissues not involved in analgesia (e.g., medullary respiratory center, hypothalamus, intestines) [32].

Four specific classes of opioid receptors have been identified: μ, κ, δ, and σ. The μ receptor seems to play a critical role in analgesia. Some evidence suggests that δ- and κ-selective compounds may produce analgesia if applied directly to the spinal cord [17,18,32,35].

Endogenous Opiates

The presence of opioid receptors within the CNS suggests that animals and humans must be able to produce opiatelike molecules to bind with them. Indeed, such endogenous opioid peptide molecules have been identified.

A variety of opioid peptides form from the breakdown of three different precursor molecules: proenkephalin-A, pro-opiomelanocortin, and pro-

dynorphin. Proenkephalin-A breaks down into enkephalins, pro-opiomelanocortin into beta endorphin, and prodynorphin into dynorphin.

Despite arising from three different precursor molecules, all endogenous opioid peptides contain a common amino acid sequence (TYR-GLY-GLY-PHE . . .). The enkephalins, beta endorphin, and the dynorphin peptides are all believed to play a role in pain modulation. A high concentration of opioid-containing cell bodies and nerve terminals are found in a variety of locations throughout the pain modulatory network. The presence of endogenous opioids in these locations suggests that they function to relieve and modulate pain. Exogenous opioid analgesics produce their analgesic effect by mimicking the action of endogenous opioid peptides in the PAG, the RVM, and the spinal cord [19–21,32].

Many physicians hold that chronic opioid usage is contraindicated for reasons other than the simple risk of addiction and severe side effects. It is thought that chronic administration of exogenous opioids will markedly inhibit the production of endogenous opioids. Some researchers argue that except for use in analgesia, endogenous and exogenous opiates have very different qualities (Table 12-2). Endogenous opiates have greater affinity for their receptors and therefore are believed to be 100 times stronger than opioids. As a result, flooding dosages of sys-

temic narcotics are required to achieve similar analgesic results to a healthy endogenous opioid production system. This argument dictates that the ideal
approach to chronic pain would be for the patient to
stimulate the production of endogenous opiates.
Indeed, exercise, proper nutrition, and some antidepressants are considered to raise the concentration
of endorphins in the CNS [36]. Despite this argument, the literature supports the fact that a subpopu-
lation of chronic pain patients benefit physically,
emotionally, and functionally from the proper
administration of exogenous opioids.

Descending Pain-Modulating Network

As noted previously, the descending pain-modulatory
network extends from the cortex to the spinal cord
dorsal horn. Opioids are thought to play an important
dual role, affecting both stimulation of this pathway
at the brain stem level and inhibition of nociceptive
transmission at the spinal cord dorsal horn.

Major sources of input to the PAG include the
hypothalamus, the frontal cortex, and the amygdala. Connections to cortical and limbic system
structures suggest that cognitive and emotional
input plays a role in pain modulation. Activation of
PAG neurons may be due to a stimulating effect of
opioid-secreting interneurons [27,37]. The PAG has
direct connections with the RVM. Serotonin-rich
neurons from the RVM send their axons via the
dorsolateral funiculus to the outer layers of the
spinal cord (Figure 12-1) [12,38,39].

The release of serotonin at the spinal cord level
is believed to inhibit pain transmission in one of
three ways: (1) direct inhibition of the second-order
pain transmission cell, (2) activation of an opioid-
secreting interneuron that subsequently inhibits the
second-order cell directly or indirectly, and (3)
inhibition of transmission of substance P from the
primary nociceptive afferents (see Figure 3-9)
[32,40–44]. Systemic opioids activate this network
by mimicking endogenous opiates at brain stem
and spinal cord levels [45].

Terminology

The definitions of four critical terms are poorly
understood by physicians, patients, families of
patients, society at large, and government agencies.
These terms are *addiction, tolerance, dependence,*
and *pseudoaddiction.* Addiction, a psychosocial
phenomenon, differs from tolerance and physical
dependence, which are due to pharmacologic and
biological properties of opioid analgesics. It must
be understood that a patient can tolerate, or depend
on, an opioid without being addicted to it. In general, the term *addiction* is used carelessly in clinical
practice. Many physicians have an overwhelming
fear of turning their patients into narcotics addicts.
This fear, in conjunction with fear of potential legal
ramifications should addiction ensue, leads to gross
undertreatment of chronic pain—whether due to
cancer or a nonmalignant nociceptive focus.
Although addiction is a potentially serious complication of opioid therapy, recent surveys suggest that
patients without a history of substance abuse present only a small risk of abuse behaviors following
the short- or long-term administration of opioids.
Only four cases of well-documented psychological
dependence could be identified among 11,882
patients without prior history of substance abuse
surveyed in the Boston Collaborative Drug Surveillance Project [46]. In a national survey of more than
10,000 patients who had no prior drug abuse and
were given opioids for burn pain, no cases of addiction were identified [47]. Finally, a survey of a large
headache clinic identified opioid abuse in only three
of 2,369 patients [48]. In the previously mentioned
clinical studies of opioids for CNMP, only 33 (5%)
of the 642 patients described developed abuse or
management problems; many of them had histories
of substance abuse [1,3–9].

As is obvious from the foregoing, the literature
suggests that the risk for development of addiction
is small. The risks for abuse behaviors can be minimized if appropriate screening procedures are used,
medications are monitored carefully, and regular
follow-up assesses drug efficacy. Finally, knowledge of certain definitions is important.

Addiction

Addiction, or *psychological dependence,* has been
defined as a behavioral pattern of drug use characterized by overwhelming or compulsive use of a
drug, the securing of its supply, and the high tendency to relapse after withdrawal [49]. More

Figure 12-1. The descending pain-modulatory network extends from the cortex and limbic system to the brain stem (periaqueductal gray region [PAG], rostroventral medulla [RVM]). Activation of PAG neurons may be the result of a stimulating effect of opioid-secreting interneurons (OIN). The PAG has connections with the RVM. Neurons from the RVM, rich in serotonin, send their axons via the dorsolateral funiculus (DLF) to the outer layers of the spinal cord. (PN = primary nociceptive afferent; T = second-order pain transmission cell.) (Adapted from PD Wall, R Melzack. Textbook of Pain [2nd ed]. New York: Churchill Livingstone, 1989;208.)

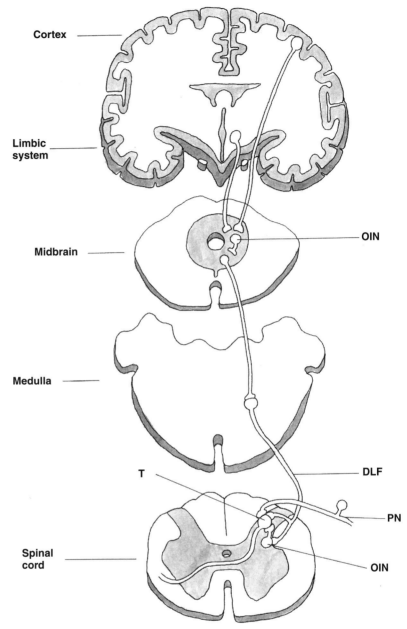

recently, the American Medical Association Task Force [50] described addiction as a chronic disorder characterized by "the compulsive use of a substance resulting in physical, psychological or social harm to the user and continued use despite that harm." Loss of personal control over drug use distinguishes the addict from the patient who is merely physically dependent. Portenoy [1] provides a defi-

nition of addiction relevant to the pain patient to whom opioid drugs are administered:

Addiction in the chronic pain patient can be defined as a psychological and behavioral syndrome characterized by: (a) an intense desire for the drug and overwhelming concern about its continued availability (psychological dependence); (b) evidence of compulsive drug use (unsanctioned dose escalation, continued dosing despite significant side effects, use of drug to treat symptoms not targeted by the therapy, or unapproved use during periods of no symptoms); and/or (c) evidence of one or more of a group of associated behaviors, including manipulation of the treating physician or medical system for the purposes of obtaining additional drugs (altering prescriptions, for example), acquisition of drugs from other medical sources or from a nonmedical source, drug hoarding or sales, or unapproved use of other drugs (particularly alcohol or other sedatives/hypnotics), during opioid therapy.

Drug Abuse

Drug abuse has been defined as the use of an agent outside socially and medically approved patterns of use in a given culture [49] or as a pattern of use that results in physical, psychological, economic, legal, or social harm to the individual or others affected by his or her use [50].

Pseudoaddiction

Addiction must be differentiated from the term *pseudoaddiction*, which refers to an iatrogenic syndrome characterized by abnormal behaviors that develop as a consequence of inadequate pain management. The natural history of pseudoaddiction includes progression through three characteristic phases including inadequate prescription of analgesics to manage the patient's pain, escalation of analgesic demands by the patient associated with behavioral changes to convince others of the pain's severity, and a crisis of mistrust between the patient and the health care team. The behavioral changes seen in pseudoaddiction can be alleviated through appropriate and timely analgesic administration to control the patient's level of pain [51].

Addiction and pseudoaddiction are behavioral phenomena. The terms *tolerance* and *dependence* refer to biological sequelae resulting from the pharmacologic properties of opioids.

Tolerance

Tolerance can be defined as the need for higher doses of an opioid over time to maintain the same analgesic effect [52]. Tolerance to various opioid

effects develops at different rates. Fatigue, nausea, and subtle cognitive dysfunction typically subside after the first 2–3 weeks of opioid therapy. Constipation may resolve over time, but it usually remains an ongoing problem, necessitating dietary changes or medical treatment. Tolerance to analgesia, the critical issue for therapy, is usually a slow process in CNMP patients with stable disease pathology. The literature suggests that patients with CNMP can usually be maintained on relatively stable doses of opioids for prolonged periods.

Dependence

Last, physical *dependence* is a pharmacologic property of the opioids, characterized by the occurrence of an abstinence syndrome (withdrawal syndrome) after abrupt discontinuation of the drug or after administration of an antagonist [50,52–54]. This term does not imply the aberrant psychological state or behaviors of the addicted or drug-abusing patient. Likewise, the term *addiction* should *not* be applied to patients who demonstrate only the potential for withdrawal [1].

Indications for Opioid Analgesic Maintenance Therapy

It is not uncommon for a physician to be presented with a patient whose quality of life, emotional status, and functional abilities have deteriorated significantly as a result of chronic pain. Often, unemployment, deconditioning, insomnia, frequent doctor or emergency-room visits, extensive diagnostic workup, and failed surgical procedures are other associated problems presenting to a physician taking on a new chronic pain patient.

It is impossible to characterize those CNMP patients for whom opioid therapy is either particularly suited or contraindicated [9]. However, certain generalizations can be made. For example, chronic opioid treatment should be considered if it can improve the patient's quality of life, decrease overall health care costs, and help patients to avoid potentially dangerous surgical procedures to alleviate pain, and if side effects from the opioids can be minimized.

After recording a comprehensive history, the physician might consider opioid therapy if it appears that the patient has an appropriate diagnosis to justify the use of chronic opioids; that reasonable conservative measures have already failed to alleviate the pain; that functional abilities, quality of life (including quality of sleep), and level of depression can be improved; and that use of the medical system (visits to emergency rooms, hospitalizations for pain management, additional or repeated medical testing) can be reduced, thereby decreasing health care costs.

Generally, researchers agree that chronic opioid therapy would not be justifiable if it further impaired function [1]. Ideally, function should improve with effective analgesia. However, if cognitive impairment, excessive sedation, and mood disturbances interfere with activity, the opioid should be switched, the dosage should be lowered and, occasionally, opioid therapy should be discontinued altogether.

Prior addiction to or abuse of prescription drugs (e.g., narcotics, benzodiazepines), alcohol, or street drugs should be viewed as a relatively strong contraindication for the use of prescribed opioids for CNMP [1,55]. If opioids are prescribed, informed consent, regular follow-up, close scrutiny of medication usage, and a contract stating that the drug will be discontinued at the first sign of abuse behavior, are often effective in keeping such patients from abusing the prescribed opioid.

It is important that any patient receive a psychological screening before starting on chronic opioid therapy. Severely depressed patients may find that opioids help them forget their worries, a setup for psychological dependence and abuse behaviors. Therefore, such patients will need to be monitored carefully.

The rapid development of tolerance with progressively escalating doses may make the use of opioids impractical. In general, the CNMP patient with unchanging pathology should remain comfortable for prolonged periods on relatively stable doses of opioids [1]. Rapid development of tolerance may be an early signal of the development of psychological dependence.

History of Opioid Preparations and Use

The use of opium dates back to antiquity. Its name derives from the Greek word for juice, as opium is extracted from the juice of the poppy, *Papaver som-niferum*. The first undisputed reference to poppy juice is found in the writing of Theophrastus. In the third century BC, Arabian physicians were well versed in the uses of opium, and Arabian traders introduced the drug to the Orient, where it was used mainly for control of dysenteries. Paracelsus (1493–1541) introduced opium to Europe in the early sixteenth century. In the eighteenth century, opium smoking became popular in the Orient. In Europe, its ready availability led to some degree of overuse.

Opium contains more than 20 pure substances known as *alkaloids*. One of the alkaloids was isolated by Serturner in 1806. He named this purified alkaloid *morphine*, after Morpheus, the Greek goddess of dreams. Another alkaloid in opium, codeine, was purified by Robiquet in 1832. By the middle of the nineteenth century, the use of pure alkaloids rather than crude opium preparations began to spread throughout the medical world [56].

By the late 1800s and the early twentieth century, opioid abuse was becoming a problem in the United States, owing to an unrestricted availability of opium, an influx of opium-smoking immigrants from the Orient, and the invention of the hypodermic needle. The intravenous use of morphine led to a more severe variety of compulsive drug abuse.

This problem stimulated researchers to look for potent analgesics that would be free of the potential to produce addiction. Such research, which continues to this day, has led to the production of a variety of synthetic and semisynthetic compounds with morphinelike qualities (meperidine, methadone), antagonistic actions (nalorphine, naloxone), and mixed actions (pentazocine, butorphanol, and buprenorphine).

Further research delineated stereospecific binding sites (receptors) for the opioids in the mammalian CNS. The discovery of opiate receptors led to the search for and ultimate discovery of endogenous opioid peptides. Over a remarkably brief period, three distinct families of opioid peptides—enkephalins, endorphins, and dynorphins—and multiple categories of opioid receptors—μ, δ, κ, and σ—were revealed [17,18,32,33,35,56–59].

Pharmacologic Properties of Opioids

The pharmacologic effects of opioids are based on their ability to bind to stereospecific opioid recep-

Table 12-3. Effects of Three Major Categories of Opioid Receptors

μ	κ	δ
Miosis	Miosis	—
Supraspinal analgesia	Spinal analgesia	—
Euphoria	Sedation	Dysphoria
—	—	Hallucinations
—	—	Delusions
Respiratory depression	Respiratory depression	Respiratory stimulation
Physical dependence	—	Vasomotor stimulation

tors (i.e., μ, δ, κ, and σ receptors). The greater the binding ability (affinity), the more potent the analgesic qualities of the drug. The putative effects mediated by three main classes of receptors were delineated by Martin et al. [60] in 1976 (Table 12-3).

The μ and κ receptors are concerned with analgesia. μ Receptors exert their effects principally at a supraspinal level. Agonist action at μ receptors results in both the analgesia and euphoria commonly associated with opioids. Other consequences of μ-receptor activity include respiratory depression, miosis, and reduced gastrointestinal motility [60].

κ Receptors exert their analgesic effect at the spinal cord level. The outer layers of dorsal horn gray matter have dense concentrations of κ receptors, although κ receptors are found within the brain. Stimulation of κ receptors causes less intense miosis and respiratory depression than does μ stimulation. Instead of euphoria, κ agonists produce dysphoria and sedation [61]. Because of these properties, κ agonists are believed to have lower potential for abuse than do opioids with strong μ affinity.

The consequences of stimulating δ opioid receptors in humans are uncertain. However, animal experiments suggest that analgesia results from δ stimulation [62,63]. Other effects mediated by δ receptors include dysphoria and respiratory stimulation [60]. Opioids affect the CNS (analgesia, sedation, euphoria, decreased hypothalamic hormone secretion, pupillary changes, depression of respiratory drive, suppression of cough, and effects on the nausea and vomiting centers in the brain stem), cardiovascular system, and gastrointestinal tract [18,64,65].

Analgesia and Mood Alteration

The relief of pain is thought to occur by activation of the opioid-mediated descending pain-inhibitory pathways. At the spinal cord level, opioids inhibit transmission of substance P from the primary nociceptors. Direct inhibition of second-order pain transmission cells also occurs [32,40–44].

The mechanism by which opioids produce euphoria, tranquility, and other alterations of mood is not entirely clear. Some believe that μ opioids activate dopaminergic neurons that project to the nucleus accumbens, resulting in opioid-induced euphoria [66,67].

In contrast to the μ agonists, κ agonists inhibit dopamine release from cells in the substantia nigra and from cortical and striatal cells. As mentioned earlier, κ agonists produce dysphoric rather than euphoric effects [68,69].

The locus ceruleus is postulated to play a critical role in feelings of alarm, panic, fear, and anxiety. Activity in the locus ceruleus is inhibited by both exogenous and endogenous opioids [56].

Effects on the Hypothalamus

Morphine acts in the hypothalamus to inhibit the release of gonadotropin-releasing hormone and corticotropin-releasing factor (CRF), thus decreasing circulating concentrations of luteinizing hormone, follicle-stimulating hormone, and adrenocorticotropic hormone. As a result of decreased pituitary trophic hormones, plasma testosterone and cortisol concentrations will decline. In women, the menstrual cycle may be disrupted. However, with chronic administration, patients develop tolerance to the effect of opioids on the hypothalamic-releasing factors, resulting in normalization of menstrual cycles in woman and circulating testosterone in men [70,71].

Pupils

Morphine and most μ and κ opioid agonists cause pupillary constriction (miosis) by an excitatory action on the nucleus of the oculomotor nerve. Pinpoint pupils signal a pathognomonic opioid toxicity or overdosage [56].

Respiration

Morphinelike opioids depress respiration by a direct inhibitory effect on brain stem respiratory centers. The primary mechanism involves a reduction of responsiveness to carbon dioxide in brain stem respiratory centers and a depression of pontine and medullary centers involved in regulating respiratory rhythmicity. Therapeutic doses of opioids depress all phases of respiratory activity (rate, minute volume, and tidal exchange) and also may produce irregular breathing. In humans, death from opioid poisoning nearly always is due to respiratory arrest [18]. Morphine and related opioids also depress the cough reflex, at least in part by a direct effect on a cough center in the medulla [56].

Nauseant and Emetic Effects

Nausea and vomiting produced by morphine and other μ agonist opioids are unpleasant, common side effects that result from the drugs' direct stimulation of the emesis center in the medulla. Certain individuals never vomit after morphine, whereas others do so each time the drug is administered. The nausea and vomiting are worse if the patient is ambulatory, suggesting a vestibular component [56]. In addition to the central actions, opioids decrease gastric motility, leading to abdominal bloating, discomfort, and increased risk of vomiting.

Cardiovascular System

Therapeutic doses of morphinelike opioids produce peripheral, arteriolar, and venous dilatation. In some patients, orthostatic hypotension and fainting may occur with changes of position [56].

Gastrointestinal Tract

In the stomach, relatively low doses of morphine decrease gastric motility, thereby prolonging gastric emptying time. Progressive gastric distention can aggravate further the centrally induced nausea and can increase the likelihood of esophageal reflux. Prolonged gastric emptying may retard absorption of orally administered medications [72].

In the small intestine, morphine diminishes biliary, pancreatic, and intestinal secretions and delays digestion of food. The viscosity of bowel contents increases as water is absorbed more completely and intestinal secretions are decreased. This effect contributes to the problem of constipation [73].

In the large intestine, four processes contribute to opioid-induced constipation: (1) Propulsive peristaltic waves are diminished or abolished in the colon; (2) the resulting delay in passage of feces causes considerable desiccation, which further retards its advance through the colon; (3) anal sphincter tone is augmented greatly; and (4) the reflex anal sphincter relaxation response to rectal distention is reduced [56,74].

Routes of Administration

Opioids can be administered through a variety of routes: oral, rectal, intramuscular, intravenous, sublingual, subcutaneous, transdermal, epidural, and intrathecal, as well as via nasal inhalation. Despite the variation in modes of opioid administration, the oral route should be undertaken in the ambulatory CNMP patient. One of the other approaches may seem indicated when certain instances arise, but the oral route should be resumed as quickly as possible.

Each patient's analgesic requirements may be different, owing to varying pathologic processes, individual perception of pain, rate of tolerance development, and the efficacy with which the medication is metabolized. To prescribe opioids properly, physicians should have a good working knowledge of the various preparations available: their strength, duration of action, common side

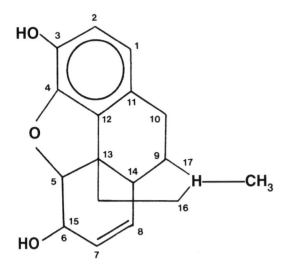

Figure 12-2. The chemical structure of morphine.

effects, typical dosages, mode of metabolism, and cost.

Morphine

Morphine remains the standard against which other opioid analgesics are measured. Morphine is a purified alkaloid obtained from opium. Many semisynthetic derivatives are made by relatively simple modifications of the morphine molecule (Figure 12-2) [56]. Morphine is available for oral, rectal, intramuscular, intravenous, sublingual, epidural, and intrathecal administration.

Protocol for Administration

For most opioids, including morphine, the effect of a given dose is less after oral than after parenteral administration, owing to variable but significant first-pass metabolism in the liver. For example, 60 mg oral morphine is required to reach blood levels similar to those achieved with 10 mg of an intramuscular or subcutaneous dose. After oral or parenteral administration of morphine, its duration of analgesic action is somewhere in the range of 4–6 hours. The drug's half-life is 2 hours and, depending on the situation, its analgesic potency may be

insufficient to control pain after only 2 or 3 hours. Therefore, patients treated with oral or parenteral morphine may require regular and frequent doses to maintain adequate analgesia [59].

Morphine is available as a slow-release oral preparation. Sustained-release morphine sulfate (SRMS) is available in 15-, 30-, 60-, and 100-mg tablets. Duration of action is in the range of 8–12 hours, so two- or three-times-daily dosing is possible. A dosage of 60 mg SRMS twice daily would be the equivalent of taking 20 mg oral morphine every 4 hours (six doses per day). Certainly, twice-daily dosing would be much more convenient.

Some key features of morphine sulfate, its sustained-release derivative, and other opioid preparations can be found in Table 12-4. Each drug has different features with respect to analgesic potency, duration of action, routes of administration, metabolism, combinations with nonopioid analgesics, receptors stimulated, side effects, and toxicities. The opioids in Table 12-4 are categorized as having mild, intermediate, or strong analgesic potency.

Side Effects

The physiologic effects of opioids have been described previously (Table 12-5). Important side effects that may interfere with opioid treatment of CNMP include respiratory depression, nausea, vomiting, constipation, sedation, and subtle cognitive impairment.

Almost all opioids produce adverse reactions, but those that do occur are generally manageable and nonhazardous [9]. Dangerous reactions, such as respiratory depression, appear rarely, if at all, in the literature about opioids and CNMP. The pain itself seems to have a stimulating effect on medullary centers for respiration. No cases of respiratory depression were recorded in a recent long-term study of 100 CNMP patients on opioids. None of 542 patients from other studies listed earlier reported respiratory depression as a significant side effect. Nevertheless, this potential complication needs to be kept in mind, particularly in patients who have respiratory compromise (i.e., chronic obstructive pulmonary disease, asthma, pneumonia, congestive heart failure, or pneumonectomy). In such cases, opioids should be titrated slowly and followed up by checking of arterial blood gases or pulse oximetry. Sleep studies might be helpful in looking for the development of abnormal respiratory patterns, sleep apnea, and decreased oxygen saturation during sleep.

A combination of other adverse reactions such as fatigue, nausea, vomiting, and dizziness may also occur in the initial phase of opioid therapy. However, these effects often subside during the course of therapy [9]. In the case of persistent nausea, one of the following suggestions might prove helpful:

- Waiting a few weeks after initiation of treatment to see whether tolerance to this side effect develops
- Switching to a different opioid that may be tolerated better
- Trying the medication either with food or on an empty stomach, as opioids produce gastroparesis, and the progressive buildup of food contents in the stomach may worsen nausea
- Regularly using low-dose metoclopramide (Reglan), which may help to promote gastric emptying if gastroparesis is contributing to the problem
- H_2 blockers
- Administering the opioid in combination with promethazine (Phenergan) or hydroxyzine pamoate (Vistaril), to decrease nausea, in addition to potentiating opioid analgesics

Prevention of constipation is obligatory for patients managed on chronic opioids. Constipation is one common side effect to which patients usually do not develop tolerance [9]. Treatment measures include adding fiber to the diet and administering stool softeners and laxatives.

Many experts are concerned that opioids might produce cognition changes that might hamper rehabilitation and cause a deterioration of functional status. However, tolerance to the subtle cognitive impairment produced by opioid drugs seems to develop rather rapidly. This effect has been demonstrated in a study of cancer patients; clinical experience in the management of these patients suggests that chronic opioid administration is usually compatible with normal cognitive and psychological functioning. Nonetheless, occasional patients report persistent mental clouding sufficient to impair function. No study has adequately assessed the long-term potential for subtle neuropsychological impairment in ambulatory patients receiving chronic opioid therapy [1,54].

Guidelines for Opioid Maintenance Therapy for Nonmalignant Pain

Documentation

The physician must have documentation of the patient's diagnoses. They should mention the manner in which the pain has affected the patient's quality of life, ability to function, sleep, and ability to engage in vocational or avocational pursuits. Usually, certain diagnoses do not warrant opioid therapy; in general, chronic low-back pain of soft-tissue etiology, myofascial pain syndrome, fibromyalgia, and headaches should not be treated with chronic opioids.

The physician should have documentation that all reasonable conservative measures have been tried and have failed (e.g., physical therapy, transcutaneous electrical nerve stimulation, psychological counseling, biofeedback, neurologic blocks, epidural steroids, nonopioid analgesics, and a pain clinic). Pain-clinic programs have become very expensive, and most place emphasis on detoxification. In select cases, a trial of opioids may provide the patient with greater comfort at a lower overall cost.

Method of Drug Administration

Three important concepts governing the use of opioids in the cancer pain population also hold true for the CNMP patient: (1) by-the-ladder, (2) by mouth, and (3) by-the-clock approaches to administration. The by-the-ladder approach to medication management of cancer and noncancer pain has been outlined by the World Health Organization [75], which states that there should be a stepwise approach to treatment of chronic pain and that one of the steps might include the use of opioids (Figure 12-3).

Every attempt should be made to give drugs orally in the ambulatory CNMP patient. One must remember that because of significant first-pass metabolism through the liver, oral opioid bioavailability will be reduced, and oral doses need to be two to three times larger than those given by injection. Occasional patients with intractable nausea and vomiting might require alternative routes (sublingual, rectal, transdermal).

The use of regularly scheduled doses (by-the-clock) should be applied in virtually all chronic opioid therapies. Most of the orally administered opioids

Table 12-4. Common Opioid Analgesics

Generic Name	Trade Name	Route of Administration (Dose)	Half-Life	Duration of Action
Mild opioids				
Propoxyphene HCl, propoxyphene napsylate	Darvon (propoxyphene HCl), Darvon Compound-65 (propoxyphene HCl, aspirin, caffeine), Darvon-N (100 mg propoxyphene napsylate), Darvocet-N (50 or 100 mg propoxyphene napsylate, 650 mg acetaminophen)	PO	6–12 hrs	4–6 hrs
Codeine	Tylenol #2 (15 mg codeine phosphate, 300 mg acetaminophen), Tylenol #3 (30 mg codeine phosphate, 300 mg acetaminophen), Tylenol #4 (60 mg codeine phosphate, 300 mg acetaminophen)	PO, IM	4–6 hrs	2–4 hrs
Pentazocine HCl	Talwin (pentazocine lactate), Talwin Compound (pentazocine HCl, 325 mg aspirin), Talwin NX (pentazocine HCl, naloxone HCl), Talacen (pentazocine HCl, 650 mg acetaminophen)	IM, SC, PO	4–7 hrs	4–5 hrs
Hydrocodone bitartrate	Anexsia 5/500 (5 mg hydrocodone, 500 mg acetaminophen), Anexsia 7.5/650 (7.5 mg hydrocodone, 650 mg acetaminophen), Lorcet 10/650 (10 mg	PO (5–10 mg [1–2 tablets])	4–5 hrs	4 hrs

Receptors Stimulated	Metabolism	Advantages	Disadvantages
Primarily μ	Liver and kidney		
Primarily μ	Liver and kidney	High oral to parenteral potency (in terms of total analgesia, codeine is approximately 60% as potent when given orally as when injected IM); abuse liability of codeine is lower than that of morphine; cough suppressant (with doses as low as 10–20 mg)	Frequent dosing necessary because of short duration of action; dosage limited by its combination with Tylenol; maximum dosage 12 tablets per day
Strong κ agonist, weak antagonist or partial agonist of μ receptors	Liver and kidney	Less abuse potential because of the μ antagonist or partial agonist effects; action at κ receptors producing an analgesic effect; parenteral abuse of the drug less likely owing to addition of naloxone (opioid receptor agonist) in Talwin NX	In higher doses, increases heart rate and blood pressure and therefore is contraindicated in patients with coronary artery disease and hypertension; irritating to subcutaneous and muscle tissues; fibrosis and contractures possible with repeated injections over long periods
Primarily μ	Liver and kidney	Antitussive qualities	Dosage limited by presence of Tylenol; short duration of action

Table 12-4. *Continued*

Generic Name	Trade Name	Route of Administration (Dose)	Half-Life	Duration of Action
	hydrocodone, 650 mg acetaminophen), Lortab 2.5, 5, or 7.5/500 (2.5, 5, or 7.5 mg hydrocodone, 500 mg acetaminophen), Vicodin (5 mg hydrocodone, 500 mg acetaminophen), Vicodin ES (7.5 mg hydrocodone, 750 mg acetaminophen)			
Intermediate opioids				
Oxycodone HCl	Percodan (5 mg oxycodone, 325 mg aspirin), Percocet (5 mg oxycodone, 325 mg Tylenol), Tylox (5 mg oxycodone, 500 mg Tylenol)	PO (5–10 mg)		4–5 hrs
Strong opioids				
Morphine sulfate	MS Contin, Oramorph SR, Roxanol, morphine sulfate immediate release (MSIR)	IM, IV, PO, SL	6–8 hrs for sustained-release morphine sulfate (SRMS); 2–3 hrs for MSIR	8–12 hrs (SRMS); 4–5 hrs (MSIR)
Methadone HCl	Dolophine, Methadone	IM, PO	15–40 hrs	4–24 hrs
Hydromorphone HCl	Dilaudid	PO (2- and 4-mg tablets), rectal (3 mg), IM, SC	2–3 hrs	4–6 hrs

Receptors Stimulated	Metabolism	Advantages	Disadvantages
Primarily μ	Liver and kidney		Dosage limited by Tylenol or aspirin (i.e., maximum of 8–12 tablets/day)
μ++, κ+, δ+	Liver and kidneys; small amounts persist in feces and urine for several days after last dose	Sustained analgesia with less frequent dosing (SRMS)	Side effects (nausea, vomiting, and constipation); cost (SRMS)
μ++, κ+	Liver biotransformation; kidney and bile excretion	Inexpensive, long duration of action—thus, useful in the treatment of addiction and detoxification; often well tolerated; good analgesia; few side effects; efficacy by the oral route	Slow titration needed until optimal dosage reached; because of drug's long half-life, increased sedation and confusion after several days owing to drug build-up with repeated doses; U.S. special controls enacted to prevent its unregulated large-scale use in treatment of opioid addiction; patient and physician resistance to use owing to association with the addict population, despite its analgesic potency
Primarily μ	Liver and kidney	Good, short-term analgesia	Short duration of action; more subject to abuse

Table 12-4. *Continued*

Generic Name	Trade Name	Route of Administration (Dose)	Half-Life	Duration of Action
Meperidine HCl	Demerol, Mepergan (50 mg meperidine, 25 mg Phenergan)	IM, IV, SC, PO	3–4 hrs	4–6 hrs
Levorphanol tartrate	Levo-Dromoran	IM, IV, SC, PO (2-mg tablets)		6–8 hrs
Fentanyl	Sublimaze, Duragesic transdermal system	IM, IV, epidural, intrathecal, transdermal (25-, 50-, 75-, and 100-µg/hr Duragesic patches)		Duragesic patches, 72 hrs; IM, IV, or epidural-intrathecal administration, 1–2 hrs

*These excitatory symptoms are due to the accumulation of normeperidine, a breakdown product of Demerol, which has a half-life of 15–20 hours and is a central nervous system excitant. Because normeperidine is eliminated by both kidney and liver, decreased renal or hepatic function increases the likelihood of such toxicity.

Sources: JH Jaffe, WR Martin. Opioid Analgesics and Antagonists. In AG Gilman, LS Goodman (eds), The Pharmacological Basis of Therapeutics. New York: Macmillan, 1990;485; and Physician's Desk Reference (48th ed). Montvale, NJ: Medical Economics, 1994.

Receptors Stimulated	Metabolism	Advantages	Disadvantages
Primarily μ	Liver and kidney		Poor oral absorption (oral-to-parenteral potency ratio lower than that of codeine); short duration of action; tremors, muscle twitches, dilated pupils, hyperactive reflexes, and convulsions possible with large doses repeated over short intervals*
Primarily μ	Liver and kidney	Less nausea and vomiting than occurs with morphine in sensitive patients; long duration of action	Possible accumulation of drug in plasma from repeated administration at short intervals
μ+++, κ+, δ+	Liver and kidney	Steady serum levels for prolonged periods with each patch; selective μ agonist, estimated to be 80 times as potent as morphine; useful for transdermal application; in epidural or intrathecal routes, less migration in the cerebrospinal fluid than morphine; potent analgesia for shorter periods	Cost of the transdermal patches; unavailable in oral form

Table 12-5. Physiologic Effects of Opioids

Central nervous system
  Analgesia
  Sedation
  Euphoria, tranquility, alterations of mood
  Dysphoria (with κ stimulation)
  Subtle cognitive impairment
  Decreased hypothalamic hormone secretion
  Pupillary changes (miosis)
  Depressed respiratory drive
  Cough suppression
  Stimulation of medullary emesis center
Cardiovascular system
  Peripheral arteriolar and venous dilatation
Gastrointestinal tract
  Prolonged gastric emptying
  Decreased biliary, pancreatic, and intestinal secretions
  Constipation

have short half-lives and short durations of action. In many patients, use of these opioids provides only 2–3 hours of effective analgesia. Therefore, an every-4-to-6-hour dose regimen will result in 1 to several hours of breakthrough pain. A four-times-per-day, as-required opioid administration schedule with weak opioids may produce a pseudoaddiction in which

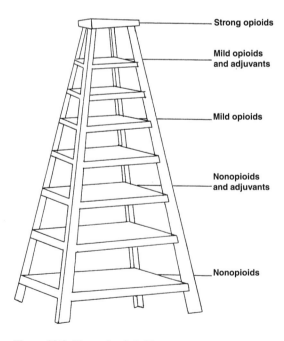

Figure 12-3. The analgesic ladder.

Labels on figure: Strong opioids; Mild opioids and adjuvants; Mild opioids; Nonopioids and adjuvants; Nonopioids

recurrent pain produces drug seeking. The discontinuous use of analgesics results in dysphoria, increased pain, and craving for pain relief. This phenomenon is prevented by administration of the opioid on a regular basis at a dose that provides for pain prophylaxis and the prevention of breakthrough pain.

A by-the-clock protocol will necessitate that short-acting opioids be given four to six times per day. With such frequent administration, dosages may be overlooked (with onset of breakthrough pain), or extra medications might be taken if confusion arises about the time of the last dose. In addition, with this protocol, physicians will be required to prescribe upward of 360 tablets per month (two tablets orally every 4 hours for 30 days), numbers that make most doctors very uncomfortable.

Longer-acting opioids (SRMS, levorphanol, methadone) can be given less frequently. This scheduling results in better and more accurate compliance by the patient, fewer pills required per month, steady analgesia, less chance of breakthrough pain, and lower cost (especially with methadone).

Psychological Assessment

A psychological screen is recommended prior to initiation of opioid treatment. Thorough evaluation of family history, social history, psychiatric history, and history of substance abuse (tobacco, alcohol, caffeine, illegal drugs) will enable the psychologist or psychiatrist to place the patient in a "potential risk for addiction" category of low, moderate, or high. Patients in the moderate- or high-risk categories still may be candidates for chronic opioid therapy. However, they need to be watched closely for abuse behaviors and rapid development of tolerance.

In addition, the presence and severity of depression is identified readily in these psychological intake reports. Appropriate counseling and medications are critical for a patient identified as having major depression so as to avoid use of opioids to "help forget about worries," a situation that can lead to higher opioid dosages than actually warranted by analgesic requirements.

The cost of medication always should be considered. Some of the sustained release derivatives are quite expensive. The physician should keep in mind that the patient may be on a given drug regimen for

Consent for Chronic Opioid Analgesic Maintenance Therapy

I, _____, consent to the use of chronic opioid/narcotic analgesic medications for the management of my chronic pain syndrome.

- I understand that a small percentage of patients on such therapy can develop psychological dependence to the opioids.
- I understand the following definitions:
  Addiction or psychological dependence refers to a set of aberrant behaviors marked by drug craving, efforts to secure its supply, interference with physical health or psychosocial function, and recidivism after detoxification.
  Tolerance refers to a decrease in the effect of a given narcotic over time.
  Dependence refers to the appearance of a withdrawal syndrome on abrupt cessation of the narcotic drug.
- I understand that the use of alcohol is not recommended while I am on chronic therapy.
- For female patients of childbearing age: I understand that a newborn will be physically dependent on opioids if these medications are taken chronically during the pregnancy.
- I agree to the medications as prescribed.
- I agree to receive my narcotic medications from only Dr. _____

_____
Date

_____
Patient (signature)

_____
Physician (signature)

Figure 12-4. Consent form for chronic opioid analgesic maintenance therapy.

an extended period, and the psychological burden of cost may have a negative impact on any analgesic benefits. Also, all patients should sign a consent form on initiation of chronic opioid therapy for non-malignant pain (Figure 12-4).

Patient Monitoring

Each CNMP patient has personal analgesic requirements, rates of drug absorption and metabolism, allergies, side effects, and history of opioid use. Therefore, analgesic requirements will vary from case to case, even if similar diagnoses are involved. If a patient is to be changed from short-acting opioids to one of the longer-acting preparations, equianalgesic dose charts should be used (Tables 12-6 and 12-7) [76,77].

In starting treatment with opioid-naive patients, low doses of weak preparations given around the clock should be used initially. Dosages should be titrated upward until the patient experiences either analgesic relief or unacceptable side effects. Frequent follow-up is necessary to evaluate the titration process in the early stages (i.e., one to two times per week).

The physician must gauge side effects versus the beneficial analgesic qualities of the particular opioid. If the patient's functional level decreases, a different drug should be substituted and, if necessary, opioid treatment should be discontinued completely and other alternatives should be found for pain management.

Often, adjuvant medications potentiate the effects of opioid drugs. Clonidine (Catapres) potentiates

Table 12-6. Equianalgesic Dose Chart for Oral Opioids

| Medication | Conversion to Sustained-Release Morphine Sulfate | | |
	15 mg bid	30 mg bid	60 mg bid
Tylenol #4 (codeine, 60 mg)	6/day	12/day	*
Oxycodone, 5 mg	6/day	12/day	*
Oral morphine	—	10 mg PO q4h	20 mg PO q4h
Hydromorphone	1 mg PO q4h	3 mg PO q4h	8 mg PO q6h
Methadone	10 mg PO bid	10 mg PO q6h	20 mg PO q6h
Meperidine	50 mg PO q3h	100 mg PO q3h	200 mg PO q3h
Levorphanol	—	2 mg PO q6h	4 mg PO q6h

*Cannot exceed 12 tablets per day owing to acetaminophen toxicity.

Table 12-7. Equianalgesic Dose Chart for Transdermal Opioids

Oral Morphine (mg/day)	Duragesic Dosage (µg/hr)
45–134	25
135–224	50
225–314	75
315–404	100

opioids, has its own analgesic qualities and, through central mechanisms, decreases sympathetic outflow, thereby minimizing withdrawal or detoxification symptoms. Tricyclic antidepressants and antihistamines may also potentiate the effects of opioids.

The prescribing physician should have thorough knowledge of the patient's overall medical condition. Opioids may be contraindicated, or lower doses required in patients with severe medical conditions, chronic renal failure or end-stage renal disease, liver disease, or in the elderly.

Once the patient has been titrated to a steady-state dosage, monthly follow-up is recommended to evaluate degree of analgesia, side effects, and functional status. Selected patients who have shown particular stability with their dosage for prolonged periods can be seen at less frequent intervals, perhaps every 2–3 months.

Abuse and Addiction

The physician must watch closely for the appearance of abuse behaviors: frequent loss or theft of medications, lying about medications being stolen or left out of town, frequent calling in early for medications, and rapid escalation of dose owing to claims of tolerance, especially after a steady-state dosage has provided sufficient analgesia for a prolonged period. Such behaviors also may be indicative of iatrogenic pseudoaddiction, and each case needs to be evaluated carefully before punitive measures (e.g., cessation of opioids, discharge from care) are taken. Patients should be referred for detoxification if addiction develops. If any concerns arise about a particular patient's use of opioids, the physician should obtain a second medical opinion, ideally from another physician with experience in the management of chronic pain [1,55]. The physician should be on the lookout for various signs of drug abuse in patients, which are outlined in Table 12-8.

Recommended Prescribing Practices

Physicians may not order prescriptions to dispense narcotic drugs for detoxification or maintenance treatment of a person dependent on narcotic drugs unless the physician is separately registered with the U.S. Drug Enforcement Agency, the Food and Drug Administration, and state department of health as being a part of a narcotic treatment program. However, a physician may administer (but not prescribe) narcotic drugs to a patient daily for up to 3 days while arrangements are being made for referral to an existing narcotic treatment program.

Adherence to state and federal regulations goes a long way in protecting a medical practice from

Table 12-8. Signs of Possible Patient Drug Abuse

Current behavior
Must be seen right away; very agitated; says "I found you in the phone book."
Makes a late afternoon (often Friday) appointment
Calls or comes in after regular hours
Must have a specific narcotic drug or other controlled substance immediately
Gives evasive or vague answers to questions regarding medical history
Reluctant or unwilling to provide reference information
Traveling through area, visiting friends or relatives, not a permanent resident
Failure to name a primary or referring physician
States that specific non-narcotic analgesics either do not work or produce allergies
Claims lost or stolen prescription needs to be replaced

Medical history
Admission of excessive use of coffee, cigarettes, alcohol, or prescription drugs
History of frequent trauma, burns, or breaks
General debilitation

Social history
Repeated automobile accidents or drunk-driving arrests
Difficulty with employment
Child abuse or severe family problems

Psychological history
Mood disturbances
Suicidal thoughts
Lack of impulse control
Thought disorders
Sexual dysfunction

Physical examination
Overt debilitation unrelated to medical problem
Physical findings disproportionate to patient's complaints
Unsteady gait
Slurred speech
Inappropriate pupil dilatation or constriction
Unexplained sweating or chills
Inappropriate lapses in conversation
Cutaneous signs of intravenous drug abuse (skin tracks, related scars overlying major veins on the neck, axilla, forearm, wrist, hand, foot, ankle), usually multiple, hyperpigmented and linear; possible new inflamed lesions
"Pop" scars from subcutaneous injections
Abscesses, infections, or ulcerations (possibly infective or chemical reactions to injections)

Source: Colorado Guidelines of Professional Practice for Controlled Substances—Physicians. Denver: Colorado Department of Health, 1993.

becoming a source of drug diversion and prescription drug abuse. Physicians can protect their practice also by safeguarding blank prescription pads, prescribing controlled substances judiciously, and being on the lookout for patient scams.

Forgery is a major source of drug diversion. Prescriptions are forged on blank prescription forms—entire pads or single sheets—stolen from physicians' offices, hospitals, and clinics. Forgers also alter legitimate prescriptions by changing the refill instructions or the quantity to be dispensed or by erasing the name of the drug prescribed and replacing it with a controlled substance.

The following list provides some specific suggestions for preventing diversion and abuse of controlled substances:

- Do not leave prescription pads in unattended examination rooms, office areas, or anywhere they can be stolen easily.
- Stock only a minimum number of pads. When not using them, store surplus stock in a secure, theft-proof drawer or cabinet.
- Report any prescription pad theft to the local police, the local pharmacy network, and the state board of pharmacy.
- Write complete prescriptions with signature and appropriate date. Include the full name and address of the patient, and physician's name, address, and telephone number.
- Do not preprint any Drug Enforcement Agency registration number on personalized prescription forms. Include a line on the form onto which a Drug Enforcement Agency number can be written as needed.
- Indicate the number of units and strengths to be dispensed by both writing the numeral *and* spelling out the number of units (e.g., 10 [ten]).
- Indicate the number of refills for the prescription. For example, if the acceptable number is zero, write "0" or "0 [zero]" in the appropriate blank.
- Never sign prescription blanks in advance.
- Do not order more than one controlled substance on a single blank; pharmacists must file prescriptions separately for scheduled drugs.
- Patiently, personally, and promptly respond to all calls from pharmacists who verify prescriptions for controlled substances. A corresponding responsibility rests with the pharmacist who dispenses the prescription order.

- Avoid prescribing, distributing, or giving schedule 2 controlled substances to a family member or to oneself except on an emergency basis.
- Use prescription pads that reveal the word *void* when photocopied, to avoid photocopy forgery.

References

1. Portenoy RK. Chronic opioid therapy in non-malignant pain. J Pain Symptom Manage 1990;5:S46.
2. Haislip GR. Impact of Drug Abuse on Legitimate Drug Use. In CS Hill, WS Fields (eds), Advances in Pain Research and Therapy, vol 11: Drug Treatment of Cancer Pain in a Drug-Oriented Society. New York: Raven, 1989;205.
3. Taub A. Opioid Analgesics in the Treatment of Chronic Intractable Pain of Non-Neoplastic Origin. In LM Kitahata, D Collins D (eds), Narcotic Analgesics in Anesthesiology. Baltimore: Williams & Wilkins, 1982;199.
4. France RD, Urban BJ, Keefe FJ. Long-term use of narcotic analgesics in chronic pain. Soc Sci Med 1984;19:1379.
5. Urban BJ, France RD, Steinberger DL, et al. Long-term use of narcotic/antidepressant medication in the management of phantom limb pain. Pain 1986;24:191.
6. Tennant FS, Uelman GF. Narcotic maintenance for chronic pain: medical and legal guidelines. Postgrad Med J 1983;73:81.
7. Tennant FS, Robinson D, Sagherian A, et al. Chronic opioid treatment of intractable non-malignant pain. Pain Manage 1988;2:18.
8. Wan Lu C, Urban B, France RD. Long-Term Narcotic Therapy in Chronic Pain. Presented at the Canadian Pain Society and American Pain Society Joint Meeting, Toronto, Canada. November 10–13, 1988.
9. Zenz M, Strumpf M, Tryba M. Long-term oral opioid therapy in patients with chronic non-malignant pain. J Pain Symptom Manage 1992;7:69.
10. Loeser JD. Pain After Amputation: Phantom Limb and Stump Pain. In JJ Bonica (ed), The Management of Pain. Philadelphia: Lea & Febiger, 1990;250.
11. Fields HL. Neural mechanisms of opiate analgesia. Adv Pain Res Ther 1985;9:479.
12. Fields HL, Heinricher MM. Anatomy and physiology of a nociceptive modulatory system. Philos Trans R Soc Lond B Biol Sci 1985;308:361.
13. Yaksh TL. Narcotic analgesics. CNS sites and mechanisms of action as revealed by intracerebral injection techniques. Pain 1978;4:299.
14. Hosobuchi Y, Adams JE, Linchitz R. Pain relief by electrical stimulation of the central gray matter in humans and its reversal by naloxone. Science 1977;197:183.
15. Richardson DE, Akil H. Pain reduction by electrical brain stimulation in man. J Neurosurg 1977;47:178.
16. Zorman G, Hentall ID, Adams JE, et al. Naloxone-reversible analgesia produced by microstimulation in the rat medulla. Brain Res 1981;219:137.
17. Chang K-J. Opioid Receptors. Multiplicity and Sequelae of Ligand-Receptor Interactions. In RA Conn (ed), The Receptors, vol 1. Orlando: Academic, 1984;1.
18. Martin WR. Pharmacology of opioids. Pharmacol Rev 1984;35:283.
19. Hughes J, Smith TW, Kosterlitz HW, et al. Identification of two related pentapeptides from the brain with potent opiate agonist activity. Nature 1975;258:577.
20. Khachaturian H, Lewis ME, Watson SJ. Enkephalin systems in diencephalon and brainstem of the rat. J Comp Neurol 1983;220:310.
21. Palkovits M. Distribution of neuropeptides in the central nervous system: a review of biochemical mapping studies. Prog Neurobiol 1984;23:151.
22. Fields HL, Basbaum AI. Brain stem control of spinal pain transmission neurons. Annu Rev Physiol 1978;40:217.
23. Mayer DJ, Price DD. Central nervous system mechanisms of analgesia. Pain 1976;2:379.
24. Baskin DS, Mehler WR, Hosobuchi Y, et al. Autopsy analysis of the safety, efficacy, and cartography of electrical stimulation of the central gray in humans. Brain Res 1986;371:231.
25. Hosobuchi Y, Adams JE, Linchitz R. Pain relief by electrical stimulation of the central gray matter in humans and its reversal by naloxone. Science 1977;197:183.
26. Abols JA, Basbaum AI. Afferent connections of the rostral medulla of the cat: a neural substrate for midbrain-medullary interactions in the modulation of pain. J Comp Neurol 1981;201:285.
27. Beitz AJ. The organization of afferent projections to the midbrain periaqueductal gray of the rat. Neuroscience 1982;7:133.
28. Mantyh PW. The ascending input to the midbrain periaqueductal gray of the primate. J Comp Neurol 1982;211:50.
29. Leavens ME, Hill CS Jr, Cech DA, et al. Intrathecal and intraventricular morphine for pain in cancer patients: initial study. J Neurosurg 1982;56:241.
30. Nurchi G. Use of intraventricular and intrathecal morphine in intractable pain associated with cancer. Neurosurgery 1984;15:801.
31. Yeung JC, Rudy TA. Multiplicative interaction between narcotic agonists expressed at spinal and supraspinal sites of antinociceptive action as revealed by concurrent intrathecal and intracerebroventricular injections of morphine. J Pharmacol Exp Ther 1980;215:633.
32. Fields HL. Central Nervous System Mechanisms for Control of Pain Transmission. In HL Fields (ed), Pain. New York: McGraw-Hill, 1987;99.
33. Snyder SH, Matthysse S (eds). Opiate receptor mechanisms. Neurosci Res Program Bull 1975;13:1.

34. Kosterlitz HW. Opiate actions in guinea pig ileum and mouse vas deferens. Neurosci Res Program Bull 1975;13:68.

35. Fang F, Fields HL, Lee NM. Action at the mu receptor is sufficient to explain the supraspinal analgesic effect of opiates. J Pharmacol Exp Ther 1986;238:1039.

36. Hooshmand H. Chronic Pain: Reflex Sympathetic Dystrophy Prevention and Management. Boca Raton, FL: CRC Press, 1993.

37. Hardy SGP. Projections to the midbrain from the medial versus lateral prefrontal cortices of the rat. Neurosci Lett 1986;63:159.

38. Bowker R, Westlund KN, Coulter JD. Origins of serotonergic projections of the spinal cord in rat: an immunocytochemical-retrograde transport study. Brain Res 1981;226:187.

39. Fields HL, Basbaum AI, Clanton CH, et al. Nucleus raphe magnus inhibition of spinal cord dorsal horn neurons. Brain Res 1977;126:441.

40. Glazer EJ, Basbaum AI. Axons which take up (3H) serotonin are presynaptic to enkephalin immunoreactive neurons in cat dorsal horn. Brain Res 1984;298:389.

41. Ruda MA. Opiates and pain pathways. Demonstration of enkephalin synapses on dorsal horn projection neurons. Science 1982;215:1523.

42. Fields HL, Emson PC, Leigh BK, et al. Multiple opiate receptor sites on primary afferent fibers. Nature 1980;284:351.

43. Hiller JM, Simon EJ, Crain SM, et al. Opiate receptors in culture of fetal mouse dorsal root ganglia (DRG) and spinal cord. Predominance in DRG neurites. Brain Res 1978;145:396.

44. Mudge AW, Leeman SE, Fischbach GD. Enkephalin inhibits release of substance P from sensory neurons in culture and decreases action potential duration. Proc Natl Acad Sci U S A 1979;76:526.

45. Fields HL, Basbaum AI. Endogenous Pain Control Mechanisms. In PD Wall, R Melzack (eds), Textbook of Pain. London: Churchill Livingstone, 1989;206.

46. Porter J, Jick H. Addiction rare in patients treated with narcotics. N Engl J Med 1980;302:123.

47. Perry S, Heidrich G. Management of pain during debridement: a survey of U.S. burn units. Pain 1982;13:267.

48. Medina JL, Diamond S. Drug dependency in patients with chronic headache. Headache 1977;17:12.

49. Jaffe JH. Drug Addiction and Drug Abuse. In AG Gilman, LS Goodman, TW Rall, et al. (eds), The Pharmacological Basis of Therapeutics (7th ed). New York: Macmillan, 1985;532.

50. Rinaldi RC, Steindler EM, Wilford BB, et al. Clarification and standardization of substance abuse terminology. JAMA 1988;259:555.

51. Weissman DE, Haddox JD. Opioid pseudoaddiction—an iatrogenic syndrome. Pain 1989;36:363.

52. Dole VP. Narcotic addiction, physical dependence, and relapse. N Engl J Med 1972;286:988.

53. Martin WR, Jasinski DR. Physiological parameters of morphine dependence in man—tolerance, early abstinence, protracted abstinence. J Psychol Res 1969;7:9.

54. Bruera E, Macmillan K, Hanson JA, et al. The cognitive effects of the administration of narcotic analgesics in patients with cancer pain. Pain 1989;39:13.

55. College of Physicians and Surgeons of British Columbia. Guidelines for Management of Chronic Non-Malignant Pain. Vancouver, British Columbia: College of Physicians and Surgeons of British Columbia, 1993.

56. Jaffe JH, Martin WR. Opioid Analgesics and Antagonists. In AG Gilman, LS Goodman (eds), The Pharmacological Basis of Therapeutics. New York: McGraw-Hill, 1990;485.

57. Bloom FE. The endorphins: a growing family of pharmacologically pertinent peptides. Annu Rev Pharmacol Toxicol 1983;23:151.

58. Akil H, Watson SJ, Young E, et al. Endogenous opioids: biology and function. Annu Rev Neurosci 1984;7:223.

59. Goldstein A. Opioid Peptides: Function and Significance. In HOJ Collier, J Hughes, MJ Rance, et al. (eds), Opioids: Past, Present and Future. London: Taylor & Frances, 1984;27.

60. Martin WR, Eades CG, Thompson JA, et al. The effects of morphine and nalorphine-like drugs in nondependent and morphine-dependent chronic spinal dog. J Pharmacol Exp Ther 1976;197:517.

61. Pfeiffer A, Brantl V, Herz A, et al. Psychotomimesis mediated by κ opiate receptors. Science 1986;233:774.

62. Millan MJ. Multiple opioid systems and pain. Pain 1986;27:303.

63. Heyman JS, Vaught JL, Raffa RB, et al. Can supraspinal delta-opioid receptors mediate antinociception? Trends Pharmacol Sci 1988;9:134.

64. Martin WR, Sloan JW. Neuropharmacology and Neurochemistry of Subjective Effects, Analgesia, Tolerance, and Dependence Produced by Narcotic Analgesics. In WR Martin (ed), Handbook of Experimental Pharmacology, vol 45: Drug Addiction I. Morphine, Sedative/Hypnotic and Alcohol Dependence. Berlin: Springer-Verlag, 1977;43.

65. Duggan AW, North RA. Electrophysiology of opioids. Pharmacol Rev 1983;35:219.

66. Wise RA, Bozarth MA. A psychomotor stimulation theory of addiction. Psychol Rev 1987;94:469.

67. Koob GF, Bloom FE. Cellular and molecular mechanisms of drug dependence. Science 1988;242:715.

68. Walker JM, Thompson LA, Frascella J, et al. Opposite effects of mu and kappa opiates on the firing-rate of dopamine cells in the substantia nigra of the rat. Eur J Pharmacol 1987;28:53.

69. Werling LL, Frattali A, Portoghese PS, et al. Kappa receptor regulation of dopamine release from striatum and cortex of rats and guinea pigs. J Pharmacol Exp Ther 1988;246:282.

70. Howlett TA, Rees LH. Endogenous opioid peptides and hypothalamo-pituitary function. Annu Rev Physiol 1986;48:527.

71. Grossman A. Opioids and stress in man. J Endocrinol 1988;119:377.

72. Duthie DJR, Nimmo WS. Adverse effects of opioid analgesic drugs. Br J Anaesth 1987;59:61.

73. Dooley CP, Saad C, Valenzuela JE. Studies of the role of opioids in control of human pancreatic secretion. Dig Dis Sci 1988;33:598.

74. Manara L, Bianchetti A. The central and peripheral influences of opioids on gastrointestinal propulsion. Annu Rev Pharmacol Toxicol 1985;25:249.

75. World Health Organization. Cancer Pain Relief. Geneva: World Health Organization, 1986.

76. Physician's Desk Reference (48th ed). Montvale, NJ: Medical Economics, 1994.

77. Dosing Conversion Reference. East Norwalk, CT: The Perdue Frederick Company, 1991.

Chapter 13
Intrathecal Opioid Pump Implantation

Jack L. Rook

Since the discovery of opioid receptors in the outer layers of the spinal cord, the intrathecal space has become a popular route for application of exogenous opioid drugs. This technique may provide potent analgesia to the suffering patient, usually with few systemic side effects. Some patients with reflex sympathetic dystrophy syndrome or other forms of chronic nonmalignant pain may be appropriate candidates for placement of an intraspinal opioid pump. Potential candidates should have tried all reasonable forms of treatment, both conservative and invasive, and found them ineffective. Trials with adequate doses of oral opioids should be attempted before opioid pump implantation. However, some patients are unable to achieve adequate analgesia via the oral route, or side effects from the opioids (nausea, vomiting, sedation, confusion, and other forms of cognitive impairment) make oral administration impractical. Such patients may benefit from placement of an opioid pump. Use of the spinal route can be justified only if it results in pain relief greater than that achieved from conventional routes associated with less troublesome or fewer unwanted effects.

Spinal Cord Opiate Receptors

In the 1970s, radioactive isotopes were used to demonstrate that large concentrations of opiate receptors were localized to the superficial spinal cord dorsal horn [1–3]. Expansion of this research led to the discovery that this region was highly sensitive to direct opiate application [4,5]. This discovery opened up an entire new field of neuropharmacologic inquiry and exploration of the great analgesic power of intraspinal narcotics [6,7].

In the superficial dorsal horn, μ and κ receptors predominate. For an opioid to be effective in producing analgesia when applied to the spinal cord, it must have agonist activity with μ and κ receptors. Opiates with both μ and κ agonist activity currently used for intrathecal application include morphine, methadone, hydromorphone, and fentanyl. Each drug varies with respect to analgesic potency and distance traveled within the cerebrospinal fluid (CSF) before exerting its effect.

Hydrophilic Versus Lipophilic Agents

An opioid's ability to be absorbed by the spinal cord has an impact on potency, duration of action, and potential side effects. The outer layers of the cord have a predominantly lipid consistency, owing to the large amount of myelin found in various ascending and descending pathways. Therefore, the absorbability of the more lipophilic (i.e., fat-soluble) agents after intrathecal injection will be greater than that of the hydrophilic (i.e., water-soluble) opioids. Of the more common opioids used for intrathecal administration, morphine is considered hydrophilic, whereas fentanyl is quite lipophilic. Methadone falls between these two

Table 13-1. Comparative Oil-Water
Solubility of Opioids

Narcotic	Oil-Water Solubility
Morphine HCl	1.42
Methadone HCl	116
Fentanyl citrate	813
Sufentanil citrate	1,778

Table 13-2. Varying Qualities of Hydrophilic
Versus Lipophilic Intrathecal Opioids

Quality of Drug	Morphine	Fentanyl
Intensity of effect	–	+
Number of spinal segments	+	–
Chance for respiratory depression	+	–
Fat solubility	–	+
Duration of action	+	–

– = lesser; + = greater.

drugs with respect to oil-water solubility (Table
13-1) [8,9].

Hydrophilic opioids such as morphine tend to
remain in the CSF for prolonged periods, migrate
cephalad and caudally in the subarachnoid space,
and result in a less intense quality of analgesia, a
longer duration of action, and a larger analgesic
area (encompassing more spinal segments) than
that of the more lipophilic agents. A potential
major problem in intrathecal administration of a
hydrophilic opioid is cephalad migration of the
drug into the brain, producing depression of respiratory centers in the medulla. If this effect occurs,
respiratory depression may be quite delayed, perhaps occurring 8–12 hours after intrathecal morphine bolus injection (owing to the drug's slow
transit within the CSF). Careful monitoring of vital
signs during early trials with intrathecal opioids is
important [8,10–13].

The more lipophilic an opioid is, the more
rapidly it will leach out of the water phase of the
CSF and enter the spinal cord. Thus, the highly fat-
soluble opioid fentanyl tends to have a rapid onset
of action, and if it is not carried very far from the
site of injection, the subsequent analgesic effect

will tend to be more intense and limited to relatively few spinal segments (Table 13-2) [8].

Anatomic Character and Pharmacokinetics of the Intrathecal Space

The spinal cord and brain are covered by two layers of tissues, the thick outer dura mater and the
thin pia arachnoid membrane, which is immediately adjacent to neural tissue. The inside of the
dura is lined with fat (epidural fat). Both membranes are vascularized, with connections to the
systemic circulation. The epidural space lies
between the dura and pia-arachnoid membrane,
whereas the subarachnoid (intrathecal) space is
bordered by the pia-arachnoid and spinal cord (Figure 13-1). CSF flows freely throughout the
intrathecal space and easily diffuses through the
pia-arachnoid membrane. Therefore, agents
injected into the epidural space permeate the
intrathecal space and vice versa.

Intrathecal opioids distribute between epidural
and intrathecal CSF, epidural fat, epidural blood
vessels, and the spinal cord (Figure 13-2). Opioids
distribute between the CSF and spinal cord according to their lipid solubility. Poorly lipid-soluble
agents spread rostrally, possibly reaching intracra-
nial structures [8].

Technique of Opioid Pump Implantation

The first step in considering implantation of an
opioid pump is to identify a potential candidate
for the device. Generally, patients with chronic
nonmalignant pain should have failed all reasonable approaches to pain management, including
optimal doses of oral opioids, before implantation
of an infusion pump. Because of cephalad migration of hydrophilic opioids, patients with chronic
intractable upper-extremity pain secondary to reflex
sympathetic dystrophy or cumulative trauma disorder can benefit from this technique.

Once an appropriate candidate has been identified, a trial of intrathecal opioids can commence.
This should be done with careful monitoring of vital
signs. During this trial, the opioid can be administered as a bolus or by drip infusion via catheter
placed into the intrathecal space. The patient should

Figure 13-1. The spinal cord and brain (central nervous system) are covered by a thick outer dura mater. The thin pia-arachnoid membrane is immediately adjacent to neural tissue. The inside of the dura is lined with epidural fat. Both membranes are vascularized with connections to the systemic circulation. The epidural space lies between the dura and pia-arachnoid membrane, whereas the subarachnoid (intrathecal) space is bordered by the pia-arachnoid and spinal cord. (Adapted from PD Wall, R Melzack. Textbook of Pain [2nd ed]. New York: Churchill Livingstone, 1989;745.)

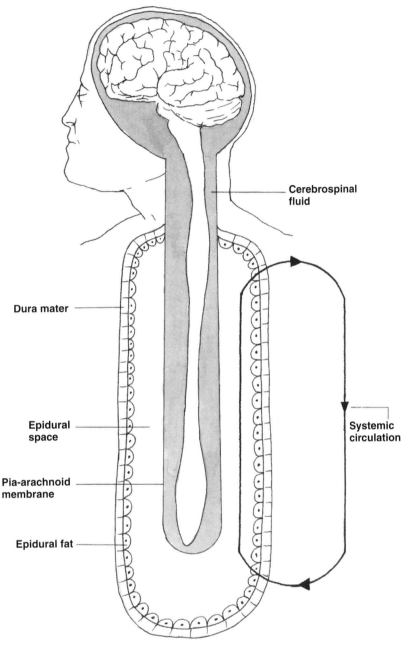

be observed for analgesic response, ability to mobilize himself or herself, and any side effects or complications. Careful observation of respiratory status is necessary for patients in poor physical condition and for those with respiratory disease. Patients with a favorable analgesic response may wish to proceed with infusion pump placement.

The next step is to provide the patient with appropriate education about the surgical procedure, potential beneficial effects, side effects and complications, and the need for regular follow-up. Postoperatively, follow-up is quite frequent, as the opioid must be titrated to an optimal dosage. Once a steady state has been reached, monthly follow-up to moni-

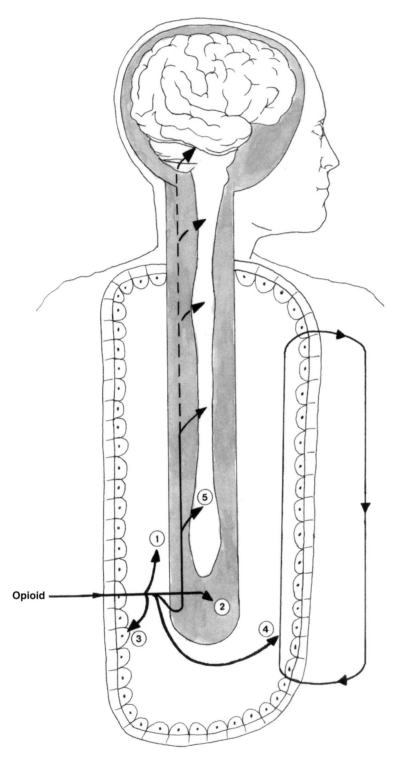

Figure 13-2. Pharmacokinetics of the epidural space. Epidural opioids distribute among epidural (1) and intrathecal (2) cerebrospinal fluid, epidural fat (3), epidural blood vessels (4), and the spinal cord (5). (Adapted from PD Wall, R Melzack. Textbook of Pain [2nd ed]. New York: Churchill Livingstone, 1989;745.)

Opioid

Figure 13-3. The Medtronic SynchroMed Infusion Pump. (Courtesy of Medtronic, Inc., Minneapolis, MN.)

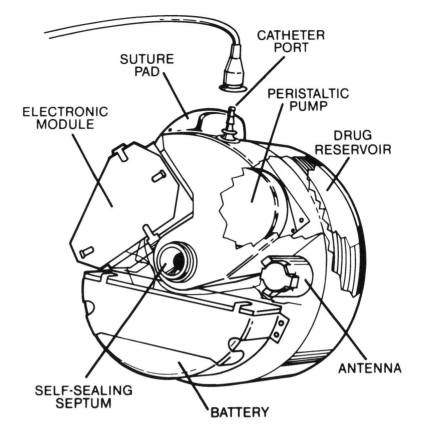

tor analgesic efficacy and to refill the infusion pump reservoir is necessary.

At this point, the infusion pump and catheter can be implanted. The opioid can be delivered by either continuous-infusion (Infusaid, Shiley-Infusaid Inc., Norwood, MA) or programmable (SynchroMed Infusion Pump, Medtronic, Inc., Minneapolis, MN) devices. Each system consists of several parts surgically implanted into the patient's body: an infusion pump, catheter, and filling port.

The infusion pump is a round, metal disc approximately 1 in. thick and 3 in. in diameter and weighing approximately 6 oz (Figure 13-3). It stores and releases prescribed amounts of medication. A computerlike external programmer can be used by physician or nurse to readjust the prescription flow rate (Figure 13-4). In the center of the pump is a raised portion that helps the treating physician to find the filling port. A self-sealing rubber septum is located in the middle of this filling port. At appropriate intervals, the physician inserts a needle through the septum to refill the pump. Last, a catheter leading from

the infusion pump delivers medication to the intrathecal space.

The infusion pump is designed to deliver a controlled amount of medication to the intrathecal space. The opioid binds to μ and κ receptors in the spinal cord dorsal horn, exerting an analgesic effect. Each pump has a memory that stores information about the infusion rate.

Because the pump is relatively small and internal, it is usually well accepted cosmetically. The device is implanted surgically, usually by a neurosurgeon. Initially, the surgeon makes a subcutaneous pocket to receive the reservoir portion of the pump and then creates a tunnel leading from the pump to the spinal canal. A catheter inserted through the tunnel connects the pump with the intrathecal space. Once the catheter and pump are in place, the wounds are closed (Figure 13-5).

After surgery, some discomfort is usually felt near the pump implantation site. Awareness of the pump soon diminishes. As the patient recovers from the procedure, the attending physician gives per-

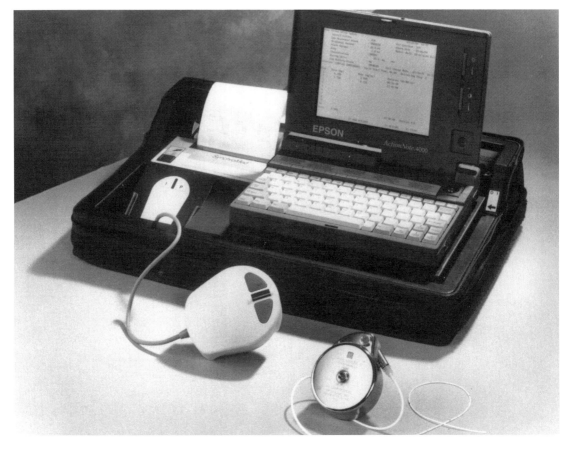

Figure 13-4. The SynchroMed infusion system from Medtronic, Inc., is the world's first commercially available implantable, programmable system. It consists of an implantable drug pump and a desktop programmer. Once implanted, the pump is programmed externally via radio signals to dispense the intrathecal opioid. Currently, only morphine is approved by the U.S. Food and Drug Administration for use in opioid infusion pumps. (Courtesy of Medtronic, Inc., Minneapolis, MN.)

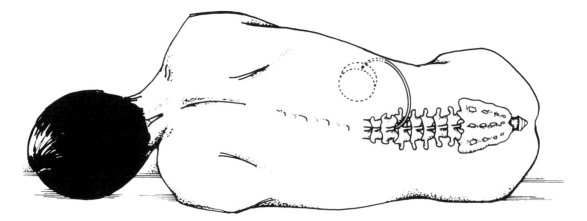

Figure 13-5. The surgically implanted morphine infusion pump. (Courtesy of Medtronic, Inc., Minneapolis, MN.)

Table 13-3. Side Effects and Complications of Opioid Pump Implantation

Complication of surgery
    Infection
Problems with the pump
    Kinked catheter
    Rundown battery
    Device component failure
Reactions to medication
    Respiratory depression
    Urinary retention
    Pleuritis
    Nausea or vomiting
    Development of tolerance

mission to the patient to resume daily activities. The patient needs regular physician follow-up indefinitely. Initially, flow-rate titration follow-up is frequent. After that, return visits may vary from weekly to monthly for refill of the pump reservoir.

The patient is instructed to (1) comply with all physician follow-up appointments; (2) watch for any swelling, redness, or pain near the incision (which may indicate the presence of infection and would necessitate prompt treatment with antibiotics, drainage, or even pump removal); (3) avoid activities that afford a chance of a blow to the pump; (4) watch for any unusual reactions to or side effects of the infused medication; (5) notify the physician in advance of prolonged vacations so that refills can be arranged; and (6) ensure that family members are aware of the device so that they can provide assistance in an emergency [14–18].

Side Effects and Complications of Opioid Pump Implantation

As with any surgical therapy, opioid pump implantation entails a slight risk for infection. If infection does occur, immediate and aggressive treatment is indicated (antibiotics, incision and drainage, and possibly removal of the unit). If treatment is not optimal, infection can spread along the catheter to the intrathecal space, possibly resulting in meningitis. Once the incision has healed, the pump and injection site require no special care, and the chances for infection are minimal, especially if proper sterile technique is used during the periodic refill injections.

Problems can occur with the unit itself (Table 13-3). The catheter could become plugged or kinked, may leak, or may dislodge. Such problems require surgical correction. The battery powering the pump will deplete every few (3–7) years. As with any complicated device, a component may fail, necessitating pump replacement [15].

Respiratory depression is the most feared side effect of pump implantation. Its onset is slow, often occurring 6–12 hours after intrathecal bolus injection. Thus, initial trials with spinal opioids, particularly in opioid-naive subjects and those with lung disease, should be done under conditions of appropriate surveillance (an intensive care milieu, backed up by appropriate apnea monitors). If delayed respiratory depression does occur, it can be treated promptly with the opioid antagonist naloxone. Surgeons should remember that the half-life of naloxone is short and that several repeated parenteral injections may be necessary [8,10–13,19].

Other potential problems with intrathecal opioids include urinary retention, pruritus, nausea and vomiting, and the development of tolerance [16].

Tolerance to analgesia varies from case to case. If it occurs, pump flow rate can be titrated appropriately. However, if tolerance develops too rapidly, requiring pump refills more than once weekly, other forms of pain control may have to be considered [8,14,20–22].

References

1. Fields HL. Central Nervous System Mechanisms for Control of Pain Transmission. In HL Fields (ed), Pain. New York: McGraw-Hill, 1987;99.
2. Atweh SF, Kuhar MJ. Autoradiographic localization of opiate receptors in rat brain, spinal cord, and lower medulla. Brain Res 1977;124:53.
3. Pert CB, Kuhar MJ, Snyder SH. Opiate receptor: autoradiographic localization in rat brain. Proc Natl Acad Sci U S A 1976;73:3729.
4. Yaksh TL, Rudy TA. Analgesia mediated by a direct spinal action of narcotics. Science 1976;192:1357.
5. Yaksh TL, Rudy TA. Narcotic analgesics: CNS sites and mechanisms of action as revealed by intracerebral injection techniques. Pain 1978;4:299.
6. Wang JK, Nauss LA, Thomas JE. Pain relief by intrathecally applied morphine in man. Anesthesiology 1979;50:149.
7. Behar M, Magora F, Olshwang D. Epidural morphine in the treatment of pain. Lancet 1979;1:527.

8. Bromage PR. Epidural Anesthetics and Narcotics. In PD Wall, R Malzack (eds), Textbook of Pain. London: Churchill Livingstone, 1989;744.

9. Kaufman JJ, Semo NM, Koski WS. Microelectrometric titration measurements of the pKas and partition and drug distribution coefficients of narcotics and narcotic antagonists and their pH temperature dependence. J Med Chem 1975;18:647.

10. Bromage PR. The price of interspinal narcotic analgesia: basic constraints [editorial]. Anesth Analg 1981;60:461.

11. Camporesi EM, Nielsen CH, Bromage PR, et al. Ventilatory CO_2 sensitivity following intravenous and epidural morphine in volunteers. Anesth Analg 1983;62:633.

12. Yaksh TL. Spinal opiate analgesia: characteristics and principles of action. Pain 1981;11:293.

13. Doblar DD, Muldoon SM, Albrecht PH, et al. Epidural morphine following epidural local anesthesia: effect on ventilatory and airway occlusion pressure responses to CO_2. Anesthesiology 1981;66:423.

14. Penn RD, Price JA. Chronic intrathecal morphine for intractable pain. J Neurosurg 1987;67:182.

15. Medtronic, Inc. Ease of Pain, Ease of Mind. The SynchroMed Infusion System—Patient Information. Minneapolis: Medtronic, Inc., April 1990.

16. Auld AW, Maki-Jokela A, Murdoch DM. Intraspinal narcotic analgesia in the treatment of chronic pain. Spine 1985;10:777.

17. Coombs DW, Saunders RL, Gaylor MS. Continuous epidural analgesia via implanted morphine reservoir. Lancet 1981;2:425.

18. Coombs DW, Saunders RL, Gaylor M, et al. Epidural narcotic infusion reservoir: implantation technique and efficiency. Anesthesiology 1982;56:469.

19. Glynn CJ, Mather LE, Cousins MJ, et al. Spinal narcotics and respiratory depression. Lancet 1979;2:365.

20. Woods WA, Cohen SC. High-dose epidural morphine in a terminally ill patient. Anesthesiology 1982;56:311.

21. Greenberg HS, Taren J, Ensminger WD, et al. Benefit from and tolerance to continuous intrathecal infusion of morphine for intractable cancer pain. J Neurosurg 1982;57:360.

22. Coombs DW, Saunders RL, Lachance D, et al. Intrathecal morphine tolerance: use of intrathecal clonidine, DADLE, and intraventricular morphine. Anesthesiology 1985;62:358.

Chapter 14
Spinal Cord Stimulation

Jack L. Rook

History

In 1967, Dr. Norman Shealy [1] published an article describing a new technique for the management of chronic intractable pain. The process used radio frequency–induced electrical stimulation of the spinal cord via electrodes implanted over the dorsal columns. This original technique was termed *dorsal column stimulation*. Although the initial concept involved stimulation of the dorsal columns, over time researchers learned that stimulation applied to the ventral surface also could be effective in relieving pain [2], and the more appropriate term *spinal cord stimulation* (SCS) came to be used to describe this technique.

The original surgical procedure was cumbersome, involving subarachnoid implantation of a monopolar electrode via laminectomy. Often, it was difficult to position the electrode, and the electrode tended to migrate, resulting in incomplete analgesia [3]. In addition, complications (e.g., infection, meningeal irritation, and spinal headaches secondary to dural leak) were more frequent than they are today.

Since that time, the field of SCS has grown immensely with major advances in various areas. Electrodes previously placed intrathecally are now placed in the epidural space, resulting in fewer complications. The open technique (i.e., surgically implanted electrodes via laminotomy) for electrode implantation has been replaced by a percutaneous technique done under fluoroscopic guidance. Elec-

trodes have evolved from monopolar to multipolar to dual multipolar leads. Multipolar electrodes cover larger areas of the spinal cord for stimulation purposes. Advances in computer technology, miniaturization of circuitry and hardware, and improvements in the biochemistry of hardware have led to more reliable and more comfortable equipment. Careful screening procedures now used result in better outcome data [4].

Although the initial concept for neuroaugmentation was for relief of pain, other uses for the technology have been identified, notably movement disorders [5–10] and peripheral vascular disease [11–15].

Pathophysiologic Considerations

A number of different mechanisms have been proposed to explain the effectiveness of SCS. Electrical stimulation disrupts pain transmission impulses traveling in fibers of the dorsal horn or anterolateral quadrant [16]. Activation of the descending pain-modulatory system in the dorsolateral funiculus causes release of serotonin, a potent inhibitor of pain transmission at the spinal cord dorsal horn. Indeed, elevated serotonin and substance P levels have been found in the cerebrospinal fluid (CSF) after spinal cord stimulation [17–19]. Stimulation of the dorsal columns results in the production of both orthodromic impulses (toward the brain) and antidromic impulses (caudal transmission within the spinal cord). The antidromic impulses travel back to the dorsal horn, possibly jamming incoming pain transmission signals at that level [20]. The orthodromic impulses travel via large dorsal column fibers to the somatosensory cortex, which perceives the stimulation as being a non-noxious paresthesia (that in the case of SCS has to blanket the painful area in order to be effective) [21–27]. This theory proposes the existence of a combination of pain block at the spinal cord level and perceived stimulation at the cortical level [4]. The fourth theory, based on the gate-control hypothesis of Melzack and Wall [28], proposes that SCS segmentally activates large-diameter afferents that inhibit second-order pain transmission cells. Therefore, a disruption of nociceptive pain transmission occurs at the level of SCS. Experimental work is continuing in an attempt to explain more definitively the exact mechanism of analgesic response created by SCS.

Patient Selection Criteria

SCS may prove helpful in treating a variety of painful conditions. However, it is important to adhere to a number of general patient selection criteria.

Characteristics of the Patient

As SCS is a costly procedure, patients must be selected carefully. If rigid criteria for selection are followed, 60–80% efficacy can be expected with spinal neuroaugmentation [25,42,44,45,55–58].

For SCS to be considered, documentation should state that all reasonable conservative pain management techniques for the patient have failed. Also, the typical prospective patient would express a desire to avoid extensive surgical procedures. Most protocols for SCS require patients to detoxify from opioid analgesics prior to consideration for the procedure. At the very least, successful stimulation in patients on opioids should lead to gradual tapering of the analgesic. SCS could be considered as an alternative to neuroablative procedures and extensive surgeries.

Psychopathologic elements contributing to or causing the pain must be determined through careful screening that includes a thorough psychological evaluation and appropriate testing (e.g., the Minnesota Multiphasic Personality Inventory, Wahler Symptom Inventory, Zung Scale, Beck Depression Index, Behavioral Analysis of Pain, McGill Pain Questionnaire). Patients with a somatoform pain disorder should not be considered for the SCS procedure. Depression, common in chronic pain, may actually lessen with successful SCS. Underlying psychopathologic components must be treated before any consideration of spinal neuroaugmentation.

The pain should not be complicated by nor contribute to any secondary gain, either emotional or financial. For some patients involved in litigation, magnified pain behaviors may be present, driven consciously or subconsciously in an effort to effect final settlement. Ideally, complicated legal issues and litigation should be resolved before implantation. Obviously, this contingency is not always possible.

Patients with drug-seeking behavior or substance abuse should be excluded from consideration until detoxification and sobriety are well established.

Last, patients must have realistic expectations regarding results from the SCS procedure. They must understand that SCS may reduce but not necessarily eliminate the pain, that SCS is not a cure for the underlying problem, that permanent implantation will be considered only if trial stimulation provides *significant* pain relief, and that careful and regular follow-up will be necessary for a postoperative period [4,29,30].

Characteristics of the Pain

The more localized the pain in the extremity, the better the response will be; a unilateral painful extremity will respond better to stimulation than both extremities. Bilateral extremity pain will respond to stimulation, but the electrode must be located in the midline. Trunk pain is not treated well by SCS. The more diffuse the pain problem, the less successful will the procedure be. Stimulation trials still may be indicated even if patients do not fulfill these criteria [4,23,29–48].

The literature supports the use of SCS in the management of peripheral causalgia and reflex sympathetic dystrophy syndrome (RSDS) [49,50]. Robaina et al. [51] used SCS for relief of chronic pain in vasospastic disorders of the upper limbs. Their study of 11 patients, of whom eight had RSDS, revealed 91% achieving good to excellent pain relief after a 27-month follow-up. The authors concluded that SCS could be used as a primary or secondary therapy after unsuccessful sympathectomy or sympathetic blocks.

Three other clinical studies on the use of SCS therapy for RSDS have demonstrated good to excellent pain relief in 85% of the patients studied (n = 26) [52–54]. Over the years, hundreds of articles about SCS have been published. More recent literature consistently reports a decrease in subjective pain intensity in the majority of patients undergoing the procedure, a decrease in their oral narcotic requirements, and an increase in their functional and working capacity. Also commonly accepted is that SCS has become an easily implemented, low-morbidity technique for treatment of properly selected intractable chronic nonmalignant pain (CNMP) patients. In benign chronic pain problems, stimulation is superior to many other methods, especially destructive surgery. It is expected that applications for SCS will continue to expand with improvements in technology and with more widespread understanding and acceptance of the methods involved [25,42,44,45,55–58].

Technique

Trial Stimulation

Trial stimulation is necessary to determine whether the patient will respond to spinal cord stimulation; to help the patient to decide whether to proceed with the implantation procedure; to avoid the needless, high cost of direct implantation of a permanent system if the quality of analgesia is insufficient or poor; and to help the surgeon to determine the optimum site for electrode positioning and optimal SCS programmable unit parameters before undertaking a permanent procedure.

Major components necessary for trial stimulation include the electrode lead (monopolar or multipolar), an extension wire, and a power source. Multipolar leads provide more precise stimulation. Permanent leads also can be used (although at greater cost) if the

anticipation is that the patient ultimately will undergo a permanent placement procedure.

The patient undergoes a trial stimulation procedure as an outpatient. An intravenous line is started, and the patient is given pretrial antibiotic coverage and is placed in the prone position. Some sedation may be used, but the patient must remain lucid and able to answer questions about the location of the paresthesias created by stimulation.

After iodophor solution preparation, the patient receives a local anesthetic-field block at the site of epidural needle insertion, which, for upper-extremity stimulation, would be the mid-dorsal back and, for lower-extremity stimulation, the upper lumbar (L1–2) area. At the appropriate interspace, a large (15- to 16-gauge) needle is inserted into the epidural space. Needle and subsequent electrode position are visualized fluoroscopically. The test lead is placed through the needle and is advanced into the epidural space. Patience is required for proper positioning of the electrode, as the electrically induced paresthesias need to cover the painful dermatomes.

For bilateral stimulation, the lead electrodes should be as close as possible to the midline (i.e., lying adjacent to the dorsal median sulcus). For unilateral stimulation, the electrode can be placed near the dorsolateral sulcus (Figure 14-1).

Pain relief is not absolutely necessary at this point. If it does occur, outcome will most likely be excellent. If it does not occur, analgesia may be achieved on an outpatient basis once optimal radio frequency–stimulation parameters are found. When appropriate paresthesias are created, the epidural needle is removed with special care so as not to dislodge the lead electrode. The electrode position is verified again with the fluoroscope. A suture fixes the lead to the skin.

After the procedure, the patient may be sent home with a temporary unit attached to the lead electrode. The lead will remain in place for 7–10 days, during which the patient will experience the electrically induced paresthesias and gauge the pain relief. Stimulator parameters may need adjustment on a daily basis. After the 10-day trial, the patient should be able to determine whether to proceed with permanent implantation. If permanent implantation is chosen, the test lead is removed, and the permanent implantation process proceeds. If per-

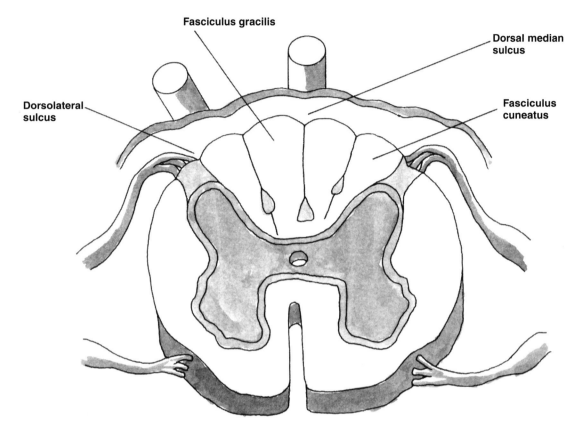

Figure 14-1. Electrode lead position. For unilateral stimulation, the electrode can be placed near the dorsolateral sulcus. For bilateral stimulation, single-lead electrodes should be as close as possible to the midline, or dual electrodes can be placed in the more lateral positions.

manent leads were used for the trial, they are left in place, and the implantation process is completed [4,29,59–63].

Permanent Implantation

Permanent implantation is performed in the operating room with strict sterile technique and antibiotic coverage. Once again, the patient will require conscious sedation. As noted earlier, the temporary lead from trial stimulation is removed; however, if a permanent lead was used initially, it is left in place, and the procedure is completed.

If a new permanent lead is required, it is inserted with the previously outlined technique, with fluoroscopic guidance and the patient's interpretation of the electrically induced paresthesias. Once optimal

lead positioning is found, the permanent lead is anchored by suture to the supraspinous ligament.

Then the patient is placed in the lateral decubitus position for implantation of the spinal cord stimulator pulse generator (SCSPG) (Figure 14-2). Possible locations for the SCSPG include the anterolateral chest for leads placed in the cervical or upper thoracic area and the abdomen or buttocks for lower-extremity stimulation leads. A large subcutaneous pocket is created for insertion of the SCSPG.

Next, a subcutaneous tunnel is created to run from the pocket to the midline back incision. An extension wire placed in the tunnel connects the lead wire to the SCSPG unit. The system is activated and tested for integrity. If stimulation is satisfactory, the wounds are irrigated, closed, and dressed, and the patient is transferred to the recovery room [4,29,64].

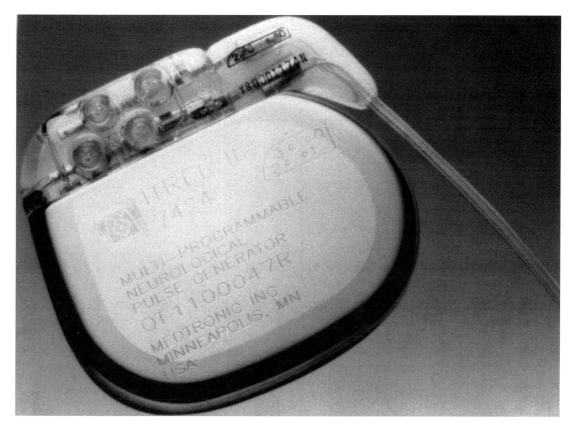

Figure 14-2. The spinal cord stimulator pulse generator. The Medtronic ITREL II pulse generator delivers electrical impulses via an insulated lead electrode. (Courtesy of Medtronic, Inc., Minneapolis, MN.)

Postimplantation Care

The SCSPG has a number of programmable parameters, and optimal settings vary from patient to patient. Such settings must be determined for each patient, through trial and error, after implantation. Some patients need very little stimulation for pain relief; others require continuous stimulation with high-voltage requirements. Certainly, this setting plays a role in battery longevity, which depends directly on the various parameters.

The programmable parameters include pulse amplitude, or intensity of the stimulus (0–10.5 V); pulse frequency (2–130 Hz); pulse width (60–450 microseconds); and stimulation cycles (on: 0.1–64.0 seconds; off: 0.4 seconds–17 minutes).

SCS units (both internally and externally controlled systems) are available from Medtronic, Inc., (Minneapolis, MN) and Neuromed, Inc., (Ft. Lau-derdale, FL) supplies an externally controlled system. The Medtronic ITREL implantable SCS system has a completely internalized pulse generator and one quadripolar lead. Stimulation parameters for the ITREL system are set by the clinician via a desktop programming console and a hand-held programmer (Figures 14-3 and 14-4).

Two available externally controlled systems are the Medtronic X-TREL (single-lead system) and Mattrix (two-lead system with independently controlled stimulation mode). With external systems, an implanted receiver receives signals from a belt-mounted transmitter. Impulses are relayed to the spinal cord via one or two insulated leads (X-TREL and Mattrix, respectively) (Figures 14-5 and 14-6).

During the early postoperative period, physician guidance is necessary for parameter adjustment of both internal and external systems. However, with external systems, the goal is for

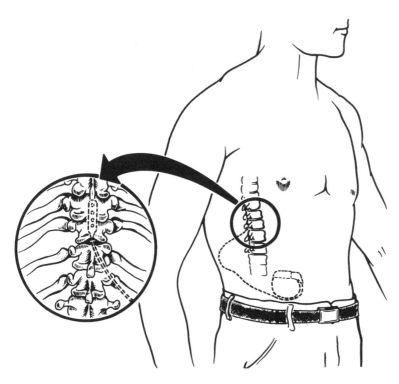

Figure 14-3. The Medtronic ITREL implantable spinal cord stimulation system has a completely internalized pulse generator and one quadripolar lead. (Courtesy of Medtronic, Inc., Minneapolis, MN.)

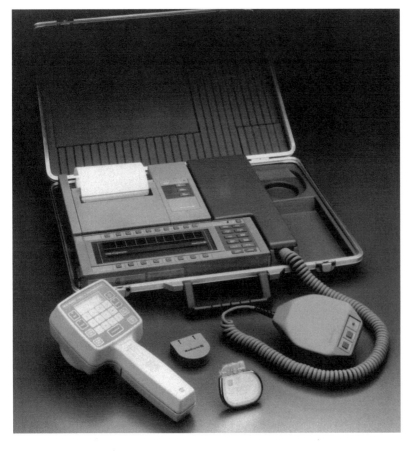

Figure 14-4. Stimulation parameters for the ITREL system are set by the clinician using a desktop programming console and a hand-held programmer (bottom left). The desktop programming console (top) also programs the pulse generator and provides printouts of information from it. (Courtesy of Medtronic, Inc., Minneapolis, MN.)

Figure 14-5. The Medtronic Mattrix neurostimulation system consists of an implantable receiver (left center), an external antenna (upper right) affixed to the skin over the receiver, a belt-mounted transmitter (not shown), and dual quadripolar lead wires. (Courtesy of Medtronic, Inc., Minneapolis, MN.)

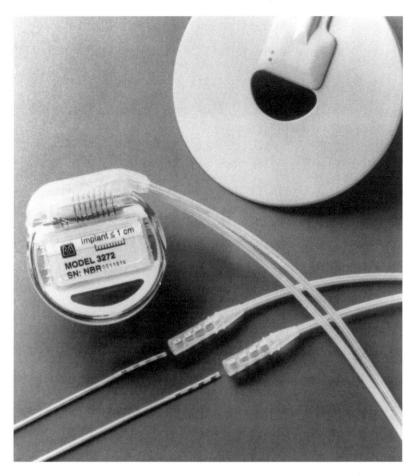

patients to become independent in turning the unit off and on and in changing parameters (amplitude, frequency, and pulse width) by using the portable external programmer.

During the postoperative period, attempts are made to find the lowest possible parameter settings that simultaneously provide pain relief and preserve battery life. Patients are encouraged to turn off or turn down the parameters of the SCSPG when pain is well controlled.

Patients should be checked regularly until wounds are well healed and sutures are removed. They are given a number of responsibilities [4,65]:

- Avoidance of stooping, bending, twisting, and lifting for the first 6–8 weeks after surgery to maintain proper electrode position during the period it is most prone to dislodge

- Avoidance of chiropractic treatment for 6–8 weeks and sparing, cautious treatments after that time
- Avoidance of wetting the transmitter (assuming use of an external transmitter device), which is not waterproof
- Avoidance of magnetic resonance imaging scans
- Gradual return to daily activities (traveling, sex, and vocational and avocational pursuits) as tolerated and based on the improved quality of analgesia

Goals of Treatment

Researchers generally agree that, when applied to appropriate patients by trained practitioners, realis-

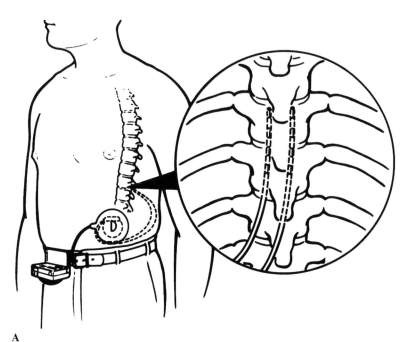

Figure 14-6. With external systems, an implanted receiver (A) receives signals from a belt-mounted transmitter (B). With the Medtronic Mattrix neurostimulation system, impulses are relayed to the spinal cord via two insulated leads. (Courtesy of Medtronic, Inc., Minneapolis, MN.)

A

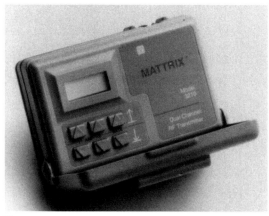

B

tic goals of treatment include 60–70% efficacy, 50–75% pain relief when efficacious, reduction in narcotic-analgesic intake, improvement in activity levels and quality of life, and elimination of need for further surgery [25,30,42,44,45,55–58].

Complications

Problems and complications associated with SCS implantation include failure, infection, lead migration, electrode damage, and battery failure. Even selecting patients through a careful screening process does not guarantee the efficacy of SCS. According to the literature, failure rates of 20–40% can be expected [25,42,44,45,55–58].

Infection, the most serious complication, occurs in 1.5–10.0% of cases [66]. It can involve the epidural space or the SCSPG pockets. Epidural infection, characterized by increasing blood pressure, fever, chills, and leukocytosis mandates aggressive treatment that includes electrode removal, appropriate cultures, and intravenous antibiotics. If infection is untreated, sepsis, spinal cord injury, meningitis, and even death can result. If infection is treated appropriately, long-term morbidity is rare, and the electrode or SCSPG can be replaced at a later time.

Lead migration is common, especially in active individuals. Cervical leads are displaced more commonly than are thoracic leads, owing to greater mobility in the cervical region. Lead migration will require opening of the back wound for repositioning of the lead.

Battery failure is inevitable over time. Continuous high-voltage stimulation will cause a more rapid drain on the lithium cell, whereas patients who turn the unit off when resting, use the lowest possible parameters (without sacrificing pain relief), and use intermittent (cycling mode) stimulation will slow battery depletion. Battery replacement requires a minor surgical procedure.

Lead fractures, although uncommon, may occur if electrodes are mishandled or traumatized during implantation. A more common occurrence is disruption of the insulating sheath around the leads with abnormal stimulatory patterns or complete cessation of stimulation. Such problems necessitate lead removal and reimplantation [4].

Conclusion

For patients with chronic nonmalignant pain or RSDS, spinal cord stimulation could represent a particularly attractive alternative to treatment options that often include living with the pain, ongoing sympathetic blockade, neuroablative-neurolytic procedures, long-term opioid intake, or further surgical attempts at correcting underlying pathologic conditions.

For the procedure to be successful in the aforementioned population, patients must be selected carefully, depression must be treated optimally, and opioids must be tapered as much as possible. Centralized disease with diffuse body pain will not respond as well as will localized causalgia pain confined to a single extremity. Success of SCS depends also on the patients' not having serious psychopathologic characteristics identified on psychological screening procedures.

For appropriate patients, SCS is a nondestructive, reversible, low-morbidity procedure. Patients can be screened for response prior to implantation of a permanent system.

References

1. Shealy CN, Mortimer JT, Reswick J. Electrical inhibition of pain by stimulation of the dorsal column: preliminary clinical reports. Anesth Analg 1967;46:489.
2. Larson SJ, Sances A Jr, Cusick JF, et al. A comparison between anterior and posterior spinal implant systems. Surg Neurol 1975;4:180.
3. Shealy CN, Mortimer JT, Hagfors NR. Dorsal column electroanalgesia. J Neurosurg 1970;32:560.
4. Robb LG, Spector G, Robb M. Spinal Cord Stimulation Neuroaugmentation of the Dorsal Columns for Pain Relief. In RS Weiner (ed), Innovations in Pain Management—A Practical Guide for Clinicians. Orlando, FL: Deutsch Press, 1993;33.
5. Cook AW. Stimulation of the spinal cord in motor neuron disease. Lancet 1974;2:230.
6. Illis LS, Oygar AE, Sedgwick EM, et al. Dorsal column stimulation in the rehabilitation of patients with multiple sclerosis. Lancet 1976;1:1383.
7. Krainick JU, Thoden U, Strassburg HM, et al. The effects of electrical spinal cord stimulation on spastic movement disorders. Adv Neurosurg 1977;4:257.
8. Siegfried J, Krainick JU, Haas H, et al. Electrical spinal cord stimulation for spastic movement disorders. Appl Neurophysiol 1978;41:134.
9. Tallis RC, Illis LS, Sedgwick EM. The quantitative assessment of the influence of spinal cord stimulation on motor function in patients with multiple sclerosis. Int Rehabil Med 1983;5:10.
10. Barolat-Romana G, Myklebust JB, Hemmy DC, et al. Immediate effects of spinal cord stimulation in spinal spasticity. J Neurosurg 1985;62:558.
11. Cook AW, Oygar A, Baggenstos P, et al. Vascular disease of extremities. J Med 1976;3:46.
12. Meglio M, Cioni B, Dal Lago A, et al. Pain control and improvement of peripheral blood flow following epidural spinal cord stimulation. J Neurosurg 1981;54:821.
13. Tallis RC, Illis LS, Sedgwick EM, et al. Spinal cord stimulation in peripheral vascular disease. J Neurol Neurosurg Psychiatry 1983;46:478.
14. Augustinsson LE, Holm J, Jivegard L, et al. Epidural electrical stimulation in severe limb ischemia. Evidences of pain relief, increased blood flow and a possible limb-saving effect. Ann Surg 1985;202:104.
15. Broseta J, Barbera J, De Vera JA, et al. Spinal cord stimulation in peripheral arterial disease. J Neurosurg 1986;64:71.
16. Gybels JM, Sweet WH (eds). Neurosurgical Treatment of Persistent Pain. Basel, Switzerland: Karger, 1989;293.

17. Basbaum AI, Fields HL. Endogenous pain control mechanisms: review and hypothesis. Ann Neurol 1978;4:451.

18. Snyder SH. Brain peptides as neurotransmitters. Science 1980;209:976.

19. Henry JL. Substance P and pain: an updating. Trends Neurosci 1980;3:95.

20. Meyerson B. Electrostimulation procedures: effects, presumed rationale and possible mechanisms of human pain. Pain Headache 1983;11:293.

21. Burton CV. Session on spinal cord stimulation: safety and clinical efficacy. Neurosurgery 1977;1:164.

22. Krainick JU, Thoden U. Dorsal Column Stimulation. In PD Wall, R Melzack (eds), Textbook of Pain. New York: Churchill Livingstone, 1989;701.

23. Kumar K, Nath R, Wyant GM. Treatment of chronic pain by epidural spinal cord stimulation: a 10-year experience. J Neurosurg 1991;75:402.

24. Nashold BS Jr, Friedman H. Dorsal column stimulation for control of pain, preliminary report on 30 patients. J Neurosurg 1972;36:590.

25. North RB, Ewend MG, Lawton MT, et al. Spinal cord stimulation for chronic, intractable pain: superiority of "multichannel" devices. Pain 1991;44:119.

26. Sweet WH, Wepsic JG. Electrical Stimulation for Suppression of Pain in Men. In WS Fields (ed), Neural Organization and Its Relevance to Prosthetics. New York: Intercontinental Medical Book, 1973;218.

27. Urban BJ, Nashold B. Percutaneous epidural stimulation of the spinal cord for relief of pain: long-term results. J Neurosurg 1978;48:323.

28. Melzack R, Wall PD. Pain mechanisms: a new theory. Science 1965;150:971.

29. North RB, Kidd DH, Zahurak M, et al. Spinal cord stimulation for chronic, intractable pain: experience over two decades. Neurosurgery 1993;32:384.

30. Medtronic, Inc. Spinal Cord Stimulation—Background and Efficacy. Minneapolis: Medtronic, Inc., 1991.

31. Law JD. Targeting a spinal stimulator to treat the "failed back surgery syndrome." Appl Neurophysiol 1987;50:437.

32. Meilman PW, Leibrock LG, Leong FTL. Outcome of implanted spinal cord stimulation in the treatment of chronic pain: arachnoiditis versus single nerve root injury and mononeuropathy. Clin J Pain 1989;5:189.

33. Ray CD, Burton CV, Lifson A. Neurostimulation as used in a large clinical practice. Appl Neurophysiol 1982;45:160.

34. Sweet W, Wepsic J. Stimulation of the posterior columns of the spinal cord for pain control. Clin Neurosurg 1974;21:278.

35. Burton C. Dorsal column stimulation: optimization of application. Surg Neurol 1975;4:171.

36. Clark K. Electrical stimulation of the nervous system for control of pain: University of Texas Southwestern Medical School experience. Surg Neurol 1975;4:164.

37. de Vera JA, Rodriguez JL, Dominguez M, et al. Spinal cord stimulation for chronic pain mainly in PVD, vasospastic disorders of the upper limbs and failed back surgery. Pain 1990;Suppl 5:81.

38. Erickson DL, Long DM. Ten-Year Follow-Up of Dorsal Column Stimulation. In JJ Bonica (ed), Advances in Pain Research and Therapy, vol 5. New York: Raven, 1983;583.

39. Hoppenstein RL. Electrical stimulation of the ventral and dorsal columns of the spinal cord for relief of chronic intractable pain. Surg Neurol 1975;4:187.

40. Long DM, Erickson DE. Stimulation of the posterior columns of the spinal cord for relief of intractable pain. Surg Neurol 1975;4:134.

41. Long DM, Erickson D, Campbell J, et al. Electrical stimulation of the spinal cord and peripheral nerves for pain control. Appl Neurophysiol 1981;44:207.

42. Meglio M, Cioni B, Rossi GF. Spinal cord stimulation in management of chronic pain: a nine-year experience. J Neurosurg 1989;70:519.

43. Nielson KD, Adams JE, Hosobuchi Y. Experience with dorsal column stimulation for relief of chronic intractable pain. Surg Neurol 1975;4:148.

44. Racz GB, McCarron RF, Talboys P. Percutaneous dorsal column stimulator for chronic pain control. Spine 1989;14:1.

45. Spiegelmann R, Friedman WA. Spinal cord stimulation: a contemporary series. Neurosurgery 1991;28:65.

46. Young RF, Shende M. Dorsal column stimulation for relief of chronic intractable pain. Surg Forum 1976;27:474.

47. Brandwin MA, Kewman DG. MMPI indicators of treatment response to spinal epidural stimulation in patients with chronic pain and patients with movement disorders. Psychol Rep 1982;51:1059.

48. Daniel M, Long C, Hutcherson M, et al. Psychological factors and outcome of electrode implantation for chronic pain. Neurosurgery 1985;17:773.

49. Hassenbusch SJ, Stanton-Hicks M, Walsh J, et al. Effects of Chronic Peripheral Nerve Stimulation in Stage III Reflex Sympathetic Dystrophy (RSD). Cleveland: Cleveland Clinic Foundation, 1992.

50. Racz GB, Lewis R, Heavner JE, et al. Peripheral Nerve Stimulator Implant for the Treatment of Causalgia. In M Stanton-Hicks (ed), Pain and the Sympathetic Nervous System. Norwell, MA: Kluwer Academic, 1990.

51. Robaina F, Dominguez M, Diaz M, et al. Spinal cord stimulation for relief of chronic pain in vasospastic disorders of the upper limbs. Neurosurgery 1989;24:63.

52. Barolat G, Schwartzman R, Woo R. Epidural spinal cord stimulation in the management of reflex sympathetic dystrophy. Stereotact Funct Neurosurg 1989;53:29.

53. Broggi G, Servello D, Franzini A, et al. Spinal cord stimulation for treatment of peripheral vascular disease. Appl Neurophysiol 1987;50:439.

54. Sanchez-Ledesma M, Garcia-March G, Diaz-Cascajo P, et al. Spinal cord stimulation in deafferentation pain. Stereotact Funct Neurosurg 1989;53:40.

55. North RB, Ewend MG, Lawton MT, et al. Failed back surgery syndrome: 5-year follow-up after spinal cord stimulator implantation. Neurosurgery 1991;28:692.

56. DeLaPorte C, Siegfried J. Lumbosacral spinal fibrosis (spinal arachnoiditis). Spine 1983;8:593.

57. Kumar K, Wyant GM, Ekong CE. Epidural spinal cord stimulation for relief of chronic pain. Pain Clin 1986;1(2):91.

58. Ray CD. Implantation of Spinal Cord Stimulators for Relief of Chronic and Severe Pain. In JC Cauthen (ed), Lumbar Spine Surgery. Indications, Techniques, Failures, and Alternatives (2nd ed). Baltimore: Williams & Wilkins, 1988;350.

59. Erickson DL. Percutaneous trial of stimulation for patient selection for implantable stimulating devices. J Neurosurg 1975;43:440.

60. Hoppenstein R. Percutaneous implantation of chronic spinal cord electrodes for control of intractable pain: preliminary report. Surg Neurol 1975;4:195.

61. Hosobuchi Y, Adams JE, Weinstein PR. Preliminary percutaneous dorsal column stimulation prior to permanent implantation. J Neurosurg 1972;37:242.

62. North RB, Fischell TA, Long DM. Chronic stimulation via percutaneously inserted epidural electrodes. Neurosurgery 1977;1:215.

63. Zumpano BJ, Saunders RL. Percutaneous epidural dorsal column stimulation. J Neurosurg 1978;46:459.

64. North RB. Spinal Cord Stimulation for Intractable Pain: Indications and Technique. In DM Long (ed), Current Therapy in Neurological Surgery, vol 2. Toronto: Decker, 1988;297.

65. Medtronic, Inc. Understanding Your X-TREL Spinal Cord Stimulation System. Minneapolis: Medtronic, Inc., 1991.

66. Law JD. The Failed Back Syndrome Treated by Percutaneous Spinal Stimulation. Presented at the American Association of Neurosurgeons Annual Meeting, 1986, San Diego, CA.

Chapter 15
Medicolegal Issues in Cumulative Trauma Disorders

Steven U. Mullens

Litigation resulting from repetitive trauma disorders or cumulative trauma disorders (CTDs) is limited primarily to workers' compensation claims, short- and long-term disability contests, and Social Security disability–supplemental security income cases. With few exceptions, these cases are tried before administrative law judges or arbitrators. This chapter discusses the dynamics of workers' compensation and the role of the medical witness in workers' compensation claims.

Some form of workers' compensation exists in virtually all of the states and, although the states may vary significantly as to the amount of benefits paid and the limitations on benefits, medical care for a recognized work injury, including CTDs, and the debate and dialogue that exist around that medical care are very similar from one state to the next. It should also be noted that the federal government has a number of different programs for workers' compensation and, although federal compensation laws may vary significantly from the state acts, constant basic issues of diagnosis, preferred treatment protocols, and methods for determining the nature and extent of impairment secondary to CTD form the battleground on which CTD workers' compensation claims are fought.

A discussion of workers' compensation starts with a review of its basic principles. Workers' compensation is legislation intended to provide work-injured employees with no-fault medical and indemnity benefits for lost time and to ensure some benefits for permanent disability or impairment once a claimant achieves maximum medical improvement. The amount of money paid for each week of lost work time is usually based on a percentage of the injured worker's average weekly income. Depending on the state in which the work-injured employee suffers the compensable injury, either the employer or the claimant may have the right to select the treating doctor.

Generally, workers' compensation is intended to provide medical care for the work-caused injury in an efficient and timely manner. The theoretic trade-off supporting the existence of workers' compensation schemes is the provision that the work-injured employee is essentially prohibited from suing the employer in the event that the injury results from the employer's negligence. This provision is called the *exclusive remedy doctrine*.

Some states have limitations on both the amount of money spent for medical care and the amount paid for temporary disability benefits. Virtually all states use one formula or another to determine the amount of permanent disability (impairment) benefits paid for a scheduled injury (an injury involving extremities or a specific organ identified in an injury schedule or catalog listed in a state's workers' compensation act). Otherwise, for injuries involving the trunk and the central nervous system, the work-injured claimant may be compensated for permanent disability on the basis of a percentage of impairment of the body as a working unit.

Some states still award permanent disability benefits on the basis of loss of earning capacity or actual vocational disability. The current trend, however, is clearly toward what is often described as a *uniform system of benefit awards* based on medical measurement of loss of function of the injured body part. This current effort is usually accompanied by the legislated adoption of such manuals as *The Guide to the Evaluation of Permanent Impairment* published by the American Medical Association [1]. This approach is encouraged by the insurance industry and self-insured employers as a way to avoid significant discrepancies in the awards being granted by various judges. In reality, the author has found that this method of compensating for work injuries usually results in an award of meager and almost meaningless benefits. Nowhere is this truer than in the case of bilateral upper-extremity injuries, such as CTDs.

If the work-injured employee and the insurance carrier (on behalf of the employer) or the self-insured employer cannot agree on disputed issues in a CTD case, the case usually ends up before an administrative law judge. Frequently, issues heard in these cases include issues of causation, degree of impairment, and the type of medical care to be provided to the claimant. Medical testimony is frequently required to resolve these issues, and the important role of the medical witnesses in these cases cannot be overstated. These workers' compensation claims usually involve no more than a few hours of hearing time, although some cases can take most of a day and, on occasion, more than a day. The treating physician and the evaluating and consulting physician called to testify in these cases are placed on the witness stand for relatively short periods. The attorneys for the respective sides usually address directly and immediately the issue in contest; therefore, adequate preparation is mandatory before one offers testimony in the courtroom.

Contested Causation

Because CTDs include maladies that produce somewhat differing symptoms and impairments and are frequently characterized as syndromes, understanding of the nomenclature and of the specific mechanics that (more likely than not) produce the claimed disorder is crucial. On cross-examination, if the medical witness does not know how a disorder developed or cannot identify the likely factors that produced the disorder, the rest of the forensic testimony cannot have much value and, in practical terms, the administrative law judge may feel that time has been wasted on the witness. That impression may jeopardize the entire case. Therefore, the medical witness must have a thorough understanding of the job routine that caused the CTD. Its history should include an exhaustive account of the last 20 years prior to the alleged onset of the disabling condition, a review of non–work-related activities that could contribute significantly to the disorder, and a full discussion of the suspect task or tasks in the job routine alleged to have produced the disorder. This inquiry may require on-site evaluation, with reliable measurements and routine demonstrated by the claimant. Some health care providers who deal with CTD–workers' compensation cases routinely send an occupational therapist or ergonomics-trained evaluator to the job site to take measurements with the assistance of the claimant. Because the disabling consequences of CTDs can be catastrophic, it may be worthwhile to pursue this evaluative process when causation is challenged by the workers' compensation insurance carrier. Possibly, the work performed by the work-injured claimant could not or did not produce the CTD. If either employer or insurance carrier concedes the existence of the patient's CTD but alleges that the disorder results from the patient's non–work-related activities, the patient-claimant must conduct adequate discovery to determine the basis for the contention that the CTD resulted from activities outside the workplace. In this context, work-injured claimants are rarely able to represent their own interests adequately in a CTD case. The insurance company is going to be represented by attorneys who try these cases daily, the rules of evidence will apply, and most administrative law judges will not assist the work-injured claimant in presenting his or her case.

In most communities, competent workers' compensation practitioners are located easily. Lawyers and health care providers routinely involved in the community workers' compensation system can usually recommend attorneys considered to be highly competent in workers' compensation matters. Physicians asked to recommend an attorney are advised to give the names of two or three considered to be competent and who concentrate on or limit their practice to workers' compensation matters. As difficult as forensic issues can be in a compensation case, nothing will aggravate the medical provider more than having to work with or be subjected to incompetent counsel. Usually, in attempting to resolve contested claims, it is best for both sides to be represented by attorneys well experienced in workers' compensation matters and expert in the issues that are presented in CTD cases. The administrative law judges who hear these cases will expect the attorneys to be prepared adequately and further will expect the medical providers, on examination and cross-examination, to provide thoughtful opinions and information. The judge depends on such preparation to issue findings of fact and order as a result of a fully developed case. When one side is clearly better represented than the other, the outcome is usually predictable. Nevertheless, these cases do have to be resolved, and it is important for the medical witness to understand that the courtroom is supposed to afford an opportunity for fair play. It is not a place wherein absolute truth is obtained in every case. It is not a place wherein the "right" result is always obtained. Because CTDs are not characterized by instantaneous, finite diagnosis, painting a complete medical picture for the administrative law judge in a relatively short period is crucial to obtaining a favorable decision regarding the compensability of the claim and the award of benefits.

Courtroom and Discovery Proceedings

Workers' compensation judges usually make one or two calendar calls (morning and afternoon) to decide which cases on the day's calendar will be heard and in what order. Although cases involving live medical testimony are usually given preference, other cases may be heard first for a host of reasons. Full-contest cases—the employer denying any liability and no benefits being paid—are usually given top priority, as are cases that have been continued from a previous date for completion of testimony.

Workers' compensation court systems usually schedule a number of cases on the morning and afternoon dockets (more cases than could possibly be heard in 1 day). This procedure is necessary because of the court's inability to predict which cases will settle shortly before the hearing date. Therefore, it is not uncommon for large groups to assemble at the beginning of each docket so that attorneys can report to the judge on the status of their cases and, if necessary, make a record as to the disposition of their cases in the event settlement has been reached. What all of this means for the physician witness is that it may be necessary to wait for extended periods before testifying. This inconvenience is an unfortunate, but sometimes unavoidable, part of the process. Therefore, the physician witness is advised to bring paperwork or reading material on the day of court appearance. It is important also for the physician witness to establish a basis for fees charged for participation in the case; that basis should be reflected in a written document known as an *engagement letter*.

The engagement letter is an agreement between the physician and the attorney representing either the patient or the insurance company. It sets forth the amount to be paid for the physician witness's participation in the case. The physician should never participate as a forensic expert witness on a fee-contingent basis. In other words, the physician's charge for services never should be based on the outcome of the case. Such arrangements invite the conclusion that the physician's testimony is purchased and biased and, therefore, inherently suspect. The physician should provide forensic services on an hourly-fee basis, regardless of the outcome of the case.

Responsibility for payment of the physician witness's fee rests with the attorney who engages the witness on behalf of a client (work-injured claimant or employer-insurance company). This principle is simple when the physician witness is not the treating physician. In that case, all services provided by the physician witness are billed directly to the attorney who has engaged the physician's services.

In cases in which the physician is treating the patient *and* is asked to testify or prepare forensic reports, that portion of the work specifically related to the forensic activity should be billed directly and separately to the attorney requesting such services. Again, in that situation and in the absence of an acceptable and comfortable working relationship with the attorney, an engagement letter should be signed.

If the claimant is pro se (*for self*, or not represented by an attorney), the treating physician who serves also as witness probably should have the patient sign an engagement letter that obligates the patient separately for that service, apart from the obligation to pay for medical services. Presenting the patient with an engagement letter could have two predictable results: It may prompt the patient to hire an attorney, and it will notify the patient that your time is money and that, although you willingly will provide requested reports and testimony, neither service is free.

The engagement letter should set forth specifically the amount you will charge for preparation of reports, testimony, and review and preparation for testimony, and your fees for travel, copy services, and waiting time in court. The letter should set forth the advance notification time required for cancellation of appointments so as to avoid a fee and the prorated amount that will be charged for any cancellation after that advance notice deadline. The engagement letter should also identify the amount to be paid in advance for the physician's witness services and whether all or part of those fees are nonrefundable. Finally, the engagement letter should note specifically that the law firm engaging the physician witness bears the primary obligation for payment of the witness's services. An additional statement in the engagement letter should recognize that in the event of nonpayment, reasonable attorney's fees and all costs of collection are included in the undertaking by the attorney requesting the witness's services.

An engagement letter is not mandatory. If a physician has a comfortable working relationship with an attorney requesting witness services, the physician surely does not require a formal agreement.

In many states, approved fee schedules for physicians' services set forth the amount the treating physician can charge for treatment *and* for testimony. Obviously, the fees charged for such services by the physician will coincide with those schedules. As an additional note, a physician treating a patient injured in another state should try to bill for services consistent with that state's approved fee schedule. Although the physician may not be paid the fee customarily charged, the inconvenience involved in chasing the patient and the patient's attorney for the "difference" usually renders any recovered funds unworthy of the effort. Given the practical realities of present medical economics, this area of practice—CTDs—and the related forensic business are sufficiently attractive financially to justify this give-and-take approach in treating and

examining CTD patients who have active legal claims in other states. As with any other industry, networking and identifying competent physician witnesses in the various states is a developing trend in CTD matters. Insurance companies long have had their favorites in every jurisdiction, doctors who most assuredly will find little or no pathologic symptoms in patients manifesting obvious and significant impairment. Surprisingly, many attorneys do not check up on such doctors and do not make an issue of the doctor's reputation before the workers' compensation judge.

The physician witness plays a specific role in court or at deposition. There are two types of depositions: discovery and evidentiary. Discovery depositions are just that: proceedings in which a deponent (the physician) under oath is asked questions about matters that may be connected either directly or only remotely to the case. *Discovery* means that the questioning attorney probably will question the physician witness's diagnosis and treatment in the case; professional education, training, and experience; method of payment for participation in the case; and past forensic-witness experience. Rules of procedure pertaining to discovery depositions have undergone major changes in recent years, and the current trend is to allow wide latitude in the scope of questions that may be asked.

Just as in live testimony, it is extremely important for the physician witness to be well prepared for a discovery deposition. That preparation means that before the deposition, the witness will meet with the claimant's attorney or the attorney retaining the witness on behalf of the patient or insurance company. The witness is advised to review diagnosis, course of treatment, future treatment recommendations, prognosis, current limitations to be imposed on the claimant's present vocational activities, and professional opinion as to whether the patient likely will suffer permanent impairment that interferes with the ability to work. A physician witness who does not know, or can only speculate about, the patient's probable future condition should advise the inquiring attorney that the opinion as to the degree or scope of permanent impairment is as yet undetermined.

The standard or legal test for admissibility of persuasive expert testimony is one of medical probability: that it is more likely than not that a particular conclusion should be reached given the underlying facts. A physician's opinion given at the time of deposition or live evidentiary testimony in court should reflect that standard.

Science, including the healing arts, prefers certainty to probability. Perhaps in recognition that the healing arts never have been an exact science, U.S. courts of law have required only that an opinion be rendered on the premise that a conclusion has a greater than 50% probability of being correct and applicable to the case in question. In other words, if it is 51% more likely that a series of facts will support a given conclusion (in the opinion of the expert), a court of law will "receive" the opinion into evidence. That does not mean that the court necessarily agrees with the opinion or anything else that a forensic witness offers. It means only that the expert's opinion will be received and considered with all the other evidence in reaching a decision in the case.

An evidentiary deposition is a deposition taken to preserve testimony for trial. In such a deposition, the forensic witness is questioned in a manner similar to that used at time of trial. The deposition transcript then is read by the judge, who considers the testimony just as it would be evaluated and weighed if the testimony were given live at the time of trial.

In a discovery deposition, objections to questions are waived except in the matter of a question's form. Objections (e.g., as to relevancy, materiality, and lack of foundation) are not allowed, on the theory that the person asking the questions should be permitted to engage in unfettered dialogue with the witness to learn more about the facts already known and to discover new information and opinions that may lead to additional information helpful to the attorney preparing the case, in the ultimate quest for the truth.

The deposition battleground has deteriorated to the point at which courts are experimenting with new systems to take the combative approach out of discovery depositions. There is a clear trend toward loosening the limitations on the type and manner of questions that can be asked, so that each question is not met with an objection and an instruction "not to answer" by the attorney whose witness is being deposed.

In any event, the physician witness's deposition, whether evidentiary or discovery, may be used at a later date for cross-examination to impeach subsequent testimony. A witness whose testimony has been taken in an evidentiary deposition still may be subpoenaed for trial, depending on the status of the case and the strategy of the respective counsel.

The easiest way to avoid being lured off track at trial is to reach an honest diagnosis, render opinions based on that diagnosis, and avoid understating or overstating the patient's status and limitations—in other words, to tell the truth.

Frequently in CTD cases, the opposing experts will agree on the underlying facts but will disagree over the conclusions to be drawn from those facts. Therefore, in such cases, it is important that the expert examine the conclusions and the analytic process that led to those conclusions. The attorney retaining the expert should be sufficiently skilled to anticipate the questions that will be asked by opposing counsel and should play devil's advocate with the physician witness regarding all the major issues that form the subject of the court contest.

The battle of the experts in CTD workers' compensation settings requires a concise, cohesive, logical evidentiary presentation. Workers' compensation judges are not unschooled in the medical issues in CTD cases. However, the actual medical mechanics behind the case in which the physician is testifying, and the clinical testing and examination results used to reach a diagnosis, should be developed and presented in no more than 20 minutes. The soft issues—prognosis (the point at which it is hoped the patient will reach maximum medical improvement) and future restrictions—usually are not relevant in determining whether the claimant suffers CTD secondary to employment. Certain questions should encompass both the deposition and the courtroom presentation of the basis for the opinion that the patient has a CTD.

- When was the patient examined?
- What history did the patient give?
- What additional questions were asked regarding non–work-related activities that might cause or contribute to a CTD?
- What is the diagnosis?
- What findings support this diagnosis?
- What tests were performed in reaching this diagnosis?
- Which of these tests are considered clinically objective, and on what basis?

Additional pertinent questions will be necessary to establish the physician witness's credentials and experience in the area. The entire presentation should not require more than 30 minutes.

Of course, in addition to having recorded an exhaustive history, the examining and treating physician will have the patient undergo diagnostic testing (see earlier chapters). It is not only important for the practitioner to keep abreast of the varying evaluation protocols employed in determining the presence or absence of CTD. It is just as important that the practitioner understand the latest theories advanced by the insurance industry. For example, it was suggested at one time that all female patients who were pregnant or taking birth control pills at the outset of suspected carpal tunnel symptoms probably suffered a condition caused exclusively by pregnancy or the pills, despite such known facts as the patient's specific work routine.

The Hearing Process

Usually, contested workers' compensation claim hearings are held in a courtroom smaller than that used for jury trials and, depending on the judge's style, the proceedings may be more informal. This atmosphere usually reflects the relatively small number of attorneys who practice in this area and who know and see one another daily before the same judges, rather than denoting merely a less formal court process than that in which juries are employed. In fact, workers' compensation administrative law judges become highly expert in assessing medical evidence. Frequently, these judges are required to decide critical issues and to render decisions that, in the aggregate, involve vast sums of money. Therefore, the health care witness should devote at least as much diligence to preparing for testimony in a workers' compensation claim as that reserved for a jury trial weighing, for instance, an automobile injury case and requiring the medical witness's opinion on all the usual issues.

In CTD cases, it may be simplest for the health care witness to start with the claimant's presenting symptoms and to work backward chronologically to develop a disorder's etiology. That factual, capsule-form presentation will provide the judge with a working synopsis. It also makes sense for the medical witness to describe the patient's condition, as that condition most impressed the examiner at the time of examination. Once the initial examination and history are presented, usually it is helpful for the medical witness to be asked to name specific symptoms or signs that were significant for the examiner in reaching a diagnosis. Because that testimony is presented right at the outset, the judge more likely will make extensive notes as to each of the symptoms or signs and the significance of each to the medical witness's diagnosis. If a symptom or sign is possible or slight, it should be described as such. It is imperative for a medical witness establishing credibility not to overstate or understate findings. If the examination findings conclusively support a medical conclusion, the witness can defend it. If the sign or symptom is mild or of questionable existence, the witness should state that opinion and move on to the other findings. No case ever is perfect, and almost no CTD patient ever presents with every symptom associated with the disorder. On cross-examination by the insurance company's lawyer, the physician witness certainly will be asked to state the significance of minimal or nonexistent findings validating a sign or symptom in reaching a CTD diagnosis. If, in fact, the witness is confident of having satisfied diagnostic criteria in the examination sufficient to establish the presence of CTD, that opinion should be stated. On direct examination, it is important for the medical witness to acknowledge and emphasize that CTD is a syndrome rather than a disease and that signs and symptoms are sufficient to support the ultimate diagnosis of CTD as scientifically and medically reliable. Obviously, the symptoms associated with full-blown reflex sympathetic dystrophy are much more dramatic and self-evident than are other maladies identified as CTDs. For that reason, the witness must offer a concise description of clinical examination findings and their probable relationship to the claimant's known work routine once testimony begins.

Establishing a specific date of CTD onset resulting from workplace activities can be a very delicate process. A significant percentage of the CTD patient population initially perceives such disorders as sore muscles, an ailment that they believe will be self-limited. As the problems worsen, many of these patients do *not* report the problem at work out of fear of losing their jobs. At that point, these patients are in a serious dilemma. On the one hand, usually they will be punished for not reporting the "work injury" immediately. On the other, everyone (employer, workers' compensation doctors, claims adjuster, administrative law judge, etc.) will subject them to some form of interrogation that very soon will translate for them into an inquisition process. Frequently, by the time such patients see an expert who makes a diagnosis of CTD, they are angry and scared, with an apparent emotional "component" added to the syndrome. Thus, care should be taken by the examiner to differentiate whether the patients' emotional response results from the manner in which they have been treated socially or stems from the disabling fact of the injury itself. Obviously, a lot of room exists for overlapping of the two causes of this emotional distress, but the distinction and discussion become important because of the patient's treatment needs. Those persons who avoid the catastrophic experience of bilateral upper-extremity CTD are fortunate indeed. The combination of the social stigma of being a workers' compensation claimant with the disorder, the workplace derision of coworkers, an employer's disbelief in a previously loyal employee, and an insurance company representative's outright suggestions of lying and malingering usually cause these patients to suffer significant emotional problems requiring additional treatment distinct from that for the work-related CTD. This familiar profile is offered so that, in reviewing the medical chart in preparation for testimony, the medical examiner can review the dynamics of a patient's situation.

Lawyers and administrative law judges in this system will want to discuss the presence or absence of objective evidence offered by the medical witness in reaching an opinion. Usually, objective evidence in this venue is viewed as being persuasive, even if such evidence supporting or ruling out a diagnosis is not conclusive. Judges are more comfortable with and impressed by show-and-tell demonstrative evidence than by elaborate medical theory. Although "red hot," cutting-edge medical theories may raise approving eyebrows at a medical conference, with rare exception, they do not count for much in the courtroom. At issue also is whether such testimony will even be allowed as reliable scientific evidence.

However, if in testifying, the medical witness can exhaust the accepted evaluation protocols with results that buttress the causation argument, the additional expert cutting-edge information is

a sort of bonus and usually will help as long as it is not exaggerated.

During cross-examination, the medical provider testifying on behalf of the work-injured claimant frequently will be asked to reveal the source of information contributing to the ultimate diagnosis of CTD. Doctors are trained to listen to their patients and are trained further to presume that patients are truthful in reporting symptoms. That presumption does not exist in the courtroom. Therefore, in recording an initial history, the examining physician should ask questions and record responses carefully about a work routine suspected of causing the symptom(s). By questioning the occupational therapist and by obtaining investigative reports and elaborate job descriptions from the employer, frequently the physician can match convincingly the facts alleged by the claimant with the information provided by the employer or the employer's insurance carrier. That type of evidence is important and persuasive.

As noted earlier, the examining and treating physician's questioning of the patient should address also the patient's non–work-related activities to determine whether such activity possibly contributed to the CTD. A patient's allegation of a performed cumulative activity should be pursued. The physician should identify and record exactly the nature of the activity: the frequency of the motion or routine in question; the position in which the patient performs the routine; the position of the arms during performance; the weight of the lifted objects; the height to or from which the objects are lifted; the amount of reaching, pulling, and overhead work involved on a daily or hourly basis; and the like. Also helpful is determining the periods of continuous work, the frequency and duration of rest breaks, and whether any exercises or stretching activities are encouraged or required by the employer. All these kinds of "facts" are relevant in the courtroom.

If the physician believes that a claimant's work produced a disabling impairment, that opinion should include a description of the activity that caused the problem. Although these comments may appear to be insultingly fundamental, the author believes that all too frequently one or both sides fail to engage in the in-depth evaluation and history required to produce definite information. This type of evidence is not only important in the case; it is evidence that will be more pleasing and usually more persuasive in the view of the administrative law judge.

Additionally, if the physician has adequate information to recommend reasonable change of workplace activity that can be accommodated by the employer, possibly the patient's work routine can be modified for successful (noninjurious) return to work. Because the parties in workers' compensation claims start out in polarized positions and the adversarial process, by definition, precludes cooperation, real-world stories of work-injured CTD claimants successfully returning to work safely are few and far between. Our high-tech society does not have much to offer the blue-collar or semiskilled employee saddled with CTD.

Documentation of the Physician Witness's Credentials and Experience

Federal (and most state) civil rules of procedure require extensive disclosure about the training and experience of expert witnesses in civil litigation. Usually, workers' compensation procedures are not as demanding, but the current trend clearly is heading in that direction. Therefore, physicians should begin assembling a dossier on themselves and should update that file appropriately on a regular (at least semiannual) basis.

Information in the file should include a brief résumé beginning with the physician's education. It should include the undergraduate, medical school, and other graduate schools attended; the place and duration of internship and residency; and a list of papers authored, courses taught, and honors received. Additionally, it should list each case in which the witness participated, the year of the case, the identity of the court in which the case was brought, the names and addresses of the attorneys representing the respective parties, and the name of the judge presiding in each case.

Most likely, the witness physician will have depositions taken in each case. In most states, it is common practice for the court reporter to provide a courtesy transcript copy of such a deposition to the medical (expert) witness. These transcripts should be retained for future use in establishing credentials.

One word of caution is in order: In most states, court reporters have a proprietary interest in the work they produce. That means that the physician witness who does not have a copy of a transcript of testimony from a case may have to ask the court reporter to prepare a copy or to grant permission to make a photocopy. Therefore, the physician is advised to keep an accurate record of the names and addresses of the court reporters who recorded testimony in each case and the name, address, and telephone number of the company employing the reporter. The easiest way to do this is to keep reporters' professional cards on file with notations for identifying the relevant case.

The physician witness should prepare notes indicating the extent of involvement in each case in which testimony was given: preparation of reports, treatment, testimony at deposition, trial testimony, or any combination thereof. The witness initially retained as an examining physician should provide a copy of this dossier-curriculum vitae to the retaining counsel.

Again, the point of the foregoing discussion is that current legal trends require complete disclosure of all forensic and academic information pertaining to the "experts." The physician should not have to scramble and reinvent the "experience wheel" for each case.

Chart Notes

Once involved in a case, the physician witness should assume that all chart notes (and correspondence) concerning the CTD claimant will be discoverable. The author has found that physicians' chart notes usually are at least partially illegible. The unprepared potential witness is guaranteed an unpleasant experience in appearing before a court reporter to read ("translate") handwritten notes into the record at deposition. The discomfort is magnified if the physician witness is asked to read scribbled notes to the jury in a civil case. Jurors find it rather difficult to take an "expert" seriously if an in-court remedial transcription course is a prerequisite to beginning a dialogue about the substantive issues in the case. Additionally, if chart notes are handwritten and difficult to read, the finder of fact possibly can become convinced, for example, that the notes said "didn't" instead of "did." The moral to this discussion is this: The witness should hire a competent medical transcriptionist to record notes dictated at the conclusion of each appointment or examination and to proofread transcribed chart notes within 48 hours of the examination. Following this protocol for all patient care will avoid the guaranteed horrendous experience that awaits the physician witness who is not fastidious in his or her preparation for court.

Narrative reports prepared from chart notes should reflect the same findings contained in the chart notes (unless, for example, the findings and differential diagnosis have, in fact, changed). Again, they should not be overstated or understated. The physician simply should state an opinion and provide the basis for that opinion.

Answering Questions at Deposition and Trial

At deposition, the nonengaging attorney questions the witness first. At trial, the witness usually is called to testify by the attorney who has engaged his or her services. After the dialogue with that attorney, the other side's attorney will cross-examine the witness. The retaining attorney will want to make the witness look competent and compassionate. The cross-examining attorney will want to make that witness look dishonest and unreliable. The witness's dialogue under direct examination usually will consist of such open-ended questions by the retaining attorney as "What were your findings?" The other side, on cross-examination, usually will ask specific questions concerning specific findings, such as, "Isn't it a fact that you would expect to find X in a patient who allegedly suffers from a condition known as CTD? And you didn't find those symptoms, did you?"

Instead of arguing with the attorney, the physician witness should answer the question truthfully: "There was some clinical indication of X, but other symptoms and findings were more profound and obvious" or (if it is supportable by the *typed* notes), "Yes, I noted on (date) that the patient presented with X" or, "No, the patient did not present with symptom X." On redirect examination, the patient's attorney can, and presumably will, ask the witness whether the absence of symptom X precludes the diagnosis. In fact, the patient's attorney may have covered this ground already on direct examination by asking the witness to list the symptoms commonly found in patients who suffer from CTD

problems, to identify those symptoms experienced by this patient, and to state whether it is significant that the patient does not present with all the signs and symptoms associated with CTD.

Remember, this forensic effort is based on probability, not on certainty. If the truthful answer to a question is "I don't know," the witness should say, "I don't know." Regardless of training and experience, the witness will, at least occasionally, be asked a question deserving of that answer.

In fact, judges and juries do not presume perfection, and a witness who professes an absolute answer to each question is not nearly as convincing as is a witness who admits to lack of knowledge or to the inability to answer or who states a preference not to engage in speculation. No case is perfect, and no witness has all the answers.

The physician witness must not lose his or her temper at deposition or in court. If the attorneys at deposition argue with each other to the point at which the witness no longer wants to participate, he or she should tell the attorneys, on the record, that the argument interferes with giving meaningful responses. This is not done to chastise and toy with the lawyers but to protect the quality of the witness's answers in the event that something has, in fact, been overlooked or if the witness has been thrown off track by the discord between the attorneys. At trial, the judge will not permit that type of behavior between counsel. The control over the courtroom makes it that much more important that at time of deposition, the witness's opinions are rendered without distortion and without only partial statement of information or opinion because of bickering between the lawyers.

Surprises should not crop up at trial. The attorney engaging the witness's services presumably will have reviewed the opposing side's case with him or her. By their very nature, CTD cases are cumulative; frequently, the general is more important than the specific in handling the patient's history and clinical presentation. Symptoms wax and wane, and findings may change (dramatically, it is hoped, with the appropriate health care). The forensic cornerstone of these cases always returns to the same focus: a comparison of the claimant's baseline condition prior to insult and the effect of cumulative trauma on the claimant. A witness comfortable with a diagnosis does not have to worry about minor matters. The best forensic witnesses are those who convey the following message: "Despite what else is said about this patient or the lack of finite diagnostic and treatment protocols for dealing with this medical problem, CTD patients suffer significantly, require treatment, and often experience significant impairment as a result of a condition. No magic amount of cumulative activity will produce the same response in all persons, just as the degree of painful response—given the same noxious stimuli—cannot be predicted in different patients. Ignoring the condition or pretending that it does not exist is scientifically unacceptable; we simply have to do the best we can with the medical knowledge currently available."

Whether in deposition or trial, the physician witness should answer the questions asked and not try to add nonresponsive extra material to help the case. The judge will not like it, and the questioning attorney may move to have such portions of the answer stricken as "not responsive" to the question. If the witness thinks information should be given in light of a question, presumably the representing attorney will ask a question on redirect examination that will allow that information to be presented in a responsive rather than a voluntary manner.

The witness should not dodge a question because the answer might seem unfavorable to the case. Not all questions can be answered favorably. However, forensic witnesses who, to buy time to think of an answer, reply "I don't understand the question" when everyone else does, can do substantial damage to that side of the case. At the same time, a witness who is asked a question that cannot be answered yes or no should characterize it as such, start with the unfavorable part of the information, and conclude with that part of the answer that helps the case or tends to neutralize the beginning of the response.

Some attorneys encourage their witnesses to look at the attorney when a question is being asked and then to address and look directly at the finder of fact in giving the answer. The physician witness may want to consider whether that posturing looks like an "infomercial" rather than expert testimony. Turning full attention to the judge (or jury) can be very effective in answering key questions on ultimate or vulnerable issues. As with everything else about testimony, the witness should be genuine rather than trying to create a false impression.

The witness should try to avoid cumbersome medical terms. The workers' compensation judge

will not be impressed. Moreover, with no real knowledge of the judge's understanding, the witness may risk only confusing the judge. Lay terms should be used whenever possible. A complex or difficult medical concept should be described as such; then the witness should explain it as simply as possible. The witness should not wait until court appearance to offer an explanation. As the witness already knows—prior to court appearance—what will be said, an answer to the anticipated difficult inquiry should be developed before testimony. The witness could try it out on lay people to ensure that they understand it. If they do, the judge will. The witness could have the lay people describe the processes (answers) back after they have heard them and should not accept noncommittal answers. The explanation given back by these listeners will help to refine and simplify the explanation that the witness will be giving in court. That refinement, in turn, might result in identifying a protocol that the witness may want to suggest to help relieve or cure a claimant's CTD symptoms.

Objections in Court

Once the physician witness is called to testify and pertinent fundamentals have been established (name, education, experience, board certification or eligibility, etc.), the retaining attorney will offer the witness's testimony as that of an expert in one or more medical specialties. The judge will accept the testimony as that of an expert in those areas for which suitable expert foundation has been established. During the course of that testimony, objections may be made by the attorneys representing the respective parties. As soon as an objection is made by an attorney, the witness should stop speaking. Usually, the judge will allow the objecting attorney to state the objection fully, may allow the other attorney to respond, and then will issue a ruling as to whether the objection is sustained or overruled. If the objection is overruled, the witness will be permitted to continue answering or to answer the challenged question. If the objection is sustained, the question either will be rephrased or the attorney will move on to a different question. In a workers' compensation proceeding, the objections most often heard in connection with expert testimony will be as follows: The question presumes facts not in evidence; foundation for the question is inadequate; the question calls for an opinion beyond the declared expertise of the witness. A question may be challenged either because it suggests the answer desired from the expert (a leading question) or because it requires the expert to speculate rather than to give an opinion based on reasonable probability in the witness's declared areas of expertise. The witness should not become involved in that discussion with the court but should remain completely silent until the judge has made a determination. Most judges then will advise the witness to answer the question or to continue answering the question. In some cases, to save time, the judge will frame the question a little differently and ask it because the court wants to hear the answer and believes the general inquiry is important for a determination of the issues. If the physician witness considers a question to be a good question but an objection to it is sustained, the answer to the next question should not begin with the answer that would have been given to the challenged question. To reply in that fashion will compromise significantly the witness's credibility as an objective expert. Additionally, a witness attempting that type of answer in the presence of competent counsel is going to be asked at length to justify that behavior. The witness will not enjoy having an attorney, on cross-examination, rephrase the question asked after the objection was sustained and then ask why the given answer really is the answer to what the witness thought was the previous question. That response will trigger inquiries as to the amount paid to the witness for appearing and the importance of winning the case. At that point, the answers to any of those questions really do not matter; the expert witness has been reduced to a testimonial plaything.

Common sense and plain speech are the most effective tools available to an expert witness. Condescension, arrogance, or any sense of "righteousness" exhibited by the expert witness severely undercuts anything that is said. Ironically, the most successful expert witnesses are those who appear to be speaking in everyday terms on a level understood by everyone in the courtroom. In reality, the law never encourages the use of complicated words or posturing on the part of expert witnesses. Expert witnesses are called *expert witnesses* because they are expected to contribute information and understanding to issues that will help the finder of fact to understand fully the issues in a case. Therefore, although not encouraged to speak in child's terms, the expert witness should use plain speech, short answers (when practical), and explanations that avoid complex terminology. The concept of disabling pain is as suspect as it is complex. Simple and logical descriptions of the mechanisms of a patient's pain or the probable absence thereof will provide the finder of fact with a comfort level both as to forensic explanation and in "reaching the right result."

The Expert Medical Witness As Viewed by the Legal Community

Defense lawyers in workers' compensation matters obviously are interested in cultivating relationships with health care providers who can guarantee to provide what euphemistically can be called *conservative* opinions on issues affecting the insurance company's financial liability. Stated differently, the insurance company's lawyers always are looking to enlarge the supply of medical witnesses who can guarantee to discount medical theories supporting findings of causation or impairment. Such attorneys seek witnesses who, if causation and impairment are established, likewise will opine that an impairment is minimal or that a claimant is exaggerating or malingering. At the same time, many perceive lawyers who represent claimants in workers' compensation matters as forever looking for adequately credentialed physician witnesses to provide ready opinions supporting determinations of extensive and permanent impairment that significantly limit a claimant's vocational abilities. The fact of the matter is that only a limited number of physicians in any community treat CTDs, and the workers' compensation judges in a community usually are acutely aware of the sympathies of the doctors who testify before them.

The author has found that, all too frequently, patients who present with significant CTD-induced impairment are dismissed by the industrial clinic physician as either suffering from an emotional problem or as simply trying to "milk" the system. In its worst form, this type of medical bias takes on an aura of unforgivable medical arrogance: The physician essentially assumes that if the patient's ailment cannot be diagnosed medically, the patient is crazy. Given the multitude of evaluation and treatment protocols suggested by the various medical specialties and subspecialties, the physician witness must keep in mind that the approach taken to the CTD clinical presentation will be influenced greatly by personal training and resulting medical bias. Additionally, expert witnesses may very much resent expressed or implied challenges to the quality of their work or their professional veracity. A witness responding to that order of stimuli in court will hurt rather than help the party requesting expert testimony and services. The witness never should be drawn into an argument in court. If the witness is insulted or patronized by inquiring counsel, a timely nod in view of the finder of fact will convey an element of self-control and maturity that will help the judge to render a decision consistent with the opinions given. At the same time, the witness should be able to admit not knowing the answer to a question. Likewise, the physician witness should be willing to admit that, for example, the working premise does not agree in total with the classic fact pattern desired. If clinical findings do not back up entirely the potential symptoms sought in support of the ultimate diagnosis, that limitation should be conceded by the witness.

The author has found that when non–mental health care providers use such terms as *functional overlay* or *symptom magnification*, such witnesses subject themselves to a much more difficult level of scrutiny by the finder of fact than do physician witnesses who comment simply that the claimant clearly presented with emotional symptoms in addition to the physical findings. The aforementioned technical terms are insurance defense creations used derisively as a "forensic wink" to tell the audience that a claimant is crazy, phony, or fraudulent, or some combination thereof. It may gratify the defense forensic witness to provide that sort of testimony; however, such an approach usually hurts the insurance carrier's cause. In the presence of competent claimant's counsel, forensic witnesses who use such terms usually become the claimant's best witnesses. If possible, invective terms and colloquy always should be avoided in expert testimony.

Repeat Performance

Most physicians who treat or evaluate CTD patients and participate as forensic witnesses in workers' compensation matters do so with some frequency. Witnesses fitting that description must be concerned about the opinion of the finder of fact toward them. Witnesses should avoid small talk with the attorneys in the courtroom, should refrain from joking with the attorneys, and studiously should avoid what might be construed as any attempt on their part to curry favor with the judge. Judges are most comfortable with repeat expert witnesses who keep their distance.

Conclusion

Participation in the workers' compensation system will afford the health care provider better insight into and understanding of the patient's experience. If the health care provider/examiner undertakes a thorough examination, avoids overstatement and understatement, simply answers the questions asked, and in essence tells the truth, the experience gained as a forensic contributor should be rewarding and professionally satisfying. The practitioner who has an overview of the dynamics of the workers' compensation system will likely become more professional in all aspects of direct health care for the work-injured CTD patient.

Reference

1. American Medical Association. The Guide to the Evaluation of Permanent Impairment (3rd ed). Milwaukee: American Medical Association, 1990.

Index